NSCA's Guide to
High School
Strength and
Conditioning

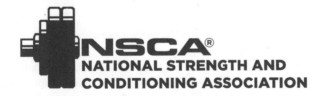

NSCA®
NATIONAL STRENGTH AND
CONDITIONING ASSOCIATION

Patrick McHenry, MA, CSCS,*D, RSCC
Mike Nitka, MS, CSCS,*D, RSCC*E, FNSCA*E
Editors

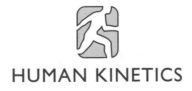

HUMAN KINETICS

Library of Congress Cataloging-in-Publication Data

Names: McHenry, Patrick, editor. | Nitka, Mike, editor. | National Strength
  & Conditioning Association (U.S.)
Title: NSCA's guide to high school strength and conditioning / Patrick T.
  McHenry, Mike Nitka, editors.
Description: Champaign, IL : Human Kinetics, [2022] | "National Strength &
  Conditioning Association." | Includes bibliographical references and index.
Identifiers: LCCN 2021010917 (print) | LCCN 2021010918 (ebook) | ISBN
  9781492599708 (paperback) | ISBN 9781492599715 (epub) | ISBN
  9781492599739 (pdf)
Subjects: LCSH: Physical education and training--Study and teaching
  (Secondary)--United States. | Muscle strength.
Classification: LCC GV711.5 .N73 2022 (print) | LCC GV711.5 (ebook) | DDC
  796.071/2--dc23
LC record available at https://lccn.loc.gov/2021010917
LC ebook record available at https://lccn.loc.gov/2021010918

ISBN: 978-1-4925-9970-8 (print)

Senior Acquisitions Editor: Roger W. Earle; **Managing Editor:** Miranda K. Baur; **Copyeditors:** Rodelinde Albrecht and Marissa Wold Uhrina; **Indexer:** Mary Hasso/Boston Informatics; **Permissions Manager:** Martha Gullo; **Graphic Designer:** Dawn Sills; **Cover Designer:** Keri Evans; **Cover Design Specialist:** Susan Rothermel Allen; **Photograph (cover):** John Coletti / Getty Images; **Photographs (interior):** © Human Kinetics, unless otherwise noted; **Photo Asset Manager:** Laura Fitch; **Photo Production Specialist:** Amy M. Rose; **Photo Production Manager:** Jason Allen; **Senior Art Manager:** Kelly Hendren; **Illustrations:** © Human Kinetics, unless otherwise noted; **Printer:** Sheridan Books

We thank Matthew Sandstead, NSCA-CPT,*D and Mel Herl, MS, CSCS,*D, RSCC at the National Strength and Conditioning Association in Colorado Springs, Colorado, for overseeing the photo shoot for this book. We also thank Gavin Berger, Lily Berger, Tim Downs, Will Robertson, Olivia Rose, and Carly Yeagle for modeling in the photos in chapter 10.

Printed in the United States of America   10 9 8 7 6 5 4 3 2 1

The paper in this book is certified under a sustainable forestry program.

Human Kinetics
1607 N. Market Street
Champaign, IL 61820
USA

United States and International
Website: **US.HumanKinetics.com**
Email: info@hkusa.com
Phone: 1-800-747-4457

Canada
Website: **Canada.HumanKinetics.com**
Email: info@hkcanada.com

E8137

Tell us what you think!
Human Kinetics would love to hear what we
can do to improve the customer experience.
Use this QR code to take our brief survey.

Contents

Credits

Figure P.1 Adapted by permission from I. Jeffreys, "Quadrennial Planning for the High School Athlete," *Strength and Conditioning Journal* 30, no. 3 (2008): 74-83.

Figure 1.1 Copyright © National Strength and Conditioning Association

Figure 2.4 Reprinted by permission from D.H. Fukuda, *Assessments for Sport and Athletic Performance* (Champaign, IL: Human Kinetics, 2019), 123. Data from G.G. Haff and C. Dumke, *Laboratory Manual for Exercise Physiology* (Champaign, IL: Human Kinetics, 2012), 305-360.

Table 2.2 Reprinted by permission from B.D. McKay, A.A. Miramonti, Z.M. Gillen, et al., "Normative Reference Values for High School-Aged American Football Players," *Journal of Strength and Conditioning Research* 34, no. 10 (2020): 2849-2856.

Table 2.6 Reprinted by permission from D.J. Szymanski and J. Vazquez, "Testing Protocols and Athlete Assessment," in *Strength Training for Baseball,* edited for the National Strength and Conditioning Association by E.A. Coleman and D.J. Szymanski (Champaign, IL: Human Kinetics, 2022), 36. Data from Szymanski et al., "Relationship Between Physiological Characteristics and Baseball-Specific Variables of High School Baseball Players," Journal of Strength and Conditioning Research 22, no. 6 (2008): 110-111; Szymanski et al., "Effect of Torso Rotational Strength n Angular Hip, Angular Shoulder, and Linear Bat Velocities of High School Baseball Players," Journal of Strength and Conditioning Research 21, no. 4 (2007): 1117-1125; Szymanski et al., "Effect of Wrist and Forearm Training on Linear Bat-End, Center of Percussion, and Hand Velocities, and Time to Ball Contact of High School Baseball Players," Journal of Strength and Conditioning Research 20, no. 1 (2006): 231-240; Szymanski et al., "Effect of Preseason Over-Weighted Medicine Ball Training on Throwing Velocity," Journal of Strength and Conditioning Research 25, no. 3 (2011): 64.

Table 2.10 Reprinted by permission from B.D. McKay, A.A. Miramonti, Z.M. Gillen, et al., "Normative Reference Values for High School-Aged American Football Players," *Journal of Strength and Conditioning Research* 34, no. 10 (2020): 2849-2856.

Figure 2.8 Reprinted by permission from D.H. Fukuda, *Assessments for Sport and Athletic Performance* (Champaign, IL: Human Kinetics, 2019), 138. Data from J. Hoffman, *Physiological Aspects of Sport Training and Performance,* 2nd ed. (Champaign, IL: Human Kinetics, 2014), 237-267.

Table 2.11 Reprinted by permission from B.D. McKay, A.A. Miramonti, Z.M. Gillen, et al., "Normative Reference Values for High School-Aged American Football Players," *Journal of Strength and Conditioning Research* 34, no. 10 (2020): 2849-2856.

Table 2.12 Reprinted by permission from J. Hoffman, *Norms for Fitness, Performance, and Health* (Champaign, IL: Human Kinetics, 2006), 58. Adapted by permission from D.A. Chu, *Explosive Power and Strength* (Champaign, IL: Human Kinetics, 1996), 171.

Figure 2.10 Reprinted by permission from D.H. Fukuda, *Assessments for Sport and Athletic Performance* (Champaign, IL: Human Kinetics, 2019), 142. Data from D.A. Chu, "Assessment," in *Explosive Power and Strength: Complex Training for Maximum Results* (Champaign, IL: Human Kinetics, 1996), 167-180, and G.R. Tomkinson, K.D. Carver, F. Atkinson, et al., "European Normative Values for Physical Fitness in Children and Adolescents Aged 9-17 Years: Results From 2 779 165 Eurofit Performances Representing 30 Countries," *British Journal of Sports Medicine* 52, no. 22 (2018): 1445-1456.xxviii Credits

Figure 2.11 Reprinted by permission from D.H. Fukuda, *Assessments for Sport and Athletic Performance* (Champaign, IL: Human Kinetics, 2019), 143. Data from D.A. Chu, "Assessment," in *Explosive Power and Strength: Complex Training for Maximum Results* (Champaign, IL: Human Kinetics, 1996), 167-180, and G.R. Tomkinson, K.D. Carver, F. Atkinson, et al., "European Normative Values for Physical Fitness in Children and Adolescents Aged 9-17 Years: Results From 2 779 165 Eurofit Performances Representing 30 Countries," *British Journal of Sports Medicine* 52, no. 22 (2018): 1445-1456.

Figure 3.5 Inti St Clair/Getty Images

Figure 3.10 John Coletti/Getty Images

Figure 3.12 Reprinted by permission from A. Hudy, "Facility Design, Layout, and Organization," in *Essentials of Strength Training and Conditioning*, 4th ed., edited for the National Strength and Conditioning Association by G.G. Haff and N.T. Triplett (Champaign, IL: Human Kinetics, 2016), 636.

Figure 3.13 Reprinted by permission from A. Hudy, "Facility Design, Layout, and Organization," in *Essentials of Strength Training and Conditioning*, 4th ed., edited for the National Strength and Conditioning Association by G.G. Haff and N.T. Triplett (Champaign, IL: Human Kinetics, 2016), 637-639. Adapted by permission from M. Greenwood, "Facility and Equipment Layout and Maintenance," in *NSCA's Essentials of Personal Training*, edited for the National Strength and Conditioning Association by R.W. Earle and T.R. Baechle (Champaign, IL: Human Kinetics, 2004), 604-606.

Figures 4.1 (p. 97 upper right), 4.17a (p. 119 upper left), 4.25d (p. 137 lower right), 4.26d (p. 139 lower right), 4.31a (p. 148), 4.36a (p. 157) Scott Sahli

Figure 8.1 Reprinted by permission from A.W. Pichardo, J.L. Oliver, C.B. Harrison, P.S. Maulder, and R.S. Lloyd, "Integrating Models of Long-Term Athletic Development to Maximize the Physical Development of Youth," *International Journal of Sports Science & Coaching* 13, no. 6 (2018): 1189-1199.

Table 8.2 Adapted by permission from R. Howard, "What Coaches Need to Know About the NSCA Position Statement on Long-Term Athletic Development," *NSCA Coach* 3, no. 3 (2014): 8-10.

Table 8.3 Reprinted by permission from J.M. Sheppard and N.T. Triplett, "Program Design for Resistance Training," in *Essentials of Strength Training and Conditioning*, 4th ed., edited for the National Strength and Conditioning Association by G.G. Haff and N.T. Triplett (Champaign, IL: Human Kinetics, 2016), 452.

Table 8.4 [a] Adapted from B. DeWeese, M. Sams, and A. Serrano, "Sliding Toward Sochi - Part 1: A Review of Programming Tactics Used During the 2010-2014 Quadrennial," *NSCA Coach* 1, no. 3 (2014): 30-36.

[b] Adapted by permission from M.C. Zourdos, A. Klemp, C. Dolan, et al., "Novel Resistance Training-Specific Rating of Perceived Exertion Scale Measuring Repetitions in Reserve," *Journal of Strength and Conditioning Research* 30, no. 1 (2016): 267-275.

Table 8.6 Adapted by permission from J.M. Sheppard and N.T. Triplett, "Program Design for Resistance Training," in *Essentials of Strength Training and Conditioning*,

4th ed., edited for the National Strength and Conditioning Association by G.G. Haff and N.T. Triplett (Champaign, IL: Human Kinetics, 2016), 439-469.

Figure 8.4 Reprinted by permission from S.J. Morris, J.L. Oliver, J.S. Pedley, et al., "Taking a Long-Term Approach to the Development of Weightlifting Ability in Young Athletes," *Strength and Conditioning Journal* 42, no. 6 (2020): 71-90.

Figure 8.5 Reprinted by permission from A. Faigenbaum, W. Kraemer, C. Blimkie, et al., "Youth Resistance Training: Updated Position Statement Paper From the National Strength and Conditioning Association," *Journal of Strength and Conditioning Research* 23, no. 5 (2009): S60-S79.

Table 8.7 Reprinted by permission from A. Faigenbaum, W. Kraemer, C. Blimkie, et al., "Youth Resistance Training: Updated Position Statement Paper From the National Strength and Conditioning Association," *Journal of Strength and Conditioning Research* 23, no. 5 (2009): S60-S79.

Table 8.8 Reprinted by permission from A. Faigenbaum, W. Kraemer, C. Blimkie, et al., "Youth Resistance Training: Updated Position Statement Paper From the National Strength and Conditioning Association," *Journal of Strength and Conditioning Research* 23, no. 5 (2009): S60-S79.

Table 8.9 Adapted by permission from A.D. Faigenbaum and J.E. McFarland, "Resistance Training for Kids: Right From the Start," *ACSM's Health & Fitness Journal* 20, no. 5 (2016): 16-22.

Table 8.10 Adapted by permission from A.W. Pichardo, J.L. Oliver, C.B. Harrison, et al., "Integrating Resistance Training Into High School Curriculum," *Strength and Conditioning Journal* 41, no. 1 (2018): 39-50.

Figure 8.6 Reprinted by permission from A.W. Pichardo, J.L. Oliver, C.B. Harrison, et al., "Integrating Resistance Training Into High School Curriculum," *Strength and Conditioning Journal* 41, no. 1 (2018): 39-50.

Table 8.11 Adapted by permission from S.L. Bertelsen and B. Thompson, "High School Weight-Training Curriculum: Course Development Considerations," *Strategies* 30, no. 3 (2017): 10-17.

Table 8.12 Source: P. McHenry (personal communication, February 20, 2020).

Figure 8.7 Reprinted by permission from A.W. Pichardo, J.L. Oliver, C.B. Harrison, et al., "Integrating Models of Long-Term Athletic Development to Maximize the Physical Development of Youth," *International Journal of Sports Science & Coaching* 13, no. 6 (2018): 1189-1199. Adapted from Granacher et al. (19a), Lloyd et al. (29a), and Lloyd et al. (29b).

Figure 8.8 Reprinted by permission from A.W. Pichardo, J.L. Oliver, C.B. Harrison, et al., "Integrating Resistance Training Into High School Curriculum," *Strength and Conditioning Journal* 41, no. 1 (2018): 39-50.

Table 8.13 Adapted from unpublished work created by Jacob Reed, PhD, CSCS. Used with permission.

Figure 8.9 Adapted from unpublished work created by Jacob Reed, PhD, CSCS. Used with permission.

Table 8.14 Adapted from unpublished work created by Jacob Reed, PhD, CSCS. Used with permission.

Figure 08.10 Reprinted by permission from A.W. Pichardo, J.L. Oliver, C.B. Harrison, et al., "Integrating Models of Long-Term Athletic Development to Maximize the Physical Development of Youth," *International Journal of Sports Science & Coaching* 13, no. 6 (2018): 1189-1199.

Table 11.1 Reprinted by permission from P. Hagerman, "Aerobic Endurance Training Program Design," in Essentials of Personal Training, 2nd ed., edited for the National Strength and Conditioning Association by J.W. Coburn and M.H. Malek (Champaign, IL: Human Kinetics, 2012), 392.

Preface

Rick Howard, DSc, CSCS,*D, FNSCA
Patrick McHenry, MA, CSCS,*D, RSCC
Mike Nitka, MS, CSCS,*D, RSCC*E, FNSCA*E

The strength and conditioning professional who works in the high school setting as a strength coach, physical education teacher, sport coach, administrator, and so on is a highly valued member of the entire strength and conditioning community. *NSCA's Guide to High School Strength and Conditioning* is the product of collaboration among many groups and individuals within the NSCA, with the primary objective being to meet high school strength and conditioning professionals where they are and provide material that supports them in their role as a strength and conditioning professional in the high school setting.

The NSCA is recognized as the worldwide authority on strength and conditioning and has long supported the high school setting as an integral and unique opportunity to motivate and inspire the entire student body, student-athletes and non-athletes alike, to be the best they can be on the field and in the weight room and as productive members of a physically literate society. This support has taken the form of creation of the high school special interest group (HS SIG), an elected position to the NSCA Board of Directors, the prestigious Strength of America Award, and the High School Strength and Conditioning Coach of the Year Award that recognizes high school strength and conditioning professionals and high school strength and conditioning facilities that not only meet but exceed industry standards.

The NSCA's Goals for the High School Professional

The NSCA's continued effort to support the high school strength and conditioning professional includes dedicated assistance in each of the four elements of the NSCA strategic plan (9):

1. *Advancing professional development* with a featured track at the NSCA National Conference and NSCA Coaches Conference, as well as presentations at regional and state NSCA events to increase exposure and address further ongoing professional development

2. *Advancing community* with continued growth in the NSCA among high school strength and conditioning professionals and increased collaboration with the long-term athletic development (LTAD) SIG (formerly called the youth SIG) in conducting conference presentations, alignment of strategies in the high school market, and sharing of resources

3. *Advancing advocacy* with a dedicated area of the NSCA website for high school strength and conditioning professionals, which includes information on the following:

- *Impact on the school:* includes why every high school needs a qualified strength and conditioning professional and the legal benefits of having one
- *Impact on the students:* includes keeping high school student-athletes safe and giving them skills that will serve them in sports, in the classroom, and in life
- *Impact on the profession:* includes creating and expanding a position for a strength and conditioning professional; best practices for full-time, part-time, and contracted positions; and hiring guidelines for high school strength and conditioning professionals
- *Impact on an existing program:* includes improving existing programs with the latest standards and guidelines, best practices for preventing sudden death, youth training and LTAD, and impact for the entire student body
- *Impact on parents:* includes information for parents such as the NSCA's 10 pillars for successful LTAD (7), keys to injury prevention, and addressing the risks of early sport specialization

4. *Advancing communication* through multiple platforms. In addition to the information provided on the NSCA website, the NSCA shares high school–specific content with other organizations such as the Inter-Association Task Force for Preventing Sudden Death (3), which included the NSCA, the American Medical Society for Sports Medicine, the National Athletic Trainers' Association, and the National Federation of State High School Associations. Articles have appeared in publications such as *Athletic Business*, Teambuildr.com, and *District Administration* magazine. High school strength and conditioning professionals and those professionals from the high school SIG and from the LTAD SIG actively participated in the development of the NSCA strategic plan and are excited to share with you this textbook that addresses all four elements of the strategic plan.

How the NSCA Board of Directors and Special Interest Groups Work Together

The HS SIG was one of the first SIGs formed and continues to be active, sharing and disseminating information specifically to help the high school strength and conditioning professional. The LTAD SIG has worked closely with the HS SIG since its inception in 2004. Originally called the Youth SIG, the name was changed in 2018 to reflect support of the NSCA LTAD position statement and subsequent initiatives, especially those for youth (children ages 6-18 years old). The integration of LTAD principles in the high school setting provides the high school strength and conditioning professional evidence-driven information to best create age- and developmentally appropriate strength and conditioning programs for freshmen as well as seniors, those who are untrained and inexperienced as well as those working to get better, and for different positions within the same sport.

The NSCA is dedicated to advancing the strength and conditioning profession around the world, so this book is intended for practitioners in a variety of settings, whether a grade 9 to 12 setting, U-15 to U-19 elite team, sports academy, or other configuration responsible for improving performance and reducing the risk of injury in the adolescent population. In concert with the NSCA mission to support and disseminate research-based knowledge and practical application to improve athletic performance and fitness, this book provides practitioners in the high school setting the information they need to apply the principles of pediatric exercise science, growth and maturation, and LTAD.

Why There Is a Need for a High School Strength and Conditioning Manual

The NSCA provides great information and resources for the high school strength and conditioning professional, and this manual includes evidence-driven information that helps the high school strength and conditioning professional be the best practitioner possible by integrating principles of sport performance, nutrition, and safe and effective program design to best benefit all student-athletes. Participation and opportunity gaps are widening in the high school student-athlete population and include fewer opportunities for low-income student-athletes (1), more student-athletes specializing too early in one sport (5), and more student-athletes dropping out of sports or never participating at all, so the need for qualified high school strength and conditioning professionals has never been greater. This book will equip readers—whether the strength and conditioning professional, physical education teacher, sport coach, or administrator—to build a solid strength and conditioning community in any setting.

Connection Between High School and Long-Term Athletic Development

The concept of LTAD has been around for centuries. Early models of LTAD created a process that laid out the development for student-athletes to go "from playground to podium" (2). Sport scientists have used a systematic approach to develop children into Olympic athletes in just about every country.

In the 1990s Istvan Balyi was one of the first coaches to popularize a series of training stages that showed the development of children and adolescents. Over the years LTAD has evolved into a philosophy and framework that is embraced around the world. This process has many iterations such as the youth development model (6) and the American development model (8); however, the general philosophy is the same.

The LTAD concept works perfectly in the American school system if physical education (PE) teachers and strength and conditioning professionals work together. Physical education, like math, science, and writing, is built off the previous information the students have learned, and the difficulty increases as the student-athlete advances through school. This spiraling curriculum allows for introduction, development, then mastery before moving on to the next phase. Each year or phase the PE teacher reviews the old information (i.e., fundamental movements or exercises) before introducing new information. A quality resistance training program should follow this model. At the beginning of each phase the strength and conditioning professional reviews the basic movement patterns, exercises, and progressions (drills) to ensure the student-athlete is ready to progress to the next level. Communication is the key to accomplishing this goal.

The high school PE teacher or strength and conditioning professional needs to work with the sport coaches and middle or junior high school PE teacher to establish a coordinated system for the exercises and drills the students have learned and worked on. This will provide a starting point so on the first day of classes the PE teacher or strength and conditioning professional has a general idea of the student-athletes' abilities and base knowledge. If a new student-athlete joins the class, a movement screen that shows basic lifting technique and running patterns can reveal where the student-athlete needs to start. The PE teacher or strength and conditioning professional then puts the new student-athlete into the four-year progression matrix (4) to develop student-athletes (figure 1).

For the high school student-athlete who plans to continue to play sports at the collegiate level, when the student-athlete is finishing high school the PE teacher or strength and conditioning professional should contact the college or university where the student-athlete will be attending to find out which exercises the athlete will be expected to perform. The PE teacher or strength and conditioning professional can then build on this information before sending the student-athlete on to the next level. If the student-athlete is not moving on to college sports they will have a solid base from which to continue their development of physical literacy. For those student-athletes moving on to the military, the PE teacher or strength and conditioning professional can help prepare the student-athlete for basic training.

Teaching resistance training as a lifelong fitness component is a focus for some high school strength and conditioning programs, other high school programs focus on resistance training for the development of the student-athlete, and others prepare the student-athlete to participate in collegiate sports. No matter the area of focus, the goal of the class is the same: all student-athletes need to learn proper technique to ensure correct motor patterns that develop lifelong movers on the path to physical literacy, while lessening the likelihood of injury during the student-athlete's high school athletic career.

The NSCA has a position paper that includes the 10 pillars for successful LTAD and how to incorporate them into a strength and conditioning program (7). Other resources are listed in the recommended reading section at the end of this chapter.

Role of Professional Standards and Guidelines

The duties of strength and conditioning professionals consist of much more than selecting exercises and prescribing sets, repetitions, and rest. The safety of all participants should be the number one concern. Throughout this book various authors will provide parameters for high school strength and conditioning professionals to refer to and use when carrying out their responsibilities to student-athletes. The NSCA *Strength and Conditioning Professional Standards and Guidelines* are referred to often (10). This document is the result of several revisions that are based on peer-reviewed scientific studies, statements from other professional associations, analysis of claims and litigation, and a consensus of expert views. This document will prepare strength and conditioning professionals to discuss with their administrators and risk management coordinator to improve their program.

The professional standard of training high school student-athletes is to incorporate the basic principles of strength and conditioning and consistently apply them to this unique population. While high school strength and conditioning

The Generic Quadrennial Plan

Freshman Year: The Foundation Level

Aim: To ensure that student-athletes have the required motor patterns to enable them to perform optimally in their sport and to enhance their performance and reduce injury risk during future stages of the performance program.

Type of cycle: This is a basic accumulative (gradual increase) cycle aimed at developing general fitness levels. Process goals dominate this stage to ensure that student-athletes target the key technique-related factors that will ensure their motor patterns have a strong foundation so as to optimize performance.

Objectives:

- To optimize muscle activation patterns and balance
- To ensure functional movement ranges and patterns
- To groove the key locomotive movement patterns
- To develop a sound base of general strength and stability
- To ensure sound technique in key resistance training activities

Sophomore Year: The Development Level

Aim: To develop the key fitness parameters of the student-athlete's sport to a level that allows trained and experienced peaking-based programs.

Type of cycle: This is another accumulative cycle, but training moves from general to more sport specific through the period. Goals follow the training objectives and become increasingly sport specific throughout this cycle in key targeted areas, such as lifting more weight, running faster, and so on.

Objectives:

- To challenge the key locomotive movement patterns and combinations until they stand up to open sport-specific challenges (e.g., a high degree of sport-specific endurance)
- To develop a high degree of overall balanced strength and stability in all of the key movement patterns
- To ensure all student-athletes have excellent grooved techniques on key resistance training exercises

Junior Year: The Performance Level

Aim: To optimize performance in sport.

Type of cycle: Performance in competition starts to be stressed. While predominantly transmutative (changeable) in nature, a small number of realization cycles can be employed in which high levels of performance in competition may be needed.

Objectives:

- To develop sport-specific strength and power
- To optimize sport-related movement, including reading and reaction to key sport-specific stimuli
- To continue to develop appropriate muscle mass for sport
- To enable the student-athlete to perform for the duration of their game through specific metabolic conditioning

Senior Year: The Peak Level

Aim: To further optimize performance in sport.

Type of cycle: This is traditionally a periodized year, in which performance in competition is stressed.

Objectives:

- To develop a high degree of sport-specific strength and power
- To optimize sport-related movement
- To optimize total performance

Adapted by permission from Jeffreys (2008).

FIGURE 1   The generic quadrennial plan.

professionals are encouraged to stay on top of trends, student-athletes are best served by being introduced to the basic principles and then having the opportunity to practice and perfect those principles throughout high school in order to best navigate the expected growth and development of this population physically, socially, and emotionally.

The word *qualified* as part of the term "qualified strength and conditioning coach" helps identify the legal responsibilities and professional scope of practice for the high school strength and conditioning professional.

"Qualified" can be subdivided into two domains. The first is called the *scientific foundations*. Having taken university-level classes (e.g., anatomy, exercise physiology, biomechanics, sport psychology, and nutrition) shows that the professional probably has a basic working knowledge to run or assist in a program. The second domain is called *practical applied*, which indicates that the strength and conditioning professional has experience in teaching exercise technique progressions; designing basic strength and conditioning programs; has organized and administered at least one program; and is knowledgeable in testing, evaluation, and goal setting. School districts are looking for candidates who have a combination of the knowledge and experience from the two domains, which may help minimize future lawsuits.

What are the legal duties and responsibilities expected of strength and conditioning professionals? All high school strength and conditioning professionals have legal duties and responsibilities to provide an appropriate level of supervision and instruction to meet a reasonable standard of care and to provide and maintain a safe training environment for the participants while under their supervision. These duties involve informing participants and their guardians of inherent risks related to their activities and preventing unreasonable risk or harm resulting from negligent instruction or supervision.

Teachers, strength and conditioning professionals, and sport coaches should be familiar with the concept of assumption of risk, meaning that the student-athlete is voluntarily participating in an activity with knowledge of the inherent risks. Athletic activities, including strength and conditioning, involve certain risks. All participants and their guardians must be thoroughly informed of the risks of all activities and be required to sign a statement to that effect. Do not let a student-athlete participate until this assumption of risk document has been signed and returned.

Another legal term is **liability**, which refers to the legal responsibility, duty, or obligation PE teachers and strength and conditioning professionals have to their classes and teams that they will take reasonable steps, for example, to prevent injury and to act prudently (but within their proper scope of practice) when an injury occurs.

Negligence is a failure on the part of an individual to act as a reasonable and prudent person would under similar circumstances. Four elements must be present for a PE teacher or strength and conditioning professional to be found liable for negligence:

1. Duties as a PE teacher or strength and conditioning professional must exist
2. A breach of a duty or duties occurred
3. Proximate cause exists (a breach of a duty is what directly caused an injury, for example)
4. Damages have resulted

Simply stated, a strength and conditioning professional is negligent if he or she is proven to have had a duty to act but failed to act with the appropriate standard of care, causing injury or damages to another person.

A **standard of care** is defined as what a prudent and reasonable person would do under similar circumstances. A strength and conditioning professional is expected to respond and act according to education, training, and certification status.

Knowing the difference between a standard and a guideline is important, because each term has different legal implications.

A **standard** is a procedure that reflects a legal duty or obligation for standard of care. (The standard statements in the NSCA *Strength and Conditioning Professional Standards and Guidelines* [10] use the phrase "must do.") The standards set forth in this professional standards and guidelines document are recognized as a legal standard of care and must be implemented into the daily operations of strength and conditioning programs and facilities.

A **guideline** is a recommended operating procedure developed to further enhance the quality of services provided. (The standard statements in the NSCA *Strength and Conditioning Professional Standards and Guidelines* [10] use the phrase "should do.") Guidelines are not intended to be standards of practice. In certain circumstances they assist in evaluating and improving services rendered.

Knowing the standards of practice and how they apply to risk management is a proactive process that should help minimize legal liability as well as decrease the frequency and severity of injuries and subsequent claims and lawsuits. While it may not be possible to eliminate all risks of injury and liability exposure in strength and conditioning settings, they can be effectively minimized by implementing sound risk management strategies. The strength and conditioning professional is responsible for drafting the risk management plan with input from others.

Applying standards of practice to the risk management process involves a four-step procedure:

1. Identify and select standards of practice that must be included.
2. Develop risk management strategies reflecting standards of practice.
3. Implement the risk management plan.
4. Evaluate the risk management plan.

While liability exposure in the strength and conditioning profession is unique to each facility, a task force has identified nine areas of concern (10). It is important to note that these nine areas are interrelated. For example, proper instruction and supervision is associated with personnel qualifications as well as facility layout and scheduling issues. Noncompliance in any one of the areas can therefore affect others and compound the risk of liability exposure and potential litigation. Furthermore, strength and conditioning professionals and their employers share these duties and responsibilities.

Collectively within these nine areas of liability exposure there are 11 standards and 14 guidelines for strength and conditioning professionals that will assist in making their facility and program safer for student-athletes. Take the time to read, study, and follow the standards and guidelines for the safety of all student-athletes in your program.

Scope and Organization of This Book

This book was written in response to the need in the high school strength and conditioning community for a resource for those working with student-athletes in the classroom and weight room. Commonly, that individual is called a *strength coach* or sometimes simply *coach*, but with the emergence of established scopes of practice, the job title has been formalized as *strength and conditioning professional*.

The high school strength and conditioning professional can have many different roles; a few common examples include:

- A PE teacher who is NSCA-certified (or working toward becoming certified) and teaches weight training classes during the day and trains the sport teams after school.

- A classroom teacher (of subjects unrelated to physical education) who trains the sport teams after school.

- A sport coach who may or may not teach a PE class but runs his or her team's strength and conditioning program.

- A personal trainer who is hired by the school to come in before or after school to train the sport teams.

The NSCA has a collection of over 30 free handouts and videos that uphold the need to hire a qualified strength and conditioning professional and explain how to launch a career in high school strength and conditioning. This material can be accessed on the NSCA's website under the "Education" tab (or search for "NSCA Tools and Resources").

The most important component of a high school weight room is the person running it. He or she needs to have the knowledge to oversee and train high school-aged student-athletes because they are not the same as college or professional athletes. The *NSCA's Guide to High School Strength and Conditioning* describes the roles and duties of a high school strength and conditioning professional, provides strength and conditioning-related resources, and presents detailed guidelines for exercise technique and program design.

Recommended Reading

Council on Sports Medicine and Fitness. Strength training by children and adolescents. *Pediatrics* 121(4):835-840, 2008.

Donnelly, JE, Hillman, CH, Castelli, D, Etnier, JL, Lee, S, Tomporowski, P, Lambourne, K, and Szabo-Reed, AN. Physical activity, fitness, cognitive function, and academic achievement in children: A systematic review. *Med Sci Sports Exerc* 48(6):1197, 2016.

Howard, R, Eisenmann, JC, and Moreno, A. Summary: The National Strength and Conditioning Association position statement on long-term athletic development. *Strength Cond J* 41(2):124-126, 2019.

Meadors, L. *Practical application for long-term athletic development*. May 2012, www.nsca.com/education/articles/practical-application-for-long-term-athletic-development. Accessed November 7, 2020.

Till, K, Eisenmann, J, Emmonds, S, Jones, B, Mitchell, T, Cowburn, I, Tee, J, Holmes, N, and Lloyd, RS. A coaching session framework to facilitate long-term athletic development. *Strength Cond J* 43(3):43-55, 2021.

Introduction:
Strength and Conditioning–
Related Professionals
in the High School Setting

Edwin C. Jones, MA, CSCS
Shawn L. Jenkins, MS, ATC, CSCS

Since 1978, the NSCA has been improving athletic performance. Many areas of strength and conditioning have expanded since its inception: Certification has evolved and is practiced in 72 countries. Colleges and universities have curricula that lead to productive careers in this profession. Through innovative school support and high school leadership, the certified high school strength and conditioning professional has evolved from a sport coach working in the weight room with student-athletes after school into classroom courses, with lifetime benefits guided by a certified professional.

NSCA's Guide to High School Strength and Conditioning draws on best practices in the field of strength and conditioning. This manual will serve as an important resource for the strength and conditioning professional and the administration in the high school environment.

The NSCA defines a Certified Strength and Conditioning Specialist (CSCS) as a professional who applies scientific knowledge to train student-athletes with the primary goal of improving athletic performance and overall health (7, 12, 18). Additional goals of a CSCS include injury prevention and minimizing recovery time from an injury (7).

Strength and conditioning professionals are an integral part of the coaching staff. They are the only coaches who interact with all student-athletes and various team sports. Training several student-athletes provides the opportunity to affect lives by demonstrating good character and leadership qualities. Interacting with hundreds of student-athletes of various ethnicities, personalities, life experiences, and socioeconomic statuses is no small task. As the strength and conditioning professional interacts with the student-athlete, they must implement methods to get maximum effort and performance. Very similar to collegiate coaching, the high school strength and conditioning professional is a very involved position and offers a great opportunity to positively affect the life of the student-athlete, possibly leading to career opportunities for the student-athlete.

In addition to developing a program and becoming familiar with hundreds of student-athletes, the strength and conditioning professional builds rapport with multiple sport coaches, the athletic director, principal, school staff, and parents. Developing healthy relationships is essential to job success.

Qualifications of a Strength and Conditioning Professional

Due to the complex nature of the strength and conditioning program, several factors must be addressed to ensure the best person is hired.

- *Certifications:* A qualified strength and conditioning professional must maintain professional certification credentialed by an independent agency. One-third of high school strength and conditioning professionals are certified by the NSCA (3, 15). Other certifications that must be obtained are first aid, cardiopulmonary resuscitation (CPR), and automated external defibrillator (AED).

- *Education:* A minimum of a bachelor's degree from a regionally accredited college or university in one or more of the scientific foundations for strength and conditioning (e.g., exercise or anatomy, biomechanics, pediatric exercise physiology, nutrition) or relevant subjects (e.g., exercise, sport pedagogy, psychology, motor learning, training methodology, kinesiology). Eighty-four percent of high school strength and conditioning professionals have degrees in physical education (PE) or an exercise science–related field (5), and as many as 50 percent have a master's degree (3).

- *Experience:* In addition to academic knowledge, experience is a valuable part of being a CSCS. Experience gained as an assistant, intern, or volunteer, preferably working with high school populations, is important when preparing for this career. Gaining this experience while in college should be the focus (3).

- *Physical requirements:* Being a strength and conditioning professional is a physically demanding job. Strength and conditioning professionals must have the strength to properly demonstrate lifting and movement skills and techniques used by student-athletes. Strength and conditioning professionals must be able to see those under their supervision. Sitting, standing, lifting and carrying (at least 50 lbs [23 kg]), reaching, squatting, climbing, kneeling, and moving equipment are other physical requirements strength and conditioning professionals must possess (10, 12).

- *Additional:* A high school strength and conditioning professional must be prepared to undergo a background check, physical, psychological test, and drug screen (10, 12).

Primary Positions or Roles

Having a certified strength and conditioning professional on staff in high schools is often viewed as a bonus or perk when it should be the norm. A strength and conditioning professional on staff is good for student-athletes, parents, and the school. The student-athlete will be under the guidance of a certified professional who will ensure certain exercises are performed correctly to minimize the risk of injury. Parents will be pleased knowing a certified professional is present to instruct and monitor their student-athlete. A strength and conditioning professional using best practices and having personal liability insurance helps mitigate liability to the school and the professional (11, 16).

The strength and conditioning professional position can be classified in five categories to meet school needs.

Split-Position Physical Education Teacher and Strength and Conditioning Professional

This individual has a unique responsibility in supporting the school's leadership while serving in two roles. The professional carries the same rights and responsibilities as an educator and will be assigned responsibilities to contribute to the overall effective operation of the school. These responsibilities, upon which the educator will be evaluated, include duty assignments (e.g., supervising students in the cafeteria, halls, or other areas in the school), preparing lesson plans to engage the student-athletes, and implementing Society of Health and Physical Educators (SHAPE)'s National Standards (13) along with NSCA *Strength and Conditioning Professional Standards and Guidelines* (11). It requires attending departmental, faculty, and system-wide meetings; serving on committees; and taking an active role in those assignments for the benefit of the school. Because of the unique skill set strength and conditioning professionals possess, they may be called upon to become involved in a variety of assignments in a leadership capacity. Whatever role is assigned, the individual must approach it as an opportunity to understand the organization of the school system and to expand the awareness of and support for the strength and conditioning program.

A primary benefit of this category is having a strength and conditioning professional who is also certified to teach PE or other classes involving the general student body, not just student-athletes. In addition to their teaching salary, a PE teacher could be paid a strength and conditioning professional stipend outside regular school hours. For some strength and conditioning professionals, teaching classes other than strength and conditioning may be undesirable, or they may have their certification without a teaching license, which would exclude them from being employed as a PE teacher. Although it is not a dedicated full-time strength and conditioning professional position, a split-position strength and conditioning professional has similar characteristics but with less strength and conditioning class load responsibilities. They interact with student-athletes throughout the day and develop relationships that foster trust and respect between themselves and student-athletes. Establishing these relationships could positively affect behaviors that help build character and the buy-in necessary to develop a good strength and conditioning program. By being on campus, the split-position strength and conditioning professional has the potential to bolster the strength and conditioning program by teaching other subjects such as health and nutrition, hosting guest speakers, and organizing field trips to promote the strength and conditioning profession.

Full-Time Certified Strength and Conditioning Professional

A full-time strength and conditioning professional is the best option when developing a high school strength and conditioning program. This individual is a full-time employee of the school. In this setting, student-athletes take strength and conditioning classes during the school day. The strength and conditioning professional trains all sport team members and other student-athletes who are assigned to the strength and conditioning program. By being on campus, the strength and conditioning professional will be able to promote the program to all sport coaches to foster relationships with student-athletes in and outside of the weight room. In addition to developing athletic skills, the full-time strength and conditioning professional will be able to develop relationships to enhance the student-athlete's character and encourage sound decision-making, which transfers into positive, lifelong development.

The long-term presence of the qualified strength and conditioning professional also facilitates relationships with school administrators and other staff. For example, a certified athletic trainer and a certified strength and conditioning professional are an effective team to promote injury prevention and recovery for the student-athletes. This is also an opportunity for the strength and conditioning professional to promote the benefits of the strength and conditioning field. The result is a greater level of respect between the two groups that will facilitate buy-in for the strength and conditioning program.

In their positions and roles, strength and conditioning professionals must fulfill the following duties and responsibilities:

- Design strength and conditioning programs based on sound scientific findings, implement baseline evaluation of student-athletes, and maintain records. In addition to student-athletes, a high school strength and conditioning professional may also train the general student body. Their sole focus may not be athletic performance but enhanced health. Therefore, the strength and conditioning professional must recognize this and design programs to meet these needs.

- Rehabilitate and train injured student-athletes. The strength and conditioning professional works in conjunction with a certified athletic trainer to design a program that will return the student-athlete to full health.

- Recommend the purchasing of exercise equipment and supplies and maintain the exercise equipment.

- Instruct and supervise work-study volunteers (9). Performing these additional duties adds to the strength and conditioning professional's toolbox and may help to grow the profession.

- Perform the duties of a full-time educator, following the guidelines of educator evaluation unless otherwise determined by the contract or administration.

Part-Time High School Strength and Conditioning Professional

A qualified part-time strength and conditioning professional on staff is more beneficial than not having one. This immediately gives the strength and conditioning program validity because a certified and knowledgeable individual will be supervising the program. Additionally, a strength and conditioning professional is available to all teams before or after school. Each team should have equal access to the weight training facility based on a predetermined schedule.

Coaching and teaching inconsistencies could occur between the strength and conditioning professional and PE teacher. The PE teacher may not be nationally certified and may possess limited knowledge and abilities in the strength and conditioning field, which could prove confusing to the students.

The position of a part-time strength and conditioning professional does have its challenges. The person is not available on campus as often as a full-time or split-position individual. The strength and conditioning professional may also only be available when a team is in season, which gives little time for interaction with student-athletes and limits the strength and conditioning professional's ability to gain buy-in to their strength and conditioning program. Typically, coaching stipends are minimal, which makes retaining a strength and conditioning professional difficult. The evaluation process will be determined by contract or the administration.

Sport Coach With Seasonal Duties in the Weight Room

The seasonal strength and conditioning professional is common at many high schools throughout the United States, particularly with football programs. Schools and sport coaches may implement this due to budget constraints.

The challenge with this category is that the sport coach may have been around for quite some time, has been successful, and is accustomed to their methods. They may supervise the strength and conditioning training program or appoint a position sport coach. In many cases, this sport coach is not a certified strength and conditioning professional and their own past experiences with resistance training in their youth may be their only strength and conditioning experience. The amount of technical experience this sport coach has in teaching correct lifting movements may be limited. An uncertified strength and conditioning professional could lead to liability issues. With this being the case, the individual sport coach with seasonal duties in the weight room must work toward obtaining a strength and conditioning certification. A sport coach benefits from this additional responsibility assignment by being a strength and conditioning professional who is tasked to only strengthen and condition the student-athletes on the team. This classification has some drawbacks, however. Ideally, this sport coach should help student-athletes on other sport teams. Assisting student-athletes from other sport teams may prove difficult because the sport coach may feel a primary responsibility to their own team. Strength and conditioning professional duties come second. The sport coach more than likely will not be available to train student-athletes not on their team. This environment could fail to build unity between student-athletes from different sport teams.

To make this experience beneficial for everyone, here are a few recommendations:

- The sport coach with seasonal weight room duties must earn a certificate through the NSCA's Foundation of Coaching Lifts course. This course addresses the need to identify correct lifting techniques and learning coaching cues and progressions to teach complex exercises safely and effectively.

- Within one year of completion of the NSCA's Foundation of Coaching Lifts course, that professional must attend the state or national clinic/conference each year for the duration of his or her employment, for additional strength and conditioning education.

- The sport coach should assist all student-athletes engaged in resistance training regardless of their sport.

After obtaining a certificate from the Foundation of Coaching Lifts course, the sport coach has a beginning knowledge of lifting techniques and progression. This course, along with continuing education, provides incentive for the sport coach to become a certified strength and conditioning professional. These recommendations address the areas of safe exercise performance under qualified supervision and enable the sport coach to safely assist all student-athletes in the resistance training facility.

Contracted Strength and Conditioning Professional or Company

Another option for a school is contracting a strength and conditioning professional from a larger company or as an individual. In this environment, a strength and conditioning professional has much more flexibility with scheduling compared to a sport coach with seasonal duties. To ensure targeted needs are met, the contract should be very specific. The flexibility of this position allows the professional to meet the needs of student-athletes from various sport teams. A company may be able to designate more than one strength and conditioning professional to a school site.

A contracted strength and conditioning professional would meet the needs of a sport team. This serves everyone knowing a certified individual will be present to oversee the strength and conditioning program. The strength and conditioning professional should implement proper program design and have the knowledge and experience to teach the exercises correctly. A contracted individual is available to train student-athletes during designated before- or after-school contracted hours. Individual student-athletes would be able to receive individualized training to focus on specified weaknesses, or the entire team could receive more training outside of the school's weight training facility. This may be an option at a company's site where updated and newer equipment is available, which can broaden the student-athletes' strength and conditioning experience.

The contracted strength and conditioning professional is not a regular and consistent presence on campus, unlike the full-time or split-position professional. Student-athletes may be engaged in other physical activities, and if the contracted strength and conditioning professional does not engage with other sport coaches or the PE teacher, over-training may occur.

This position makes it much more difficult to connect and build trust with student-athletes. The contracted strength and conditioning professional will need to use innovative ways to build buy-in to the resistance training program. Buy-in also applies to the coaching staffs and physical educators. This unfamiliarity could be a barrier to the program's progression. Strength and conditioning professionals hired through a company may not always send the same strength and conditioning professional, which would add further unfamiliarity. Although the strength and conditioning professional is certified, the company may send one who is not as experienced in the field of strength and conditioning. To avoid this scenario, it is recommended to add a stipulation in the contract that the strength and conditioning professional must have previous experience working with high school student-athletes in the high school setting. This way, the school will know it is receiving a strength and conditioning professional who is certified and has the requested experience.

High School Strength and Conditioning Professional's Role in Interacting With Others

Strength and conditioning professionals need the assistance of student-athletes, colleagues, supervisors, and community to effectively deliver the program; effective leadership requires interaction with all stakeholders. Collaboration, communication, and relationships are consistently listed collectively as key elements for a successful program in schools and school systems. Creating a successful program requires effective communication (14), which is communication between two or more persons where the intended message is successfully delivered, received, and understood (6). The following sections identify and provide insight to enhance communication skills with colleagues, the leadership of the organization, and the community.

Physical Educator

Whether interacting with 200 student-athletes or few athletic department personnel, the one skill a strength and conditioning professional must possess is the ability to communicate clearly and confidently, which includes being a great listener.

Among the traits necessary for success as the high school strength and conditioning professional are teaching ability, communication skills, relationship-building skills, empathy, and the ability to promote success. Many other skills are needed, but relationship building and the ability to promote success are relevant to open lines of communication between the physical educator and the strength and conditioning professional. As relationships with colleagues build, informal discussions on lesson planning, delivery of instruction, organization, and reflective teaching practices place the educators in a continual learning and sharing cycle. Best practices approach learning as a continual process. Through attending conferences and clinics, the team can jointly elevate the PE and strength and conditioning programs.

Before an employment interview or reporting to the assignment at the school, it is necessary for the strength and conditioning professional to research and understand the organizational structure of the school and the PE department. It is imperative for the new strength and conditioning professional to listen and understand what has previously been established when launching the program. Coming into a new school environment, it is beneficial for the PE department members and school leadership to share the rules and procedures to provide effective instruction. Mentors are often assigned to new strength and conditioning professionals to assist with the adjustment to the school environment and to provide daily support to address specific concerns. The department will meet to discuss strategies to improve student performance in class. It will be beneficial to the PE department for the strength and conditioning professional to share the strategic plan of action to improve the health and confidence of the student-athletes in the general population of the school.

Student-athletes benefit when the PE teacher and strength and conditioning professional are made aware of each other's resistance training program. They must also communicate regarding injuries sustained during training. In a joint effort, both should make exercise and physical fitness such a positive experience that student-athletes will want to make it a lifelong commitment.

Sport Coach

The high school strength and conditioning professional's relationship with the sport coach is one that can be directed toward team progress and confidence. In this relationship, communication and respect are crucial factors (6). The strength and conditioning professional must have a firm understanding of the physical attributes a sport coach desires for players and the training necessary to develop them. The strength and conditioning professional's task is to implement safe measures while enhancing a student-athlete's strength and sport performance and preventing injury.

Before training begins, a thorough, well-organized strategic plan should be developed by the strength and conditioning professional with some input from the sport coach. This is needed to identify the strengths and weaknesses of the team. The pretest assessment combined with the sport coach assessment will provide the basis for initial training. With this data, the strength and conditioning professional can design a program that will improve the overall physical and mental condition of the student-athletes. Improvement will be shown directly through the daily progress and posttesting. This information is valuable to the sport coach, who is actively involved in the complete process of the team's strength and conditioning improvement. The success of the sport coach's interaction with the strength and conditioning professional is based on the joint effort of the student-athletes, which is guided by the strength and conditioning professional with the encouragement and full support of the sport coach. The strength and conditioning professional, with formal education and experience in the strength and conditioning field, and the sport coach must have mutual respect and humility for each other to ensure the program's success. The young men and women of the program have advocates for their safety, and their parents are assured of professionals working in the best interest of their child's well-being.

Athletic Director

Depending on whether the strength and conditioning professional is a full-time professional or a split-position PE and strength and conditioning professional, the strategic plan remains intact for the classes. The five basic student-athlete benefits of the strength and conditioning program for the general population are to improve health, improve confidence, reduce injuries, improve long-term athletic development, and improve athletic performance. Always keeping these student-athlete benefits in mind will serve as the basis for a sound fundamental strength and conditioning program as the strength and conditioning professional communicates with student-athletes, parents, the athletic director (AD), administration, and community representatives.

The AD and the strength and conditioning professional's interaction will be based on one of the five professional positions in the career ladder. As a full-time professional in the school under the leadership of the principal, the strength and conditioning professional should obtain an organizational chart from the principal. Whether the direct supervisor is the assistant principal, PE department chairperson, or AD, the strength and conditioning professional should clearly understand the chain of command in the organization. It would be advantageous to provide periodic updates to the direct supervisor on the progress in the strength and conditioning professional's learning environment. To initiate dialogue with the AD, invite them to observe the training sessions and have open communication concerning the program. This is also a great opportunity to educate the AD about the strength and conditioning professional's duties and provide an active understanding of the program. This will be important for when it is time to request resources and support.

The AD's job is to ensure that programs are operating safely to avoid liability issues, as well as to manage the budget, oversee staffing and scheduling, and other responsibilities. Knowledge of those responsibilities are beneficial as the strength and conditioning professional navigates through the coordination of AD interactions. When designing a resistance training program, the strength and conditioning professional must analyze it for any unsafe practices that could potentially harm the student-athlete.

Principal

Communication with the principal is important to keep the leadership abreast of the program's progress. From the first contact with school leadership, it is imperative that the full-time strength and conditioning professional and split-position physical educator and strength and conditioning professional clearly display the following: positive attitude, dependability, professionalism, organization, and evidence of daily preparation for class. Additionally, the strength and conditioning professional should volunteer to open the educational environment for visits as a model classroom. When challenges occur, the ability of the strength and conditioning professional to handle adversity is helpful for the school leadership. These are components of effective professionalism that translates into trust to assist the strength and conditioning program and the organizational structure of the school. As the relationship develops, the open lines of communication will assist the operation of the school and the advancement of the program when the need arises for support. To gain complete support for the program, the strength and conditioning professional should request the opportunity to provide a visual presentation on the program benefits during a faculty meeting.

Parents

The most common ways that strength and conditioning professionals can stay in contact with student-athletes' parents are notes, emails, and telephone calls. A positive message will lay a solid foundation for a good relationship. Starting with the first contact with a parent, the message should communicate the benefits of the program to the student-athletes and the school very clearly. During the school year, parent and community relations may be increased with a request for the opportunity to provide a visual presentation on the program benefits. This may occur at a parent–teacher association, booster club, or board of education meeting and through various school system–approved media resources. To effectively support the visual presentations, the strength and conditioning professional should maintain an updated portfolio of the ongoing accomplishments of the student-athletes and the program (14). These methods of communication will be helpful to support the general communication methods of school-developed progress reports and report cards.

Benefits of a High School Strength and Conditioning Program

Perhaps the most long-lasting benefit of a strength and conditioning program is overall health. Consistent exercise combats many health-related issues (6, 7, 9); decreases the risk of injury (7); and minimizes injury recovery time (7), which ultimately results in increased muscular strength, power, and endurance required for sport performance.

A strength and conditioning professional must be familiar with the long-term athletic development dynamics of resistance training for youth (8) and understand the age-appropriate, developmental stages of the student-athlete and how to design a resistance training program that yields positive results (2, 8). The strength and conditioning professional prepares young men and women for their sport through the design and implementation of a specially structured program to help reduce the frequency and severity of sport-related injuries.

A well-designed strength and conditioning program develops stronger, faster, and more powerful individuals, compared to those who do not participate in such a program (1). Any sport coach would want this type of student-athlete on their team. Additionally, this program could provide the student-athlete with increased confidence via positive body changes and competence with movement, which could prove advantageous against the competition (8, 17).

A sport coach may develop the best game plan ever seen, but if the team's student-athletes are not strong, fast, quick, agile, and conditioned at a high level, the execution and success of this plan will be hindered. A strength and conditioning professional or sport coach has the training and expertise to enhance those athletic components (5, 7).

Hiring a strength and conditioning professional who has earned the title by way of academics, certification, and experience offers several benefits. One benefit is to avoid or mitigate the school's liability in the area of strength and conditioning. A qualified strength and conditioning professional will develop procedures to limit potential risks (4, 11, 16).

Having a qualified strength and conditioning professional on staff brings professionalism (15) in that the sole purpose of the position is to design and implement strength and conditioning programs to develop the student-athlete's strength, athleticism, and lifelong healthy practices (5, 7, 18). The strength and conditioning professional will also address physical and mental demands of sport through the strength and conditioning program, which also has been shown to minimize injuries (2, 7, 11, 16).

A strength and conditioning professional on staff provides the opportunity for the sport coach to focus on their day-to-day sport duties. Hiring a strength and conditioning professional specifically designated to design and implement a resistance training program will make this transition possible. This action eliminates putting the program under the supervision of someone who may be uncertified and unqualified. A strength and conditioning professional is trained to meet the needs of all student-athletes.

Physiological and Psychological Effects of Strength and Conditioning

It has been hypothesized that resistance training can cause harm, especially in youth. This is incorrect, and, in fact, weight training has been shown to have positive effects when under the supervision of a certified strength and conditioning professional (2, 7, 16). The job of a strength and conditioning professional is to enhance a student-athlete's physical ability to become stronger, faster, and more agile (6, 12). Participating in a sound and supervised strength program also offers psychological benefits. Resistance training has been found to improve physical self-perception (9), decrease anxiety and depression (10), and encourage physical activity that, when it is continued into adulthood, decreases risk of chronic diseases (5, 7).

Schools must understand that having a strength and conditioning professional on staff is not only desirable, but a necessity. If the school is unable to hire a full-time strength and conditioning professional, there are other options, as described earlier in this introduction. It must be done for the sake of the student-athlete's safety and the school's liability. The key to a successful program is the supervision of a strength and conditioning professional who has the knowledge and experience to design and properly apply the program, making it a positive experience for all involved.

Conclusion

Despite budget constraints and other challenges, strength and conditioning professionals are needed in all high schools. The cost of one liability issue can pay for the salary of several professionals, highlighting the importance of the proactive rather than the reactive approach. The strength and conditioning professional on staff limits and helps to protect a school from these issues (11, 16). To meet program implementation, a high school has a choice of five classifications of strength and conditioning professional models.

In addition to designing programs to enhance sport performance (5, 7, 18), the strength and conditioning professional improves the health of all student-athletes, which has lifelong benefits (7, 11). Whether the challenge of implementation is budget or knowledge, it is possible to present the facts to leadership so that the program will be on its way to implementation.

The confidence gained through reaching goals from personal challenges transfers into academic and career opportunities. Adhering to the guidelines and regulations when hiring a certified strength and conditioning professional is the best choice for any athletic or PE program.

1

Curriculum and Class Structure and Guidelines

Anthony S. Smith, PhD, CSCS,*D, NSCA-CPT,*D, TSAC-F
Bruce R. Harbach, MEd, CSCS,*D

Physical education combines knowledge from various domains including human performance characteristics, learning goals, teaching techniques, facilities, and equipment to create an effective and efficient learning environment. These domains should be included as part of the physical education (PE) curriculum. A curriculum is a plan for what will be taught, how it will be organized, how classroom space and equipment will be managed, and what students are expected to know. Physical educators apply scientific principles to pedagogical content knowledge to prepare adequate unit and lesson plans as part of the curriculum. The inclusion of strength and conditioning is not different than any other topic in PE.

This chapter identifies the scope and sequence of tasks and activities that physical educators can use when implementing strength and conditioning into the curriculum. The process begins by aligning the goals and objectives (or outcomes) of the PE program with the vertical stakeholder team including other teachers, school administrators, and community members. Sample curriculum plans for PE and strength and conditioning are presented with details of class operations, rules, and policies. At the end of the chapter, readers should be able to justify the implementation of a strength and conditioning program into the PE program at their schools.

Development of a Vertical Stakeholder Team

Successful high school strength and conditioning curricula and programs are ones that meet the specific needs of student-athletes and multi-sport student-athletes in the school. As high schools continue to recognize the importance of an evidence-based strength and conditioning program, many high schools find themselves in a position to create and manage both a PE program and a strength and conditioning program (28). Being able to design a district-wide strength and conditioning curriculum will give teachers and sport coaches the opportunity to introduce the program piece by piece at the middle or junior high school and high school level (28).

Just as a quality PE program should provide guidelines for appropriate instruction, strategies and concepts, skills and techniques, challenging and meaningful content, and program and student-athlete assessment, so should a quality strength and conditioning program. School districts and PE teachers usually have the freedom of making content decisions concerning lifetime activities, skills, knowledge, and values. Those decisions on course content could be based on the SHAPE America (formerly known as the American Alliance for Health, Physical Education, Recreation and Dance, or AAHPERD) National Standards and Grade-Level Outcomes framework (2, 25) and its sequence, safety concerns, and specific skill requirements (2, 25).

Several methods can be used to design strength and conditioning programs, which may include sport-specific group and individual training. Each method should have a distinct and specific guideline according to the program goal (2). With the increasing rise in popularity of resistance training programs, it is imperative that the vertical stakeholder team (i.e., school districts, school administrators, school boards, teachers, and communities) examine how classes are being taught and administered (2).

Although strength and conditioning curricula vary from school to school, it is wise to refer to the NSCA *Strength and Conditioning Professional Standards and Guidelines* when developing or reviewing a high school strength and conditioning curriculum, because this document will identify areas of liability concerns (20).

Strategic Planning to Include a Full-Time Strength and Conditioning Program

The clear underlying vision for strength and conditioning at the scholastic level from the perspective of the NSCA is that every school district that sponsors extracurricular athletics should have a certified strength and conditioning professional meeting the needs of all of the student-athletes associated with the program. Creating a strength and conditioning position can be challenging for a school district because the value of a full-time position may not yet be understood. Comparatively, athletic directors (ADs) and athletic trainers have only become full-time positions in most school districts over the last 10 to 15 years. These positions still may not be full time in some areas of the country. To reach the NSCA's vision for strength and conditioning in scholastic athletics, school professionals may have to use a strategic planning approach to convince district officials to make a commitment to a full-time professional.

Steps in Strategic Planning

1. Identify stakeholders who will influence the decision.
   a. Students, health and physical education (HPE) faculty, parents, coaches, administrators, financial managers, professional associations, and school board
2. Gather data.
   a. Needs analysis for student-athlete performance standards and injury-prevention data
   b. Risk management plan: Identify risks within the program that can be mitigated by a full-time strength and conditioning approach

    c. Qualitative and quantitative data from stakeholders highlighting the value of a full-time strength and conditioning program

    d. Identify and access NSCA resources

3. Sell the vision: How is this idea in the best interest of the district's students?

    a. Using key stakeholders (such as parents, coaches, student-athletes, teachers, and administrators) as assets, the most crucial aspect of strategic planning is to sell the vision to key decision makers in the district. In this case, key decision makers are typically the superintendent and school board. In some cases, strategic planning decisions may be underestimated due to the complexity of tabled athletic initiatives in upcoming contracts, for instance, so it can be challenging for a strength and conditioning professional to be considered for top salary ranges within the contact metrics involving length of season and number of student-athletes in each sport.

4. Identify funding sources.

    a. Most school districts conduct five-year plans that outline changes in practice and financial commitments via capital improvements, curricular changes, or new initiatives. All streams of revenue will be included. Once the vision is sold, work with the business manager and superintendent to insert the funding for the full-time position into the five-year plan. Ideally the full-time position will be incorporated into the professional teachers' association's collective bargaining agreement.

5. Evaluate the data.

    a. Evaluation is an important aspect of the strategic planning process. Once the full-time program is implemented, the strength and conditioning professional and the administration should maintain contact with parents, student-athletes, coaches, and school board members so they can illustrate the value of the school district's commitment. Reinforcement is often done through the collection and dissemination of student-athlete, team, injury, injury-prevention, and performance data. This data reinforces the district's decision and builds credibility for the strength and conditioning program so the program has the support to grow in the future.

The strategic planning process is a tool to reach every scholastic program in the country. It should be a goal to have a full-time, NSCA-certified professional who meets the needs of all student-athletes. School systems are publicly funded organizations with many needs and moving parts. School districts generally have three separate power centers: the school board, superintendent, and professional teachers' association. While a strategic planning process is not always required to reach the vision, it is seldom sufficient to simply share an idea like hiring a full-time strength and conditioning professional with decision makers and have it come to fruition. It generally takes a team approach with a long-term vision to make large-scale changes in a school system.

Building Level

Designing a resistance training and conditioning curriculum can be a daunting task. Selling a strength and conditioning program and the need for such a program to school administrators can be even more challenging. Strength and conditioning professionals are essential for every high school. PE teachers may have a strong knowledge of the curriculum content, but designing the curriculum can be challenging. When designing a strength and conditioning course many elements require a deeper understanding of resistance training protocols (2). *Essentials of Strength Training and Conditioning* suggests a two-stage process that includes an evaluation of the requirements and characteristics of the sport and an assessment of the athlete (26). Grade level, workout environment safety, proper teaching techniques for exercises, proper supervision, and maturity and experience levels of student-athletes are considerations to present to administrators (2).

When constructing a strength and conditioning program, it is helpful to keep in mind where the program is now and what the program will look like with the curriculum implemented. When first starting a program analysis, develop an inventory of the PE and strength and conditioning equipment already at the school, and list other required equipment. Contact local equipment companies to develop a quote for equipment and a possible floor plan that may be needed to support the program and curriculum. Working with local companies may be a beneficial way to receive equipment at a discounted price and develop a relationship with equipment dealers (28). By compiling and presenting detailed information to school stakeholders, administrators will be able to see an overall plan, cost, and value of the program. The curriculum should be performance based, and all student-athletes will need to demonstrate knowledge, skill development, and competency in all areas of the program (2, 28).

District Level

Worldwide fitness trends reflect the popularity of fitness and strength and conditioning classes in high schools (2). Resistance training activities have proven beneficial to youth. Increases in muscular strength and endurance, increased bone mineral density, increased motor coordination, maintenance of a healthy body weight, decreased body fat percentage, and decreased depression (27) are all benefits of a well-designed strength and conditioning program (22).

Some factors should be considered when putting together a high school strength and conditioning program with district stakeholders (19, 22, 28). Those considerations include the following:

- Space and equipment available for training
- Length of time for classes or training sessions
- Class and practice schedules
- Class size and student-to-teacher ratio
- Number of student-athletes training at once
- Experience and age of student-athletes
- Injured student-athletes in class
- Number of training days, classes, or periods in a week

Much of what is done in the strength and conditioning program should be designed to be integrated with student-athlete goals, school goals, and the school district's mission while maintaining academic emphasis, promoting physical literacy, and driving student-athletes toward athletic excellence (15). Goal setting with student-athletes can serve as both a motivation and an inspiration (1). Student-athletes have various reasons for resistance training, such as increasing body weight, reducing body fat, increasing sport performance, improving overall appearance, and gaining confidence. Using specific, measurable, achievable, relevant, and time-based (SMART) goals to track the program and its progression is a good way to observe the program's effectiveness for each student-athlete (1). Realistic goals are important for student-athlete progress in the program, and the teacher or strength and conditioning professional and student should meet on a periodic basis to determine short, intermediate, and long-term goals (1). Figure 1.1 explains the benefits of a strength and conditioning professional at the high school level (21).

Benefits of a Qualified Professional

Benefits to the Students

1. Reduce injuries: A qualified strength and conditioning professional can play a pivotal role in preparing young athletes for sport and thereby minimize or offset the incidence and severity of sport-related injuries common to young athletes. (29, 30, 31, 32, 33)

2. Improve long-term athletic development: A qualified strength and conditioning professional understands the many variables that go into designing training age–appropriate programs, and can produce more positive results. (34, 35, 36, 37)

3. Improve performance: Athletes who participate in a well-designed strength and conditioning program typically will be faster, stronger, more powerful, move more efficiently, and be more athletic than they would be without it. (29, 37, 38, 39, 40)

4. Improve confidence: Athletes who invest time in strength and conditioning tend to develop confidence through changes in their body composition and increased physical literacy, as well as the knowledge that the development that occurs as a result of their training can give them an advantage in competition. (41, 42, 43)

5. Improve health: In addition to increasing muscular strength, power, and muscular endurance, regular participation in a youth resistance training program has the potential to influence many other health- and fitness-related measures, and can play an important role in alleviating many health-related conditions. (29, 40, 44, 45)

Benefits to the School

1. Limit liability: A qualified strength and conditioning professional can help limit your school's liability and implement procedures that support risk management. (30, 32, 44, 46, 49)

2. Increase professionalism and safety: For the same reason schools require a certified athletic trainer to work with their injured athletes or a certified lifeguard on pool decks, the same should be true for the coach who is designing and supervising the strength and conditioning program. (46, 47, 48)

3. Extra coach on staff for all sports: A strength coach allows the sport coach more time to focus on the day-to-day practice schedule while the strength coach oversees the strength and conditioning of the team. (44)

4. Due diligence: A qualified strength and conditioning professional on staff demonstrates due diligence in properly equipping athletes for the physical and mental demands of a particular sport and establishes a greater commitment to injury prevention. (50)

5. Gender equity: A qualified strength and conditioning professional on staff assists an athletic department with implementing strength and conditioning programs that are gender specific. (50)

FIGURE 1.1 Benefits of a qualified professional.

Community Level

A high school strength and conditioning program should incorporate values of the community that prepare students to carry on individual fitness and strength programs beyond their high school days (15, 22). Relationships between the high school strength and conditioning professional and community programs are essential, and communication between the two is critical to create buy-in for programs that are sound and research driven (4). Strength and conditioning professionals have a product that is of value to parents, school boards, administrators, faculty, and community members, all of whom will benefit and gain an understanding of the impact a sound strength and conditioning program can have on student-athletes (4).

Marketing a strength and conditioning program to parents and the community about program values and the relationship they have with increased athletic success will not only benefit the student-athlete but also the whole community. Asking for feedback from the community can be helpful. A community forum provides the opportunity for the community to ask questions, provides details about the program, and establishes lifelong healthy physical activity patterns among children and adolescents (4, 15, 22). Community leaders can provide resources and access to parks, gyms, and other facilities that can enhance the health and fitness of children and adolescents outside the classroom. This can be done with parent meetings; weekly emails on student-athlete progression in the classroom, athletic field, or weight room; or an informational website or email link that the community can access. Selling strength and conditioning programs through the local media (e.g., radio stations, newspapers, websites, television stations, and social media) can be excellent means of not only promoting the program itself but also promoting the student-athletes involved in the program and their accomplishments (15, 22).

Schools that have the facilities but sometimes lack qualified personnel to monitor extracurricular activities and strength and conditioning programs can work with community resources to expand after-school programs by providing additional programs, camps, and clinics supervised by qualified personnel (28). Communities can promote year-round strength and conditioning programs, which can be one of the most effective strategies for reducing injuries, improving motor skills, establishing healthy and active lifestyles, decreasing diseases associated with sedentary lifestyles, and establishing positive habits that can continue throughout adulthood (4).

Examples of Common Strength and Conditioning–Related PE Curricula

The purpose of a curriculum is to guide educators on the development, implementation, and assessment of students and the program (17, 18, 24). This is done by creating a framework that establishes a scope and sequence, program goals and objectives, and content areas. SHAPE America has an established framework for teaching PE that includes National Standards and Grade-Level Outcomes (25). Most states have aligned their PE programs with the SHAPE America National Standards with some modifications to the Grade-Level Outcomes. Even with modifications, states include strength and conditioning, fitness, wellness, and health content throughout each grade level to help students become physically literate (18, 24, 25). The scope and sequence found in the SHAPE America framework includes five standards and topics from three different educational domains or objectives: psychomotor (physical skills), cognitive (why and when), and affective (values).

Psychomotor objectives are the primary outcomes found in PE and include all physical skills that are taught: basic movements, dance and rhythmic activities, individual and team sport skills, lifetime activities, and fitness activities. Each of these psychomotor topics is also developed with cognitive and affective objectives in mind. Student-athletes knowing why a skill is learned and when to use a skill falls under the cognitive domain, while learning to value skills and exhibiting responsibility in the gym is found in the affective domain. An aspect unique to PE is that each lesson taught contains objectives from all three domains. Many sport coaches already incorporate components of the cognitive and affective domains when working with players to build better student-athletes through individual and team sport practices and development.

An established goal or outcome identified by SHAPE America is for high school student-athletes to create a strength and conditioning program (25). Creating a workout program involves knowledge, values, and skills related to strength and conditioning. In order to design a strength and conditioning program, the goal should be for student-athletes to perform various skills and appropriate techniques for a variety of resistance training activities; they should also demonstrate knowledge of sport science principles and movement concepts (25). Along with psychomotor and cognitive skills, student-athletes can be taught how to behave safely in a gym environment while applying best practices in both policies and classroom rules (25). The importance of using appropriate weights and exercises designed to meet personal goals can be exhibited by student-athletes choosing the appropriate level of challenge.

SHAPE America established a project team that created a comprehensive Instructional Framework for Fitness Education in Physical Education (SHAPE 12), which suggests what student-athletes should know and understand in relation to fitness for various grade levels, ranging from pre-kindergarten to college. It includes eight categories of fitness knowledge that cover the three domains of learning and proposes specific topics to be covered through progressions. Some of the topics covered include health-related fitness concepts, maintaining physical activity, creating a fitness plan, benefits of physical fitness, and assessment. Many of these topics are already taught in PE and health education courses, making the transition to a strength and conditioning curriculum less complicated. Outside of the framework presented by SHAPE America, some already-established curriculum models can incorporate strength and conditioning content. These curriculum models include the sport education model, personalized system of instruction, and teaching personal and social responsibility (TPSR) models of instruction (18). Each of these models has been researched, tested, and performed in a variety of PE settings with great success, and are briefly reviewed here.

The sport education curriculum model is like sport coaching. Teaching units are created so that content that is usually delivered from coach to player is now controlled by other student-athletes and peers. The teacher mainly acts as a guide, helping student-athletes to understand the material and work with each other to practice new skills and ideas. This curriculum model attempts to educate student-athletes in all aspects of the sport education domain by allowing them to be involved in the design, implementation, and assessment of the curriculum. Student-athletes are active participants and work in cooperative learning environments that enhance student-athlete responsibility and personal experiences in the sport. A curriculum of this design is usually developed prior to the semester of implementation, and the teacher creates the framework for the student-athletes to follow.

A personalized system of instruction is a curriculum model that allows each student-athlete to progress at their own rate, using a preprogrammed sequence of skills and learning tasks. A characteristic of this curriculum model is that student-athletes read prepared materials on the topics and watch videos depicting organization and management of the skills along with techniques for performance. Student-athletes are introduced to performance standards and criteria for self-assessment, leading to the completion of one task before engaging in the next task. This model has a psychomotor objective priority with some applications in cognitive and affective learning. A benefit of this type of curriculum is that teachers are given more freedom from long, tenuous instruction time to large groups and instead provide specific instruction and feedback to individuals and small groups at various developmental stages using differentiated instructional methods. Again, this curriculum model is designed and developed by the teacher prior to the start of the semester. Student-athlete choice allows every student-athlete to work and practice at a pace that is reasonable to their abilities and interests.

Not all curriculum models for PE focus on the psychomotor domain. The TPSR model is focused on the affective learning domain (18). Considering the interaction between student-athletes that exists during PE, and specifically during strength and conditioning events, the TPSR model provides opportunities for student-athletes to learn both personal and social responsibility. Student-athletes learn that skill and knowledge are not isolated topics but can and should be taught and learned in conjunction with each other. Personal and social responsibilities such as following directions, helping others, and learning to value and appreciate other ideas and concepts are all embedded in the TPSR model and are aligned with concepts taught in high school team sports. This model is used in school settings where leadership and innovation are highlighted as curriculum components.

The establishment of a strength and conditioning curriculum plan can use the concepts of an established framework and a specific curriculum model. Initial development and inclusion of a framework aligned with standards, either national or state, can show administrators, teachers, sport coaches, and student-athletes what content is to be taught and learned. A variety of frameworks and models have demonstrated positive results for student-athlete learning in PE, though most are aligned with the National Standards and Grade-Level Outcomes established by SHAPE America (25). Preparing student-athletes for lifelong physical activity, including components of strength and conditioning, are a significant aspect of every curriculum model in PE. The models described in this chapter reflect ideas and protocols that specifically include resistance training and skill-related health concepts that can be transferred from the PE classroom to the sport world as needed.

Provided in this chapter are sample curriculum plans for untrained and inexperienced, intermediate, and trained and experienced courses. The skills and knowledge included in each curriculum plan builds on the materials from previous courses and is aligned with the SHAPE America National Standards and Grade-Level Outcomes (25). These curriculum plans are intended only to show strength and conditioning professionals and PE teachers how content can be organized and presented during the semester. Each example is based on a 90-minute high school curriculum with classes five days a week for 16 weeks. Each day includes materials from the psychomotor, cognitive, and affective domains of learning. Following each curriculum plan is a list of the Grade-Level Outcomes that are taught during the semester. Including various outcomes from all three domains is a great way to impress principals and school administrators to show that PE classes, specifically strength and conditioning courses, are comprehensive in nature and are important in the overall education process. Included with each curriculum plan is a sample week-long class schedule with ideas for skills to be practiced, knowledge to be taught and learned, and pro-social behaviors to incorporate during PE class.

Examples of Training or Exercise-Based Classes

The following section demonstrates how strength and conditioning can be embedded into the physical education curriculum. Using the framework recommended by SHAPE America (2), all three domains of learning (psychomotor, cognitive, and affective) should be included within a lesson. Student-athletes need to learn more than just proper exercise technique (psychomotor domain); they also need to learn how to work out with others in the gym, follow gym rules, and support each other during workouts (affective domain) as well as learn fitness terminology, how the human body moves, and how to structure workouts and programs based on their individual needs and desires (cognitive domain).

PE teachers and strength and conditioning professionals commonly have various levels of experienced and skilled individuals in class so they need to be prepared for different types of programming instruction. Tables are presented that illustrate a general workout weekly plan and a curriculum plan for beginning, intermediate, and advanced student-athletes. The curriculum guide includes lesson plan options for psychomotor, cognitive, and affective objectives from the SHAPE America framework (2) to demonstrate how all three learning domains can be included in each lesson.

Introduction to Strength and Conditioning: Inexperienced and Untrained Student-Athlete Curriculum

Student-athletes need to learn about the body, basic principles of training, and how to perform skills, so a beginning course should include all these concepts. A high school class that meets daily for 90 minutes is the basis of this format: eight two-week units with three training days and two academic days to learn about terms, ideas, and concepts of strength and conditioning. See table 1.1 for an example of topics to be covered in the first week of an inexperienced and untrained curriculum.

TABLE 1.1   Week One: Sample 90-Minute Class Schedule—Inexperienced and Untrained Student-Athlete Curriculum

Monday	Tuesday	Wednesday	Thursday	Friday
Introduction to the class: syllabus, schedule, rules, protocols	Notes about flexibility and range of motion Video about sit-and-reach test Sit-and-reach test Dynamic stretching routine	Notes on gym etiquette Dynamic stretching routine Introduction to lower body body-weight-only exercises Worksheet on exercise and stretch names	Dynamic stretching routine Introduction to upper body body-weight-only exercises Static stretching routine	Video on total body workout routine Dynamic stretching routine Total body workout using only body weight

Table 1.2 gives an example of a 16-week untrained and inexperienced strength and conditioning class with objectives.

To align the proposed strength and conditioning curriculum and unit plan, table 1.2 provides examples from the SHAPE America National Standards and Grade-Level Outcomes for psychomotor, cognitive, and affective learning domains (25). The objectives selected for this unit plan demonstrate that each lesson can include material from all three learning domains, as suggested by SHAPE America. Each cognitive and affective domain can be used, enhanced, or exchanged for any number of other outcomes for any specific class or lecture.

The code for each outcome includes a standard number, 1 through 5, educational level (H for high school, M for middle school, E for elementary school), and a progressive level (indicated by L1 or L2). See the SHAPE America handbook for additional outcomes that can be used (25).

Psychomotor Objectives

S1.H3.L1 Demonstrates competency in 1 or more specialized skills in health-related fitness.

S2.H1.L1 Applies the terminology associated with exercise and participation in selected individual-performance activities, dance, net/wall games, target games, aquatics and/or outdoor pursuits appropriately.

S2.H2.L1 Uses movement concepts and principles to analyze and improve performance of self and/or others in a selected skill.

Cognitive Objectives

S3.H1.L1 Discusses the benefits of a physically active lifestyle as it relates to college or career productivity.

S3.H6.L1 Participates several times a week in a self-selected lifetime activity, dance or fitness activity outside of the school day.

S3.H7.L1 Demonstrates appropriate technique in resistance training machines and free weights.

TABLE 1.2   Inexperienced and Untrained Strength and Conditioning Class Example

Week	Psychomotor objectives	Cognitive objectives	Affective objectives
1	Dynamic warm-up procedures and basic exercises	Flexibility	Observe rules and etiquette
2	Basic exercises	Safety and spotting	Evaluate peers
3	Upper body exercises	Anatomy	Analyze barriers
4	Lower body exercises	Anatomy	Respect others
5	Total body exercises	Terms and principles	Use best practices
6	Routines and programming	Terms and principles	Use best practices
7	Self-testing	FITT principle	Solve problems
8	Self-selected workouts	FITT principle	Solve problems
9	Max weight projections	Program design	Select and participate in physical activity
10	Self-selected workouts	Program design	Select and participate in physical activity
11	Personalized program routine	Logging exercises, sets, and reps	Select and participate in physical activity
12	Personalized program routine	Logging exercises, sets, and reps	Select and participate in physical activity
13	Unilateral options, lower body	Unilateral training concepts	Choose appropriate challenge
14	Unilateral options, upper body	Unilateral training concepts	Choose appropriate challenge
15	Exercising with different equipment	Value of different training equipment	Choose appropriate challenge
16	Exercising with different equipment	Benefits of different training equipment	Choose appropriate challenge

FITT = Frequency, intensity, time, and type

S3.H9.L1 Identifies types of strength exercises and stretching exercises for personal fitness development.

S3.H12.L1 Designs a fitness program, including all components of health-related fitness, for a college student and an employee in the learner's chosen field of work.

Affective Objectives

S4.H2.L1 Exhibits proper etiquette, respect for others and teamwork while engaging in physical activity and/or social dance.

S4.H3.L1 Uses communication skills and strategies that promote team or group dynamics.

S4.H4.L1 Solves problems and thinks critically in physical activity or dance settings, both as an individual and in groups.

S4.H5.L1 Applies best practices for participating safely in physical activity, exercise and dance.

S5.H3.L1 Selects and participates in physical activities or dance that meet the need for self-expression and enjoyment.

Introduction to Strength and Conditioning: Intermediate Student-Athlete Curriculum

Entering the intermediate level of the curriculum, student-athletes should have a basic understanding of foundational weight resistance movements. Intermediate strength and conditioning classes provide student-athletes an opportunity to design and implement longer training programs during the semester while enhancing knowledge in several topics related to health and fitness. Student-athlete learning includes knowledge of why and how movements and programs are aligned. The core movements listed in table 1.3 are recommendations; however, the authors suggest using the most appropriate core exercises for the program.

During the intermediate student-athlete curriculum (and, later, the trained and experienced curriculum), student-athletes can be safely introduced to testing. Traditional 1-repetition maximum (1RM) testing for strength and power movements is not highly recommended because untrained and inexperienced and some intermediate individuals may not have mastered adequate lifting techniques, especially for near-max exercises, leading to increased risk of injury. The preferred method of max testing is the **criterion repetition maximum** (CRM) testing protocol (14). In this method, the final score, or grade, for a max test is based on using proper technique when performing the near-max exercise. This type of evaluation tool aligns with the assessment protocols promoted by SHAPE America (25). Research indicates that 1RM testing can be acceptable in some cases; however, the training status and skill level of the individual and direct supervision of a qualified strength and conditioning professional are necessary components of the evaluation process (13, 14). See table 1.3 for an example of topics to be covered in the first week of an intermediate curriculum.

A 16-week intermediate strength and conditioning class example with objectives is presented in table 1.4.

TABLE 1.3   Week One: Sample 90-Minute Class Schedule—Intermediate Student-Athlete Curriculum

Monday	Tuesday	Wednesday	Thursday	Friday
Introduction to the class: syllabus, schedule, rules, protocols Video of comprehensive workout program and routine	Video of max test technique for deadlift and bench press Dynamic stretching routine Deadlift test Bench press test	Video of max test technique for push press and squat Dynamic stretching routine Push press test Squat test	Notes on program design principles Worksheet to estimate sets, reps, and % max for deadlift and bench press Introduction to assistance exercises for these movements	Worksheet to estimate sets, reps, and % max for push press and squat Introduction to assistance exercises for these movements

Table 1.4 provides examples from the SHAPE America National Standards and Grade-Level Outcomes for psychomotor, cognitive, and affective learning domains so as to align the proposed strength and conditioning curriculum and unit plan (25). The objectives selected for this unit plan demonstrate that each

TABLE 1.4   Intermediate Strength and Conditioning Class Example

Week	Psychomotor objectives	Cognitive objectives	Affective objectives
1	Introduction to the weight room/max testing	Program development and design for a 2-day push–pull routine	Exhibit proper etiquette, respect for others during physical activity
2	Program development and design for a push–pull 2-day routine	Dimensions of health and wellness	Analyze the health benefits of a self-selected physical activity
3	Core/assistance exercises	Health-related fitness testing	Apply best practices for participating safely in physical activity, exercise, and dance
4	Core/assistance exercises	Health-related fitness testing	Apply best practices for participating safely in physical activity, exercise, and dance
5	Core/assistance exercises	Skill-related fitness testing	Apply best practices for participating safely in physical activity, exercise, and dance
6	Core/assistance exercises	Skill-related fitness testing	Identify the opportunity for social support in a self-selected physical activity
7	Core/assistance exercises	Program development and design for a 4-day routine	Assume leadership role in a physical activity setting
8	Max testing (CRM)	Nutrition basics	Employ effective self-management skills to analyze barriers
9	Program development, 4-day split	Sport nutrition	Accept differences between personal characteristics and the ideal body images in the media
10	Core/assistance exercises and plyometrics	Plyometric techniques	Choose appropriate challenge to experience success
11	Core/assistance exercises and plyometrics	Developing agility and quickness skills	Choose appropriate challenge to experience success
12	Core/assistance exercises and agility drills	Developing speed	Choose appropriate challenge to experience success
13	Core/assistance exercises and agility drills	Injury prevention	Analyze the health benefits of a self-selected physical activity
14	Core/assistance exercises and speed development	CPR/first aid	Analyze the health benefits of a self-selected physical activity
15	Core/assistance exercises and speed development	Flexibility and rehabilitation	Apply best practices for participating safely in physical activity, exercise, and dance
16	Max testing (CRM)	Relationships among physical activity, nutrition, and body composition	Exhibit proper etiquette, respect for others during physical activity

lesson can include material from all three learning domains, as suggested by SHAPE America. Each cognitive and affective domain can be used, enhanced, or exchanged for any number of other outcomes for any specific class or lecture.

Psychomotor Objectives

S1.H3.L1 Demonstrates competency in 1 or more specialized skills in health-related fitness activities.

S2.H1.L1 Applies the terminology associated with exercise and participation in selected individual-performance activities, dance, net/wall games, target games, aquatics and/or outdoor pursuits appropriately.

S2.H2.L1 Uses movement concepts and principles to analyze and improve performance of self and/or others in a selected skill.

Cognitive Objectives

S3.H6.L1 Participates several times a week in a self-selected lifetime activity, dance or fitness activity outside of the school day.

S3.H7.L1 Demonstrates appropriate technique in resistance training machines and free weights.

S3.H7.L2 Designs and implements a strength and conditioning program that develops balance in opposing muscle groups and supports a healthy, active lifestyle.

S3.H9.L1 Identifies types of strength exercises and stretching exercises for personal fitness development.

S3.H11.L2 Develops and maintains a fitness portfolio.

S3.H12.L1 Designs a fitness program, including all components of health-related fitness, for a college student and an employee in the learner's chosen field of work.

S3.H12.L2 Analyzes the components of skill-related fitness in relation to life and career goals and designs an appropriate fitness program for those goals.

S3.H13.L1 Designs and implements a nutrition plan to maintain an appropriate energy balance for a healthy, active lifestyle.

S3.H13.L2 Creates a snack plan for before, during, and after exercise that addresses nutrition needs for each phase.

Affective Objectives

S4.H1.L1 Employs effective self-management skills to analyze barriers and modify physical activity patterns appropriately as needed.

S4.H1.L2 Accepts differences between personal characteristics and the idealized body images and elite performance levels portrayed in various media.

S4.H2.L1 Exhibits proper etiquette, respect for others and teamwork while engaging in physical activity and/or social dance.

S4.H3.L1 Uses communication skills and strategies that promote team or group dynamics.

S4.H3.L2 Assumes a leadership role in a physical activity setting.

S4.H4.L1 Solves problems and thinks critically in physical activity or dance settings, both as an individual and in groups.

S4.H4.L2 Accepts others' ideas, cultural diversity, and body types by engaging in cooperative and collaborative movement projects.

S4.H5.L1 Applies best practices for participating safely in physical activity, exercise and dance.

S5.H1.L1 Analyzes the health benefits of a self-selected physical activity.

S5.H2.L2 Chooses an appropriate level of challenge to experience success and desire to participate in a self-selected physical activity.

S5.H3.L1 Selects and participates in physical activities or dance that meet the need for self-expression and enjoyment.

S5.H4.L1 Identifies the opportunity for social support in a self-selected physical activity or dance.

Trained and Experienced Strength and Conditioning Programming: Trained and Experienced Student-Athlete Curriculum

This curriculum is for trained and experienced individuals, usually those with at least one full year of training experience. The 16-week semester is divided into four units focused on strength development and power. The first unit introduces the trained and experienced concept of the push–pull angle (PPA) program and introduces a new set of exercises each week to be practiced. In the second unit student-athletes use the exercises and techniques in the first unit to organize and plan a workout routine leading into a max testing week. The third unit introduces Olympic lifts and assistance exercises for each Olympic lift. In the final unit student-athletes develop a training program based on their strength, power, and personal goals. See table 1.5 for an example of topics to be covered in the first week of a trained and experienced curriculum.

Table 1.6 represents a 16-week trained and experienced strength and conditioning class guide and objectives.

TABLE 1.5 Week One: Sample 90-Minute Class Schedule—Trained and Experienced Student-Athlete Curriculum

Monday	Tuesday	Wednesday	Thursday	Friday
Introduction to the class: syllabus, schedule, rules, protocols Video on the PPA training program	Notes on living a physically active lifestyle Video of push exercises and max testing procedures Dynamic stretching routine Max testing for 1-2 push exercises	Notes on rules and etiquette in the gym Video of pull exercises and max testing procedures Dynamic stretching routine Max testing for 1-2 pull exercises	Notes on program design for PPA programs Video of angle exercises and max testing procedures Dynamic stretching routine Max testing for 1-2 angle exercises	Static stretching routine Introduction to assistance exercises for each training day

TABLE 1.6   Trained and Experienced Strength and Conditioning Class Example

Week	Psychomotor objectives	Cognitive objectives	Affective objectives
1	Introduction to PPA training exercises after fitness test for cardiovascular endurance	Discuss benefits of a physically active lifestyle; health- and skill-related fitness components	Rules and etiquette in the gym
2	New exercises in the PPA program	Identify the structure of muscle and fiber types related to development	Safety and spotting
3	New exercises in the PPA program	Identify the structure of muscle and fiber types related to development	Work with a partner
4	New exercises in the PPA program after tests for muscular strength and endurance	Identify types of strength exercises and the best order of participation	Employ effective self-management skills to analyze barriers
5	Individual program workouts	Analyze and apply technology and social media as supportive tools	Accept others' ideas, cultural diversity, and body types
6	Individual program workouts	Participate several times a week in a self-selected lifetime activity	Select and participate in physical activity
7	Individual program workouts	Participate several times a week in a self-selected lifetime activity	Select and participate in physical activity
8	Max testing	Develop and maintain a fitness portfolio	Choose appropriate challenge
9	Introduction to Olympic lifts	Design a fitness program based on fitness scores, personal goals, and equipment	Use communication skills and strategies that promote group dynamics
10	Olympic lifting techniques; peer evaluation using a rubric	Identify different energy systems	Identify the opportunity for social support in physical activity settings
11	Olympic lifting techniques; peer evaluation using a rubric	Participate several times a week in a self-selected lifetime activity	Apply best practices for participating safely in physical activity
12	Olympic lifting techniques; peer evaluation using a rubric	Demonstrate appropriate technique for evaluation by instructor	Apply best practices for participating safely in physical activity
13	Individual program workouts	Design a strength and conditioning program	Employ effective self-management skills to analyze barriers
14	Individual program workouts	Design a strength and conditioning program	Apply best practices for participating safely in physical activity
15	Individual program workouts	Design a strength and conditioning program	Analyze the health benefits of a self-selected physical activity
16	Max testing	Develop and maintain a fitness portfolio	Choose appropriate challenge

Table 1.6 provides examples from the SHAPE America National Standards and Grade-Level Outcomes for psychomotor, cognitive, and affective learning domains so as to align the proposed strength and conditioning curriculum and unit plan (25). The objectives selected for this unit plan demonstrate that each lesson can include material from all three learning domains, as suggested by SHAPE America. Each cognitive and affective domain can be used, enhanced, or exchanged for any number of other outcomes for any specific class or lecture.

Psychomotor Objectives

S1.H3.L2 Demonstrates competency in 2 or more specialized skills in health-related fitness activities.

S2.H1.L1 Applies the terminology associated with exercise and participation in selected individual-performance activities, dance, net/wall games, target games, aquatics and/or outdoor pursuits appropriately.

S2.H2.L1 Uses movement concepts and principles to analyze and improve performance of self and/or others in a selected skill.

Cognitive Objectives

S3.H7.L2 Designs and implements a strength and conditioning program that develops balance in opposing muscle groups and supports a healthy, active lifestyle.

S3.H8.L2 Identifies the different energy systems used in selected physical activity.

S3.H9.L2 Identifies the structure of skeletal muscle and fiber types as they relate to muscle development.

S3.H12.L2 Analyzes the components of skill-related fitness in relation to life and career goals and designs an appropriate fitness program for those goals.

S3.H13.L2 Creates a snack plan for before, during, and after exercise that addresses nutrition needs for each phase.

Affective Objectives

S4.H1.L1 Employs effective self-management skills to analyze barriers and modify physical activity patterns appropriately as needed.

S4.H2.L1 Exhibits proper etiquette, respect for others and teamwork while engaging in physical activity and/or social dance.

S4.H3.L2 Assumes a leadership role in a physical activity setting.

S4.H5.L1 Applies best practices for participating safely in physical activity, exercise and dance.

S5.H2.L2 Chooses an appropriate level of challenge to experience success and desire to participate in a self-selected physical activity.

Common Classroom Policies, Rules, and Procedures

General school policies have been established to keep students and staff safe. Attendance, absences, tardiness, dress code, and grading policies are a few of the rules and procedures that schools already have instituted. School administrators have established these guidelines for an effective learning environment so students can feel safe and secure during the day and therefore learning can take place. Teachers may have different approaches to how their classrooms are run; however, the weight room is a different entity simply because of the environment in which the student-athlete is learning. Weight room policies and classroom procedures that have been reviewed and approved by the administration are essential for the safety and well-being of student-athletes and should be consistent with the expectations of the strength and conditioning program. To maximize student-athlete training, weight room safety guidelines, procedures, and class rules should be established to ensure student-athletes can train safely and efficiently. Some general weight room safety guidelines may include the following (5, 16, 26):

- Wear proper exercise attire as established by the teacher and school policy (e.g., clean shirt, shorts, socks, athletic shoes).
- Warm up prior to working out. General and specific warm-up methods are preferred.
- Always use collars on bars to prevent the weights from sliding off.
- Use capable spotters when doing certain free weight exercises.
- No student-athlete trains on their own during class. Student-athletes must be in a group or with a partner.
- Clean equipment after each use using prescribed weight room cleaners.
- Lift using proper technique. Use appropriate weights that enable correct performance of the exercise.
- Only use bumper plates on platforms.
- Do not drop bars or weights, and do not lean or place weights against or on equipment or benches.
- Keep chalk use to a minimum in the designated areas. Clean and sweep up the area after use.
- Load and remove weights from bars evenly so the bar will not tip.
- Remove all weights from bars, place collars on bars, and restack weights on proper weight horns when exercise is completed. Leave the weight room in better shape than you found it.
- Keep the facility clutter free, and keep weights off the floor.
- Report broken or damaged equipment to the teacher.
- Be respectful to the teacher and classmates.
- Do not prop open doors to the weight room.
- Return workout sheets to the proper folder or file at the end of class.
- Advise the teacher of injuries when arriving to class or any injuries sustained during class.
- Know where the emergency action plans are posted, and refer to them when necessary.

- Failure to follow the above safety guidelines may result in dismissal from the facility and loss of weight room privileges.

These safety rules and information have been established in order to protect student-athletes and others from injury. Post these safety guidelines in the resistance training facility in several clearly visible areas for everyone to see. Safety procedures, proper technique, functional equipment, and proper instruction and supervision are important aspects of a sound strength and conditioning program (7).

Teachers and school administrators should set in place school policies and rules to ensure strength and conditioning classes run smoothly and so that if an issue arises, everyone knows what to do and how to address it. Building a sound strength and conditioning program can tie directly to these procedures and guidelines (5, 6). Safety guidelines and class rules should be in place to help student-athletes avoid injury and harm, help the class run at a teachable pace, avoid problems ahead of time, understand the principles and purpose of training, and contribute to student-athletes' long-term athletic development (5). The following are basic principles for running a safe and efficient strength and conditioning class. Keep in mind these principles can vary from school to school based on the school district's policies, available facilities, class size, and so on (7, 29).

- *Space available:* Consider how much space and how many students the facility can handle safely (20).
- *Equipment:* This allows the choice of exercises in the strength and conditioning program.
- *Time:* Instructional time based on sets, repetitions, tempo, and rest will determine how many exercises student-athletes can perform in the allotted period. Entire course time (i.e., number of classes and number of weeks) can affect the entire program and should be planned out in advance after reviewing the academic schedule.
- *Class size:* NSCA standards suggest a 15:1 student-to-teacher ratio for a high school strength and conditioning class (20).
- *Program design:* The scope and sequence aligned with state standards and outcomes determines the extent of the content provided related to program design.

Because the resistance training facility is unique in nature, determining and establishing class rules at the beginning of the year (i.e., during the first week of class) and periodically reviewing them throughout the year will clarify expectations of the class and create a safe learning environment for all student-athletes. Classroom strength and conditioning rules should be posted in the facility and locker rooms where they can be clearly observed by all student-athletes (5). Student-athletes should be reminded of the safety rules as they continue to train in the facility. Classroom rules and expectations for establishing an efficient and effective classroom environment may include the following (5, 16, 23):

- Be dressed on time for class.
- A shirt (no cut offs or sleeveless), athletic shoes, socks, proper shorts, or other appropriate athletic attire is required for class and training. Students must abide by this dress code for class.

- Bring proper materials to class if needed (strength manual, workout sheets, calculator, etc.).
- Log all exercises, sets, repetitions, and weights on the workout sheet.
- Remove all jewelry, watches, loose necklaces, earrings, and bracelets before coming into the facility. Lock valuable and personal belongings in a locker or bring them to the weight room for storage.
- Cell phone use is prohibited during class per school policy. Cell phones, headphones, earbuds, and so on are not allowed when lifting free weights but may be used on cardio equipment for listening to music only, with the teacher's approval.
- No objectionable music.
- No food or drink is allowed in the facility. Exceptions may be plastic water bottles approved by the teacher.
- No bullying, horseplay, unsafe activity, profanity, or offensive language.
- Use only equipment that the teacher has demonstrated or approved for use.
- Submit medical excuses or absent-from-class notes. Attend a make-up session arranged with the teacher.
- No leaving the facility without permission from the teacher.
- Do not adjust the stereo or sound system unless given permission by the teacher.
- Dismissal at the end of class will be given by the teacher.
- Remain in the locker room or common area until the end-of-class bell rings.

Instructor Supervision

Proper supervision of the resistance training facility and the student-athletes involved in the strength and conditioning class is critical. Demonstrating proper technique with an emphasis on safety will enable student-athletes to achieve proper instruction, therefore reducing the injury factor and chance for liability issues (26). The teacher should always have a clear view of the facility and be able to instruct and communicate effectively to student-athletes during workouts (1). The weight room should always be supervised by a qualified teacher, and no student-athletes should be allowed in the weight room without the presence of a qualified teacher (19). Both the student-athletes and teachers share responsibility for maintaining a safe environment (19). Principles of supervision include the following (3):

- Always be actively present in the facility.
- Be prudent, careful, and prepared.
- Be qualified.
- Be vigilant.
- Inform student-athletes of safety and emergency procedures.
- Know the health status of student-athletes in the class.
- Monitor and enforce rules and regulations.
- Monitor and scrutinize the environment.

Adequate floor space in the facility to perform exercises is paramount. Standard 3.1 in NSCA *Strength and Conditioning Professional Standards and Guidelines* states (20):

> Strength and conditioning activities should be planned, and the required number of qualified staff should be present, such that recommended guidelines for minimum average floor space allowed per participant (100 ft²), minimum professional-to-participant ratios (1:10 junior high school, 1:15 high school), and number of participants per barbell or training station (up to 3) are applied during peak usage times (20).

Inadequate instruction or supervision is often the main cause of athletic injuries (3) and supervision of students is a priority. In addition to the principles of supervision listed above, instructor guidelines for supervising a resistance training facility are as follows (8, 9, 10):

- Do not let students into the facility without a teacher present.
- Be visible to all student-athletes, and be able to observe the entire facility.
- Move about the weight room, instructing along the way.
- Arrange the weight room equipment so all student-athletes and instructors can move freely about the aisles.
- Keep track of class time so student-athletes can change clothes at the end of class.
- Monitor student-athletes as they are working. Make corrections or adjustments to workouts if necessary.
- Display daily workouts and goals on a whiteboard, chalkboard, computer, or video monitor for student-athletes and administrators to observe.
- Write daily objectives of the class (e.g., "The student will be able to . . .") where they can be seen by everyone.
- Follow the approved teaching progression for each exercise.
- Demonstrate or show a video of each primary exercise and how to perform the exercise using correct form and technique.
- Design workout programs, cards, or sheets for student-athletes, and have them keep a folder or file for all class materials and handouts.
- Lead by example, and be consistent in enforcing rules.
- Keep student-athletes on task, and make sure workouts are followed and weights logged for each exercise.
- Keep the facility clean. Straighten up and put items in place after each class in preparation for the next class or team in the facility. Clean up any trash, spills, or slick spots.
- Notify the maintenance staff, AD, or administrators if there is damage to mirrors, flooring, windows, doors, or any equipment, and place a "Do not use" sign on damaged equipment.
- Explain and review grading procedures.
- Keep accurate daily, weekly, and semester records.

Standard 3.1 in NSCA *Strength and Conditioning Professional Standards and Guidelines* gives additional information on proper program supervision and facility management (20).

Conclusion

Much of what is done in strength and conditioning programs should be designed to integrate with the mission of the school and school district while striving for athletic excellence and personal health for each student-athlete. Physical educators without a strong resistance training background may find course design implementation challenging. Having administrative support and community involvement is critical to the success of any strength and conditioning program. A properly designed and implemented strength and conditioning course at the high school level can be one of the most beneficial courses taken by student-athletes, leading to a lifetime of health and fitness. Not only is the design and content of the course of primary importance, but so is the way in which it is presented to the student-athletes. Proper scope and sequence should be followed for student-athletes to retain basic knowledge of how to design and put into practice a resistance training program designed to meet their personal goals.

While in high school, students may have the option of enrolling in a resistance-training class. That strength and conditioning course must provide a thorough foundation and instruction for student-athletes to master various exercises, use proper lifting techniques, gain knowledge of sport science, and be able to design an effective strength and conditioning program. Following the proper protocols of design, instruction, safety, rules, and procedures are all important aspects of the course. To have the greatest effect on student-athlete outcomes, teacher knowledge along with continuing education about class structure, course design, and proper supervision must be a priority. Based on program goals and objectives, policies and procedures should be developed to guide student-athletes and instructors to ensure a safe training environment.

The contents of this chapter provided a detailed framework for which strength and conditioning coaches can implement a strength and conditioning program through the PE program on campus. The program can and should be aligned with the current athletic program, coaches, student-athletes, players, school administrators, and community. Strength and conditioning professionals can use the materials found in the book to plan, organize, and administer a highly efficient and effective strength and conditioning program both in and outside of the classroom.

2

Class Scheduling, Planning, and Assessments

Gary S. McChalicher, EdD, CSCS, USAW, CAA
Brandon Peifer, MA, CSCS

Strength and conditioning has become common in high school athletics, mostly in an extracurricular fashion outside of the school day. Individuals who historically facilitate training for student-athletes range from well-intended but uncertified sport coaches to NSCA-certified strength and conditioning specialists (CSCS). As the physiological and psychological benefits of strength and conditioning become more apparent to leadership at the high school level, more high school programs are working to incorporate NSCA-certified staff to appropriately train athletes. While some high school programs may prefer to relegate strength and conditioning programs to outside of the school day, many high school programs will recognize the value of embedding strength and conditioning programs into the curricular day as a stand-alone program or through the health and physical education curriculum.

Curricular and Extracurricular Strength and Conditioning Programs

The physiological and psychological benefits of strength and conditioning for student-athletes are well-documented (24). While this chapter will provide helpful information about high school strength and conditioning to all industry professionals, the benefits of a well-organized strength and conditioning program may be even greater at the high school level when it is embedded into the school day with the physical education curriculum. Increased benefits of an embedded program include the following:

1. Access to a strength and conditioning program by non-athletes
2. Physical education paradigm shifts from general physical activity to data-based performance measurables for all students
3. Access to professional staff who have adequate background to become a CSCS
4. Opportunity for vertical curriculum alignment through elementary levels to support a valid long-term athletic development model
5. Increased training consistency
6. Increased student availability
7. Benefit of continuous curricular evaluation and staff development resources

The purpose of this chapter is to identify and outline instructional frameworks that professionals can use to embed strength and conditioning into the curricular day and to discuss various strength and conditioning assessments that will cultivate a data-rich program to support the curricular strength and conditioning program. The examples of curricular frameworks include three class schedule possibilities and an outline of necessary components for curricular lesson plans. While certain class schedule frameworks are more optimal than others, this chapter will provide resources for professionals to adapt and maximize all class structures. Scholastic educational leaders are increasingly data driven to deliver instructional best practices. The reliance on data to support student learning may have a negative effect on physical education when programs fail to produce quantitative measures that illustrate student growth and justify the program's expense. Scholastic resources are limited by federal, state, and local budgets. The allocation of financial resources often is determined by initiatives that produce data on student performance. The strength and conditioning assessments outlined in the chapter will provide assessments that professionals can implement to collect data on content literacy, student movement, and student performance.

It is important to compare and contrast the curricular approach to strength and conditioning with the extracurricular approach prior to discussing optimal class structure, lesson plans, and assessment data. As previously mentioned, the framework for high school strength and conditioning will be different at every school. Strength and conditioning programs at some schools may be informal in that they are coordinated by a sport coach who has some experience with training but is likely uncertified. Informal strength and conditioning roles are often uncompensated and not equally offered to all sports within the school. While this framework is still common, it poses severe risk management and Title IX compliance issues. Strength and conditioning at the high school level may also be categorized as an extracurricular activity, in which case sport coaches are often stipend positions within the school district's collective bargaining agreement for professional staff. Extracurricular stipend-based strength and conditioning professionals may offer a more consistent program across all sports and may also be certified; however, their stipends most likely do not qualify as full-time employment. This may result in low job security and high turnover rates.

Schools may also outsource strength and conditioning services through the athletic department's budget or a booster club's budget. Outsourced strength and conditioning programs typically access strength and conditioning professionals in the local community. While outsourced strength and conditioning contracts between schools and professionals will vary depending on the scope of training, these strength and conditioning professionals may be certified by a professional organization and include scholastic training in their full-time training portfolio. Outsourced strength and conditioning professionals may be a better solution than stipend-based extracurricular programs because the strength and conditioning professional is likely employed full time independently of the school and certified; however, this framework still may not provide equal opportunities to all sport programs and generally does not provide opportunities for non-athletes.

The optimal framework for extracurricular strength and conditioning is for schools to provide a full-time, certified strength and conditioning professional to work with all athletes. While a full-time strength and conditioning professional is still fairly rare, especially in public schools, it still may be difficult for a single full-time strength and conditioning professional to meet the needs of all in-season and out-of-season sport teams during the week. Scholastic programs can have athlete numbers ranging from 500 to over 1,000 participants, dependent on the size of school and the number of sports offered. The full-time extracurricular strength and conditioning model requires the professional to coordinate training for all participants outside of the school day, which can be a challenge given the aforementioned factors.

It is relevant to discuss the overarching objective for high school strength and conditioning professionals when analyzing the differences between a curricular and extracurricular approach. The differences should be examined through two different lenses: the professional and the student-athlete. Ideally, the high school strength and conditioning professional should be a full-time employee with the minimum of a bachelor's degree and certification by a nationally accredited organization like the NSCA. The NSCA CSCS credential should be considered the gold standard for strength and conditioning certification. The goal for every strength and conditioning professional should be to interact with all of the student-athletes at least minimally, not just select teams or individuals. It is understood that schools may undergo a slow progression from an informal strength and conditioning framework to a full-time, certified framework. An essential component of the rationalization for the need of a full-time professional is equal access to strength and conditioning for all student-athletes.

Curricular programs may use a certified health and physical education (HPE) teacher who is also a certified strength and conditioning professional. Combining the role of an HPE teacher and a certified strength and conditioning professional can be an ideal way for schools to commit to a full-time strength and conditioning solution, because it combines a traditional full-time teaching role with job functions that fit within most existing HPE curriculum frameworks. In most states, if the strength and conditioning class counts toward physical education graduation credit, the strength and conditioning professional will also have to be a state-certified HPE teacher. It is likely most physical education and teacher education bachelor programs provide the necessary coursework covered in the two sections of the CSCS exam (i.e., scientific foundations and practical/applied), so certified HPE teachers should be adequately prepared to take the CSCS exam.

Curricular strength and conditioning programs may be focused on the school's student-athletes, or they can be open to all students. Curricular strength and conditioning programs focused on athletes exclusively may do so because of limitations related to teacher availability or perhaps short-sightedness on behalf of the department leadership. It may be logical to initially focus on the school's student-athletes when embedding strength and conditioning into the school day due to the student-athletes' familiarity and to offset time dedicated to training outside of the school day. The ability to conduct strength and conditioning during the day should provide student-athletes with more flexibility with their time after school and offer a more consistent training program to all sports.

Curricular strength and conditioning classes during the school day are a giant step for schools, especially if the strength and conditioning professional is a full-time employee. The most likely issue with offering strength and conditioning classes only to student-athletes stems from the school's academic schedule. Most school administrators develop the master course schedule around the school's core academic courses and fill in elective courses and partial-credit courses once the core academic schedule is completed. This method of scheduling may create obstacles to maximizing student-athletes' ability to take strength and conditioning classes if the classes are only offered one or two periods per day. However, a school that has the personnel and the foresight to offer strength and conditioning classes every school day, throughout the day, will create many more opportunities for both student-athletes and non-athletes to take advantage of the program.

The most positive aspect of embedding a strength and conditioning program into the HPE program for all students has been the progress of the non-athletes and the recognition HPE departments have received for their pursuit of data-driven physical fitness growth for all students. A comprehensive strength and conditioning program for all students represents a shift in HPE from an emphasis on physical activity to an emphasis on data-based performance measures. This paradigm shift will result in the following benefits for the program and school:

- Students will have goal setting opportunities, making HPE instruction more relevant to the learner.

- HPE teachers can illustrate fitness growth and conduct qualitative and quantitative analysis to support the need for HPE in schools.

- The fitness-based curriculum will feature strength and conditioning principles that begin in the elementary level and increase in complexity and scope annually through the 12th grade.

- An HPE-based strength and conditioning program may result in generating interest in non-athletes to try, or return to, scholastic sports.

- An HPE program that offers strength and conditioning to all students will be more likely to accommodate more student-athletes during the school day.

Curricular strength and conditioning during the school day has several other benefits in addition to providing opportunities for non-athletes, increasing training opportunities for student-athletes, and shifting to a data-based HPE model. Curricular strength and conditioning also supports the overarching education-based athletics model that connects scholastic athletics and educational values. When determining whether to use an extracurricular approach or a curricular approach, one should also consider access to existing school district resources and the ability to fit into an existing school district framework.

Proposing a new strength and conditioning program that requires hiring an additional full-time staff member can be a challenge in public school districts because they are public entities, supported by taxpayer dollars. Budgets are typically handcuffed by personnel-related expenses, and available funding is typically fixed or tied to local tax increases. In addition, extracurricular positions in athletic departments are often part-time stipend positions in nature. It may be easier to add full-time extracurricular staff in a private school, but private schools make up a very small percentage of the high school student attendance across the nation. It may be easier for schools to embed a strength and conditioning professional in the school day than to hire an additional full-time position outside of the school day if schools can use an existing HPE teacher or fill an open HPE teaching position with a certified HPE teacher who is interested in strength and conditioning.

Upon embedding a strength and conditioning program into the school day through the HPE department, the long-term athletic development model (LTAD) provides an excellent guide for vertical alignment of strength and conditioning principles. The concept of LTAD has increased in popularity and refers to best practices for practical, functional, and sequential skill development (18). To HPE educators, the existing LTAD model as it is discussed basically represents an ideal scope and sequence for a K-12 HPE curriculum. Embedding strength and conditioning into the existing HPE curriculum vertically gives professionals an opportunity to reach all youth at the appropriate ages (3-14) for LTAD. The reality of the LTAD model is that many youth will not have the opportunity for focused skill development during the crucial ages if they are not exposed to it in school HPE. It is unlikely that an extracurricular approach to strength and conditioning will be able to focus on vertical applications of strength and conditioning and LTAD with students ages 3 to 14.

HPE departments, like all curricular programs, have existing resources for annual curricular evaluation and professional development. Schools that support an extracurricular strength and conditioning framework may be able to financially support staff development, but it would be an additional cost for the athletic department to absorb. From an HPE curricular perspective, these resources are typically budgeted annually and include the following:

- Funds available for conference attendance
- Dues toward professional organizations and certification
- Paid time for curriculum writing and evaluation
- In-house staff development and collaboration through the year
- Tuition reimbursement for collegiate coursework

One of the NSCA's objectives is to service all high school student-athletes across the nation with certified strength and conditioning professionals. Much like the introduction of certified athletic trainers to all high school athletic programs in the 1980s and 1990s, individual schools will support new strength and conditioning programs as they are able. Many schools may have to start with a certified stipend-paid sport coach and eventually build the program to feature a full-time extracurricular strength and conditioning professional or a certified strength and conditioning professional that is also a certified HPE teacher.

Class Scheduling Options and Examples

Several effective scheduling methods exist for strength and conditioning classes during the school day. Realistically, the strength and conditioning class structure during the school day will be a reflection of the overall school schedule. Strength and conditioning professionals must understand that the school leadership has many reasons for the school's schedule, and optimizing strength and conditioning classes may not be a priority. Strength and conditioning professionals should have conversations with the chairperson of the HPE department and school administration to advocate for the class schedule that will optimize the impact with students while advancing the overall mission of the school. For the purpose of gaining an accurate organizational perspective, a school's class schedule considers the following:

- Leadership's overarching philosophy on how to best educate students
- Leadership's available staff for the students in the school and to effectively run the building
- The number of electives the school offers to students; increased electives require more schedule flexibility

A building's class schedule will most likely be a balance of the aforementioned factors. Sometimes a school schedule is built around something as simple as the cafeteria schedule to ensure all students and staff have adequate lunch time. Administratively, there are generally two philosophies on how to best design class schedules to educate students. Some school leaders prefer shorter classes through the day that meet throughout the school year. This is referred to as *traditional scheduling*. Other school leaders prefer longer classes during the day that occur daily but only last for one-half of the year, or a single semester. This is commonly referred to as *block scheduling*. A block schedule gives students fewer class options during the day—typically four classes—and a traditional schedule typically gives students seven classes during the day. Building administrators occasionally use a modified block schedule that allows the core curricular classes to take advantage of the longer, more condensed block framework while the elective courses use a more spread out, traditional approach. Modified block schedules typically only exist when building resources are sufficient to facilitate the many moving parts of a school day. The length of the school day will vary from school to school. No federal regulations exist on the maximum length of the school day; rather, most scholastic regulations occur at the state level.

As previously stated, the ideal strength and conditioning class or physical education class may be a minor consideration for school leadership when designing a class schedule. Strength and conditioning professionals should be prepared to advocate to all stakeholders for a schedule that may be optimal; however, strength and conditioning professionals should be prepared to work within their constraints and still achieve maximum results. The ideal class schedule will be dependent on several factors; however, it is believed that a strength and conditioning professional's primary objective should be to reach as many students as possible throughout the school day.

Factors affecting the ideal strength and conditioning class schedule include the following:

- Availability of the strength and conditioning professional
- Inclusion of athletes only or all students
- Co-ed or homogeneous groupings
- Ideal training frequency and duration
- Student-to-teacher ratio (i.e., a ratio of 15:1 [32])
- Facility constraints (i.e., 100 sq ft per student [32])

Traditional Schedule

A strength and conditioning professional should be able to work within any of the scheduling parameters outlined, and it is likely the strength and conditioning professional will not have input into the decision. Each schedule has unique benefits. The traditional, block, and modified frameworks all have unique benefits, and all can be used successfully. The most common may be traditional schedules, with seven academic periods throughout the day for students. Teachers will likely teach five or six classes during a traditional schedule in addition to a planning period and a lunch period. The class periods in a traditional schedule will range from roughly 42 to 50 minutes, dependent on the school. One consideration is how the school characterizes HPE classes. In most schools, HPE classes are generally a half-credit class. If that is the case, that means the strength and conditioning professional will have each class every other day for a full year, or every day for a semester.

Generally, the length of class time in a traditional schedule can be a challenge for most strength and conditioning professionals, especially when considering students lose another 5 to 10 minutes when given time to change attire. This framework can still be extremely effective if the strength and conditioning professional is able to maximize time. When evaluating the strengths and weaknesses of the schedule variations for traditional-schedule, half-credit HPE classes, contributor Gary McChalicher has found that the half-credit framework of meeting every day for a semester works best. While the class lengths are shorter than desirable, meeting daily optimizes training frequency, giving the strength and conditioning professional ample time to program for all phases of student-athlete performance over the time given. It is recommended that strength and conditioning professionals embed days for speed and agility development, active recovery, and metabolic training when working with student-athletes daily in a traditional schedule. This class framework is also beneficial because students can take a second half-credit strength and conditioning class as an elective for the second half of the school year to maintain training throughout the school year. The school would have to allow students to take HPE classes as an elective. Actual class size will be affected by the size of the training facility and the appropriate training ratios as outlined by the NSCA: a ratio of 15:1 for student-athletes to strength and conditioning professionals at the high school level (32). However, school administrators may schedule more than the recommended ratio in each HPE class. The strength and conditioning professional should work with the administration to meet the needs of the school and students while ensuring a safe learning and instructional environment. The size of the facility will be the greatest determining factor when determining reasonable class sizes. A teacher will generally teach five periods per day in a traditional schedule. Over the course of a school year, a teacher who exclusively teaches strength and conditioning can accommodate 150 students using the NSCA recommended ratio; however, actual class sizes may be larger.

Block Schedule

A block academic schedule typically uses four class periods a day, with each period lasting between 80 and 90 minutes. Teachers typically teach three classes each day in a block schedule. Block differs from traditional scheduling in that a full-credit class meets every day for a semester. HPE classes are typically considered a half-credit class, which means the class meets every other day for the semester. Though block scheduling will generally facilitate class three days in a six-day cycle, the block format allows strength and conditioning professionals to facilitate more thorough workouts, with more time for warm-up, cooldown, and group instruction during the class. When comparing the actual training minutes available between a traditional schedule meeting every day and a block schedule meeting every other day over a six-week cycle, the available time for training is virtually the same. A block schedule does provide a slightly better framework for training because the class length is longer and provides built-in rest days between workouts. Though a strength and conditioning professional certainly can optimize the traditional schedule framework that meets daily through the six-day instructional cycle, it is possible for student-athletes to get burned out if they are not used to training. Block scheduling also provides an opportunity for more students to take advantage of the curricular strength and conditioning program. A teacher who teaches strength and conditioning full time can teach six sections of strength and conditioning each semester. If a teacher can accommodate 15 students per class, a strength and conditioning program can service 180 students during the school year. As previously stated, it is likely that a strength and conditioning professional may have more than the NSCA recommended student-athlete-to-professional ratio. Some HPE classes across the nation may have ratios in the 20:1 to 30:1 range.

Modified Schedules (Includes Modified Several-Period and Alternating Block Schedules)

A modified class schedule can look vastly different between school districts. The underlying premise of a modified schedule is to provide block schedule period lengths for core academic classes and shortened periods for elective courses and HPE. An administration may also flip that framework, assigning core classes to full-year schedules and electives and HPE to semester schedules. Schools may use a modified block schedule if they have sufficient staffing and want to maximize elective offerings to students. A key factor allowing administrators to offer a modified schedule is adequate staffing to support the schedule. Regardless of the modified framework, HPE teachers' schedules will likely fall within the parameters outlined in the traditional schedule framework or the block schedule framework.

Optimal Framework

The ideal schedule framework will vary by strength and conditioning professional, although the block framework is optimal because it can reach more students and features longer periods in an alternating day format. Regardless of the schedule framework, the strength and conditioning professional's goal should be to maximize the number of students throughout the class. It is recommended that the strength and conditioning professional support open classes for all students and resist the urge to push school administrators to schedule classes in homogeneous groupings by experience level or sport. One of the greatest attributes of a strength and conditioning class is that it is easily differentiated by ability; this is also one of the best-selling points to administrators. Similar to a standard strength and conditioning program one may find in the private sector or after the school day, the strength and conditioning professional can easily manage inevitable differences in ability levels through differentiation of movements and in-workout groupings by ability. Conversely, pushing administrators to schedule classes homogeneously by ability, sex, or sport may alienate the strength and conditioning professional in the eyes of the administration because it will require the administrator to consider too many variables during the master scheduling process. It is recommended that strength and conditioning professionals advocate that HPE classes be allowed to be taken as elective courses. It is contributor Gary McChalicher's experience that opening strength and conditioning classes so they can be counted toward HPE graduation credit and also serve as electives will grow the program due to popularity. McChalicher's school now has two strength and conditioning professionals, who both teach full schedules that are only strength and conditioning oriented. This occurred due to the overwhelming popularity of the strength and conditioning courses; a high percentage of the school's student-athlete and non-athlete population wanted to take the strength and conditioning classes as an elective annually, in addition to taking the course as their HPE graduation requirement. McChalicher's school designated a second HPE teacher in the department to exclusively teach strength and conditioning classes, and this support included financially contributing to the teacher's certifications and continued professional development.

Another question that arises when examining the optimal framework for curricular strength and conditioning is to determine which grade levels should be prioritized when scheduling. It is possible that the building schedule may dictate that certain grades have HPE during specific periods (e.g., 9th grade students have HPE period 1, 10th grade students have HPE period 2, and so on). In this case students of each grade may be scheduled for strength and conditioning based on interest, athletic team membership, or through prerequisites. Schools and students are best served when all students have access to the benefits of curricular strength and conditioning. However, even if a curricular strength and conditioning program prioritizes athletes, a fully scheduled block framework can accommodate 180 students per year, and a fully scheduled traditional framework can only accommodate 150 students per year, with a single strength and conditioning professional.

Regardless of how building administration schedules HPE, the HPE department may have to develop a priority list to determine the students who receive the class. At times, upperclassmen and underclassmen may be scheduled to take HPE during the same periods. There is merit to prioritizing upperclassmen or to prioritizing underclassmen, albeit for different reasons. The reality is that a curricular strength and conditioning program staffed by a single strength and conditioning professional may not be able to reach the needs of all students or student-athletes during the school day. Even with a curricular program, schools should still offer after-school strength and conditioning opportunities for students with schedules that cannot accommodate strength and conditioning class year-round.

The merit of prioritizing upperclassmen is that the students may be more mature both physically and emotionally for training. They may be more motivated and more coachable and require less redirection during training. Upperclassmen may also be more confident in pushing themselves past their comfort zone during training. The merit of prioritizing underclassmen is to reach them earlier in order to develop a culture of training. Underclassmen may generally be less confident in their physical abilities at the start of training; however, they may also be more raw and less encumbered by bad habits. It is the authors' view that the importance of developing a culture of training in early ages cannot be understated. Ideally, these students have had the benefit of a vertically aligned strength and conditioning curriculum and should have developed solid foundations of movement. Underclassmen may not have the means to access after-school training opportunities, while upperclassmen may generally have a better opportunity to do so once they come of age to drive. Most importantly, prioritizing underclassmen develops a culture of continuous self-improvement at an earlier age. Having to prioritize is difficult, and strength and conditioning professionals naturally want to accommodate all. By developing a culture with underclassmen, the program will put upperclassmen who have been properly trained during previous years of curricular strength and conditioning in a position to take ownership of their personal fitness goals with adequate after-school activities if they are not able to fit curricular strength and conditioning in their schedules.

Lesson Plan Guidelines and Examples

A lesson plan for a curricular strength and conditioning class and a workout program for a typical strength and conditioning workout will look very similar from a 30,000-foot view. The same programming elements and considerations exist; however, the lesson plan in the curricular setting should have minor additions that support the strength and conditioning professional's planning considerations expected of educators.

Traditional strength and conditioning programming elements of a curricular lesson plan include the following:

- Appropriate warm-up and cooldown
- Considerations for preseason, in-season, postseason, and off-season student-athletes
- Appropriate periodization
- Considerations for the metabolic demands of specific sports
- Exercise selection and progression
- Scaling considerations for each exercise relating to student-athlete ability level
- Desired volume and intensity prescriptions for each exercise

Additional components of a curricular lesson plan that should also be identified in the school's curriculum map for the class include the following:

- A statement identifying the essential learning for each day
- Identification of the direct instruction skill component for each day as reflected in the curriculum
- Identification of state and national HPE standards that the lesson satisfies
- Guidelines for adaptive considerations for special education students

The additional components of a strength and conditioning lesson plan may seem daunting to the inexperienced strength and conditioning professional; however, these elements of a lesson plan are typically nonnegotiable for all curricular courses. These components of the lesson are what give strength and conditioning courses a distinct advantage over traditional game-style HPE classes. Strength and conditioning courses offer a higher level of relevance to the student-athlete because the student-athlete can set personal performance goals in line with the content.

A key difference between traditional strength and conditioning and curricular strength and conditioning is the strength and conditioning professional's explicit role in providing student-athletes with the tools to facilitate their lifelong personal fitness initiatives. The statement that identifies the essential learning for each day should be a higher-level thinking opportunity that prompts student-athletes to connect an element of that day's workout to their personal performance goals or to their understanding of how their body adapts to the training plan for lifelong application. As a strength and conditioning professional, it should be easy to develop higher-level thinking statements that relate workout elements to personal performance goals or lifelong personal fitness initiatives.

Identification of the direct instruction component is simply that day's point of emphasis for the workout. This could be the introduction of a new movement or the review of a previous movement. Ideally, the strength and conditioning professional will informally assess student-athletes daily and then review the components of movements where student-athletes need help during this time. The essential movements introduced and reviewed in the lesson plan should mirror the movement progression outlined in the strength and conditioning curriculum. The identification of new movements or the review of previous movements prior to a training session typically occurs in any strength and conditioning setting; the strength and conditioning professional breaks down points of emphasis for a particular movement using a direct instruction tactic of "I do," "we do," and "you do." The direct instruction component also provides or reiterates specific cues for the student-athletes, geared to achieve a specific result of the movement.

A simple instructional progression strength and conditioning professionals can use when determining the proper direct instruction component for a lesson is listed next.

1. What do I want my student-athletes to know and be able to do?
   a. The progression for essential movements should be identified vertically from K-12 in the strength and conditioning program curriculum.
2. How does the strength and conditioning professional know when student-athletes have mastered a movement?
   a. What formative and summative assessment strategies should the strength and conditioning professional use to determine this?
      i. Formative assessments are informal snapshots of student-athlete progress during training sessions.
      ii. Summative assessments may be considered a test of some type that relates to the movement or activity.
3. What area of direct instruction is ideal for student-athletes when they get it?
   a. Does the strength and conditioning professional prescribe enrichment activities related to that movement, or does the strength and conditioning professional move on to the next movement?

4. What area of direct instruction is ideal for student-athletes when they do not get it?

    a. While conducting formative assessments, the strength and conditioning professional notices that student-athletes are generally not responding appropriately during certain cues of the back squat.

        i. At this point in time, the strength and conditioning professional should review the specific aspect of the back squat the student-athletes are having an issue with prior to the next training session that involves the back squat.

        ii. Review or evaluate the student-athletes' posture and range of motion.

        iii. Identify possible variations of the squat movement that may be more appropriate due the student-athletes' physical needs or limitations.

Connection to State and National Standards

Learning standards can be found for virtually all curricular courses in K-12 public education. Standards exist at the national and state levels; however, national and state standards are rarely identical. HPE educational standards are outlined by SHAPE America (27), and state standards for each curricular course can be found within each state's department of education. SHAPE America has five overarching standards that are broad enough for school districts to interpret and outline their preferred progression. A well-written K-12 strength and conditioning curriculum will certainly meet the needs of SHAPE America's National Standards and should be an extension of state standards, which should have valuable initiatives of a progressive nature through the grade levels. These initiatives should provide staff development through state and regional clinics and should encourage school districts' support of individual professional development.

The National Standards developed by SHAPE America (27) follow:

1. The physically literate individual demonstrates competency in a variety of motor skills and movement patterns.

2. The physically literate individual applies knowledge of concepts, principles, strategies and tactics related to movement and performance.

3. The physically literate individual demonstrates the knowledge and skills to achieve and maintain a health-enhancing level of physical activity and fitness.

4. The physically literate individual exhibits responsible personal and social behavior that respects self and others.

5. The physically literate individual recognizes the value of physical activity for health, enjoyment, challenge, self-expression and/or social interaction.

A key point to consider when examining the desired learning outcome of standards is what the educator wants the student to know and be able to do upon graduation from the 12th grade. To determine an appropriate progression for learning through grade levels, the educator should map backward from the 12th grade through the start of schooling in kindergarten. This is an example of a vertically aligned curriculum. Educators should apply research-based, age-appropriate activities for each grade level. For example, a barbell back squat may not be appropriate for a fifth grader, but a bodyweight squat is appropriate. It is important for the strength and conditioning professional to recognize that the learner's ability to "demonstrate," "apply," "exhibit," and "recognize" will vary and increase by grade level. When examining SHAPE America's first standard, a student's "demonstrated competency" of a motor skill or movement pattern should consider age appropriateness and reflect the value of experience, while practicing differentiation for the varying populations. "Demonstrated competency" will be more advanced as the student progresses in age.

Goal Setting and Student Differentiation

A well-run strength and conditioning program is an ideal curricular program for HPE because the content is easily individualized and differentiated for the learner. Our nation's educational system has been increasingly moving toward an individualized approach by measuring each student's yearly growth in all subjects, in addition to requiring proficiency on standardized tests. Physical education has been behind this curve because data collected on student performance is rare, especially in a game-oriented HPE culture. In the eyes of some educational leaders, a lack of data on student performance in HPE may result in a diminished perception of the importance of HPE. The reality is that today's adolescents may face more challenges in health and wellness than any other time in history. Levels of childhood obesity are up, leading to a host of physical health issues, and emphasis on the emotional wellness of adolescents has increased. HPE teachers are on the front lines of the physical and emotional challenges youth are facing. A data-driven approach in HPE can help today's HPE teachers secure the support and funding to face the challenges affecting our youth.

The strength and conditioning professional can easily facilitate a goal-setting framework in the curricular setting. If dealing with student-athletes, the strength and conditioning professional can work with the student-athlete and sport coach to set measurable goals related to the student-athlete's performance in the training facility and on the field and use applicable examples that involve injury reduction as well as skill acquisition and mastery. The essential learning for the student-athlete that comes from the goal-setting piece occurs when the strength and conditioning professional has each student-athlete commit to goals in writing and facilitates ongoing evaluation of those goals. The strength and conditioning professional can just as easily facilitate goal setting with non-athletes. When discussing goals with non-athletes, their measurables may be less quantitative than a student-athlete's, like, "I want to be in better shape" or "I want to be stronger." This is an opportunity for the strength and conditioning professional to have rich conversations with both student-athletes and non-athletes to outline the progression of training and how it relates to them reaching their goals. The strength and conditioning professional can also lean on the results from screening methods as outlined later in this chapter to guide each student-athlete's training progression. Ultimately, the training program of the non-athlete will focus on improving structural balance, body composition, and metabolic performance.

A strength and conditioning professional in the curricular setting should have a battery of tests to assess student-athletes' muscular strength, power, agility, speed, and aerobic endurance after a program cycle. If the strength and conditioning professional is training both student-athletes and non-athletes, assessments used may vary by group. These tests are valuable because they produce quantitative data. Quantitative data is powerful because they illustrate growth over time on measurable factors that the HPE department can relate to improvements in overall physical health. Strength and conditioning professionals can also use qualitative interviews or surveys to assess the impact of strength and conditioning on student-athletes' emotional wellness. The basis of qualitative interviews or surveys could be centered on the results of student-athletes' personal goal-setting process.

The goal-setting and data collection process is a multiphased process that will take time for the strength and conditioning professional to master. The most important, and perhaps the most time-consuming, phase of the process is creating reports that appropriately communicate the outstanding things that student-athletes achieve to parents and administrators. Testing time in strength and conditioning is always exciting for the student-athletes; they enjoy setting new records on the school's record boards or reaching their personal goals or benchmarks from regional or national standards. Witnessing their excitement when they surpass the expectations they had for themselves is always just as exciting for the strength and conditioning professional. It is just as important for parents and administrators to get excited about the student-athletes' achievements; this is also how the strength and conditioning professional can build the program. The strength and conditioning professional should find ways to connect the excitement of the student-athletes to parents and administrators and provide parents and administrators annual reports of student-athlete progress. Strength and conditioning professionals may cultivate excitement and understanding of the strength and conditioning program in the following ways:

- Use social media to connect parents, sport coaches, teachers, and administrators to the program.
- Create annual reports for sport coaches, administrators, and the school board highlighting quantitative and qualitative data from student-athletes.
- Conduct anonymous surveys with student-athletes that assess levels of participant satisfaction, then share information with administration and the school board in the annual report.

By taking extra steps to share data about student performance with parents, sport coaches, administrators, and the school board, the strength and conditioning professional will illustrate to all stakeholders the value of a performance-based HPE program. This will help the strength and conditioning professional and the HPE department gain support for developing the ideal vertically aligned program.

The premise of differentiation in the classroom is based on the idea that student-athletes are unique and deserve an opportunity to learn and grow at their particular level. Educators increasingly reject a one-size-fits-all educational system or an educational system that teaches to the middle in hopes that the trained and experienced learner, as well as the untrained and inexperienced learner, equally benefit from the instruction. Differentiation in strength and conditioning is intuitive and natural. It would be obvious while teaching a squat movement that everyone on a sport team or in a strength and conditioning class will be on different levels. Each student-athlete may have different physical abilities as well as different levels of experience with training. A simple form of differentiation for the squat would be to assign work sets of 15 repetitions of bodyweight squats to an untrained and inexperienced student-athlete and to assign work sets of 5 repetitions of a back squat to an intermediate-level student-athlete. Differentiation naturally occurs in strength and conditioning through the following factors:

- Program goal
- Program type (untrained and inexperienced, intermediate, trained and experienced)
- Exercise selection (involving the use of variations or movement development progressions)
- Exercise volume
- Exercise intensity
- Daily, weekly, and monthly volume

A strength and conditioning professional will easily be able to differentiate all of these factors for each student-athlete, basing the assessment of the student-athlete's abilities off preprogram formal or informal screening, informal discussions with the student-athlete, or information from the sport coach or athletic training staff. Connecting with school administrators on vital nuances of instruction such as differentiation will give the strength and conditioning professional increased credibility and support as the program builds. It will be evident to the school leadership that the curricular strength and conditioning program is fully invested in improving the health and well-being of all students.

Sample Lesson Plan Templates

Lesson plans for curricular strength and conditioning classes will be very similar, regardless of the class schedule framework. The main difference between a lesson plan for the traditional and block framework will be the extra time per class period that the block schedule allows. While block scheduling provides more time per class period, a traditional schedule will meet more frequently if it is a half-credit class that meets for one semester. Strength and conditioning professionals in a curricular setting must remember to allocate time in their lesson planning before and after training sessions for student-athletes to change clothes.

As depicted in figure 2.1, essential descriptive elements of a lesson plan include the following:

- Unit and movements that correspond to curriculum progression
- The same language as outlined in the curriculum
- Identification of standards with which the lesson connects
- Overarching essential student-athlete learning for the lesson
- Direct instruction: movement introduction or movement review
- Warm-up activity
- Exercise selection and progression
- Exercise volume and intensity
- Exercise differentiation: needs dependent on class roster
- Cooldown activity
- Formative or summative assessment used

Lesson Plan Template

Teacher Name: _____ Date: _____ Period: _____

Unit: _____ Corresponding Standards: _____

Essential Student Learning: _____

Warm-Up Activity: _____

Movement Introduction or Review: _____

Exercise Selection and Progression:

Exercise 1:	Exercise Alternative (a):	Exercise Alternative (b):
Exercise 2:	Exercise Alternative (a):	Exercise Alternative (b):
Exercise 3:	Exercise Alternative (a):	Exercise Alternative (b):
Exercise 4:	Exercise Alternative (a):	Exercise Alternative (b):
Exercise 5:	Exercise Alternative (a):	Exercise Alternative (b):
Exercise 6:	Exercise Alternative (a):	Exercise Alternative (b):
Exercise 7:	Exercise Alternative (a):	Exercise Alternative (b):
Exercise 8:	Exercise Alternative (a):	Exercise Alternative (b):

Note: Add details for volume and intensity where appropriate.

Cooldown Activity: _____

Formative or Summative Assessments: _____

From *NSCA's Guide to High School Strength and Conditioning*, edited for the National Strength and Conditioning Association by P. McHenry and M. Nitka (Champaign, IL: Human Kinetics, 2022).

FIGURE 2.1 Lesson plan template.

Considerations for Adaptive Lesson Planning

The National Consortium for Physical Education for Individuals with Disabilities (NCPEID) is an organization that works to improve the quality of physical education and recreation for students with disabilities (23). NCPEID developed 15 national standards to ensure adaptive physical education was developed by a Certified Adaptive Physical Educator, a credential that educators can receive by passing the nationally certified exam. Curricular strength and conditioning professionals should consider obtaining the credentials to work with adaptive populations because there is a deficit of appropriate adaptive physical education in many schools. Strength and conditioning professionals can use materials like low step-up boxes, lighter large-style medicine balls, fitness bands, fitness games, and even kettlebells with the incorporation of bodyweight exercises to produce well-rounded fitness sessions for adaptive populations.

Effective Strength and Conditioning–Related Assessments

As discussed throughout this chapter, the value of data for the curricular strength and conditioning professional cannot be understated. The following forms of data are vital to the curricular strength and conditioning professional.

1. Movement pre-assessments and screening to identify baseline levels and movement deficiencies in student-athletes
2. Strength pre-assessments to determine baseline levels
3. Metabolic, speed, and agility pre-assessments to determine baseline levels
4. Movement post-assessments
5. Strength post-assessments
6. Metabolic, speed, and agility post-assessments
7. Participant numbers broken down by sex, sport, and grade
8. Satisfaction survey data from student-athletes
9. Qualitative data from student-athletes reflecting evaluation and application to goal-setting process and impact on health and wellness

Needs Analysis

This collection of data is vital to the strength and conditioning professional's effectiveness with the student-athletes. This data is also a key component of the strength and conditioning professional's effectiveness in cultivating support and resources for the program over time to reach the long-range goal of developing a K-12 vertically aligned curriculum with the addition of more strength and conditioning professionals.

The facilitation of testing during the school day may be easier with assistance from such people as the athletic training staff and possibly sport coaches. If additional help cannot be secured, the strength and conditioning professional may have to enlist members of the class to take turns filling administrative roles like recording times. Outside of the curricular setting, the athletic training staff can be particularly valuable in assisting with data collection from sport teams after school. Much like how athletic trainers collect baseline tests for head injury information, the athletic training staff can also be used to collect movement screen data on a randomized basis with sport teams in an attempt to find common themes across sexes or sport teams. The results from these procedures can be reinforced if injury data is available to explore additional identifiable trends.

It may initially be overwhelming for a new strength and conditioning professional to conduct a needs analysis and roll out new testing protocols. It is important for strength and conditioning professionals to structure a simple and consistent testing protocol. Do not try to conduct every test that is available or relevant; rather, determine what tests and progression work. Strength and conditioning professionals should try to keep their testing periods concise and space testing periods appropriately throughout the school year, so the student-athletes have adequate time for their bodies to produce physiological adaptations. When mapping out the semester, strength and conditioning professionals should consider breaks in school so student-athletes are not testing after a long break or during demanding academic periods. Check the school calendar for in-service days, exams, and holidays.

It is very important for strength and conditioning professionals to exercise extreme caution during the pre-assessment process when working with untrained student-athletes. It may be prudent to implement a preparatory or pre-training period before testing. Use simple bodyweight assessments or low-weight, high-repetition conversions if unsure about a student-athlete's ability to conduct a movement. Safety must remain a top priority, so strength and conditioning professionals should always remain mindful of mechanics and consistency before focusing on intensity with all students. Pre- and post-assessments should correspond to the needs of the sport when dealing with student-athletes. For a classic example, testing a mile run may not be the best assessment when working with offensive linemen. In addition, assessments should mirror the work that is performed during the lessons. Using the mile run again as an example, strength and conditioning professionals should not use the 1-mile run as a test if the curriculum does not consistently include aerobic conditioning. The outline of assessments found later in the chapter represents sample tests that can be used, but it should not be considered an exhaustive list. A qualified strength and conditioning professional should be familiar with a battery of assessment options for any situation.

Strength and conditioning professionals must remember to celebrate post-testing with the student-athletes. The student-athletes get excited to reach their goals or break records. Strength and conditioning professionals can use testing time to reinforce the culture they are trying to build by communicating and celebrating the student-athlete's accomplishments. Professionals should consider dedicating walls in the training facility to posting records and setting goals. The use of a leader board for various measurables gives student-athletes a visual goal and serves as an important motivation tool.

Once the strength and conditioning professional feels comfortable with the data collection and an efficient data dissemination process, the professional can then find ways to take the data further to support the strength and conditioning program. The data on pre-assessments and screens should be maintained and grouped by sex, age, sport, and sport type. This will allow the strength and conditioning professional and the athletic training staff to find common themes in the data and create warm-up or prehabilitative plans for sport teams based on common deficiencies. This data should be shared with sport coaches so they are aware of unique athlete deficiencies as well as broad-based needs among the team. The strength and conditioning professional and athletic training staff can produce videos for the athletes and the sport coaches that illustrate the warm-up progressions and discuss the nuances of each movement so the warm-ups can be facilitated as a team in practice. This team approach will cultivate continuity of service for the athletes between the strength and conditioning program and the athletic training department and should help reduce certain types of injuries.

Classroom Written Tests

It may not be intuitive for the strength and conditioning professional to facilitate written assessments in a strength and conditioning class. However, the written assessments will connect elements of educational foundations that are outlined in the lesson plan's essential student-athlete learning for each day. A vast majority of written assessments should focus on content literacy and higher-level application and evaluation of the student-athlete's work toward personal goals. Content literacy means ensuring the student-athletes understand the terms associated with training. *Volume, intensity, metabolic demands, periodization, program design, eccentric,* and *concentric* are a sample of terms that all people interested in strength and conditioning should be familiar with and be able to apply. The process of evaluation and application in the strength and conditioning class gives student-athletes an opportunity to gain a greater understanding of the process so they can apply it for themselves later in life. One of the overarching student-athlete-centered objectives of this class is to provide student-athletes with real-world skills that allow them to facilitate their own fitness through their life. The written assessments give student-athletes an opportunity to demonstrate the ability to do this.

One way strength and conditioning professionals can implement written assessments is through journaling. Tracking training progress is an important skill, and prompting the student-athletes to journal can help create positive habits relative to training that can also give them an opportunity to evaluate their work. Other ways strength and conditioning professionals can implement written assessments are through online discussion blogs, summative tests or quizzes, or informal periodic homework assignments that ask student-athletes to evaluate their level of effort in relation to their personal goals.

Movement Assessments

Movement assessments are useful tools that can provide the strength and conditioning professional with a snapshot of student-athletes' movement strengths and limitations prior to training. Data collected from movement assessments should inform the strength and conditioning professional's programming decisions. Strength and conditioning professionals should avoid conducting movement assessments too often, because student-athlete familiarization with the assessment may skew the data and consume valuable training time. Assessments can be periodically conducted during the training process to measure improvements in movement. Movement assessments should occur one or two times per year. It is good to obtain a baseline movement screen of student-athletes upon the start of training, much like ImPACT test baselines for the assessment of head injuries.

Strength and conditioning professionals can analyze movement screen data individually or as subgroups. Movement screen data that illustrates common traits among sex or sport teams will inform the strength and conditioning professional's training methodologies and can be applied to on-field team activities like warm-ups or conditioning.

Conducting movement assessments with an entire team, or class, can be very time consuming. Successful testing protocols will require the strength and conditioning professional to be highly organized and to communicate expectations clearly to student-athletes during the process. It is recommended that the strength and conditioning professional structure the time for student-athletes, providing alternate activities for student-athletes while others are being assessed so they are not left with idle time. It is also recommended that the strength and conditioning professional seek assistance during testing to supervise students and possibly help with testing protocols. For example, the school's athletic trainer or a sport coach may be available to assist with testing.

The functional movement system (FMS) created by Gray Cook (7) provides a comprehensive screening tool that is comprised of seven movement patterns that can be used to evaluate a student-athlete who does not have a current issue or musculoskeletal injury. As examples, the deep squat test evaluates the stability and mobility of the student-athlete's ankle, knee, and hip joints, while providing an opportunity to assess core integrity; the shoulder mobility screen demonstrates the range of motion a student-athlete has in both shoulders as well as scapular stability and thoracic spine mobility; and the trunk stability test is used to assess the ability of the student-athlete to stabilize the core when force is applied distally to the body. (*Note*: the FMS screen should be performed as a whole—meaning all seven tests—as the data that was gathered to create this effective screening tool and overall system was based on the full collection of tests.)

Basic Performance Assessments

Performance assessments provide the strength and conditioning professional a snapshot of a student-athlete's ability before and after a training cycle. The assessments provide data that ideally illustrate the abilities of a student-athlete that connect in some way to the physiological demands of the activity. The strength and conditioning professional should always connect performance assessments to the physiological demands of the activity for which the student-athlete is training. For example, a test for upper body strength may not be the most relevant assessment for a soccer player, and a test for muscular endurance may not be the most relevant assessment for an offensive lineman. Performance assessments can be conducted more frequently than movement assessments because an element of assessment familiarity on behalf of the student-athlete should promote a more accurate performance snapshot; however, performance assessments should generally only occur before and after an 8- to 12-week training cycle. Testing for performance too often or having athletes attempt maximal-effort tests too often in the training cycle should be avoided. Excessive maximal-effort testing may promote injury and also decrease physiological adaptations due to inappropriate training intensity and training volume.

Strength and conditioning professionals should also consider testing protocols prior to the immediate start of the sport season. It is important for the strength and conditioning professional to find the proper balance of testing to formally assess student-athlete progress, reinforce the team's culture of training, illustrate the achievement of student-athlete goals, and promote the student-athletes' transition to the sport season as healthfully as possible. To mitigate these concerns, strength and conditioning professionals may elect to schedule preseason testing a couple weeks prior to the official start of sport practice. The strength and conditioning professional may also work with the sport coaches to define a battery of performance tests that are lower impact in nature prior to the start of the season.

Strength and conditioning professionals should work to incorporate a goal-setting framework with student-athletes in conjunction with performance assessments. Goal setting with student-athletes should occur during the first week of the training cycle. Assessing performance with student-athletes can be a powerful moment that reinforces elements of goal setting, work ethic, and social support. A strength and conditioning professional's ability to harness and reinforce these elements during assessment time may lead to greater buy-in and culture development in the training facility. It is also important to share and celebrate team and student-athlete accomplishments at the conclusion of the posttraining assessment period. Strength and conditioning professionals can provide reports to sport coaches, update assessment leader boards, and point out team and student-athlete accomplishments on social media. Each of these post-assessment activities will cultivate enthusiasm among the student-athletes and reinforce the culture of the training facility.

Similar to movement assessments, performance assessments are time consuming. The strength and conditioning professional must be organized and effectively communicate instructions. This is especially true in the weight room when student-athletes are conducting maximal-effort attempts. Spotting guidelines should be described and demonstrated (see chapter 4 for specific details) immediately prior to maximal-effort testing, and the strength and conditioning professional should check for student-athlete understanding of the procedures and prescribe progression protocols for increasing resistance. In addition, it will be extremely helpful for the strength and conditioning professional to seek assistance during assessment time to help organize and supervise student-athletes and to collect performance data.

The assessments presented in this chapter do not represent an exhaustive list; rather, strength and conditioning professionals should research assessments that best fit their facility, training methodologies, and the physiological needs of their student-athletes.

Performance Assessment Finder

Speed and Acceleration Test

Purpose

The purpose of this test is to assess acceleration and speed.

Equipment

- Cones
- Stopwatch or timing system
- Measuring tape

Setup

Measure 40 yards (37 m) with a measuring tape on an athletic surface, and clearly mark the start and finish lines (figure 2.2).

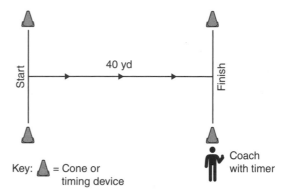

FIGURE 2.2   Speed assessment setup.

Protocol

1. Student-athletes should be led through a warm-up activity and dynamic stretching.

2. Review starting procedures with the student-athletes, and allow for a few low-intensity practice runs.

3. Student-athletes should assume a beginning position in a three- or four-point stance to ensure that they are in an optimal position to accelerate (figure 2.3).

4. On an auditory signal or on the student-athlete's first movement, start the clock. (Timing systems will do this automatically.)

5. Allow for at least 2 minutes of recovery time before another attempt.

6. The best times should be recorded to the nearest tenth of a second.

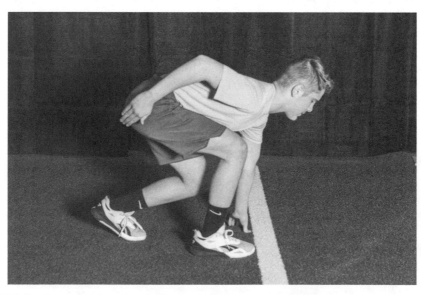

FIGURE 2.3   Speed assessment three-point beginning position.

Coaching Tips

- Coach student-athletes on proper starting technique.
- If using a stopwatch, clearly instruct the student-athletes on whether timing will begin with an auditory signal or if their movement will start the clock.
- Allow for long rest intervals (at least 2 minutes) between tests to limit fatigue.
- Be sure student-athletes are not fatigued when implementing this test (19).

Descriptive Data

See figure 2.4 for the 40-yard (37 m) sprint time classifications.

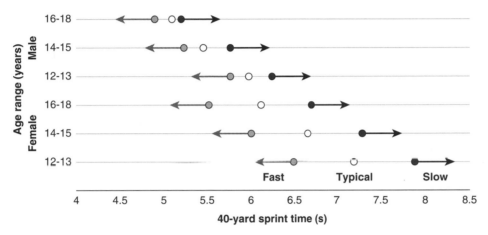

FIGURE 2.4   Forty-yard (37 m) sprint time classifications for youths aged 12 to 18 years: fast—70th percentile; typical—50th percentile; slow—30th percentile.

Reprinted by permission from Fukuda (2019, p. 123).

Pro-Agility Test

Purpose

This test is also known as the 5-10-5 shuttle or the 20-yard (18 m) shuttle; it is used to assess quickness, agility, and ability to change direction.

Equipment

• A field or a dry, nonslip, flat surface with three parallel lines that are all 5 yards apart (figure 2.5)

- Stopwatch or timing system
- Cones (if needed)
- Tape (if needed)
- Measuring tape (if a marked field or surface is unavailable)

Setup

Clear the testing area of any potential hazards, and be sure the surface is safe for student-athletes to run and change direction. Next, be sure that excessive background noise would prohibit the student-athlete from hearing instructions and the signal.

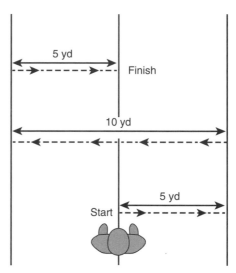

FIGURE 2.5   Pro-agility (5-10-5) assessment setup.

Protocol

1. The student-athlete should stand over the center line with one foot on each side of the line and assume a stance with the left hand lightly touching the center line (figure 2.6).

2. On the starting signal, the student-athlete should explode out of the beginning stance and sprint 5 yards (4.6 m) to the line on the left and touch with the left hand. The student-athlete should immediately turn and sprint 10 yards (9 m) to the line on the far right and again touch the line with the right hand. Finally, the student-athlete should sprint through the center line to end the drill.

3. Stop the clock when the student crosses the center line at the end of the test. Timing systems that work with this test should automatically display the time.

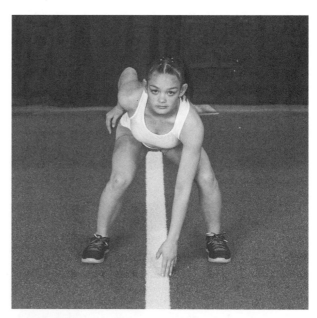

FIGURE 2.6   Pro-agility (5-10-5) assessment beginning position.

4. Each student-athlete should be given two attempts. Record their times to the nearest hundredth of a second.

Coaching Tips

• If a lined field is unavailable, tape on a floor or cones can be used to mark the three parallel lines.

• Be sure to take time to teach and practice the drill so that student-athletes fully understand the procedure. This will help ensure results that reflect each student-athlete's ability.

• Remind student-athletes that their time will not be recorded if they do not touch each line with a hand.

• Keep criteria of hand contact consistent.

• Student-athletes should be reminded to sprint through the finish line to ensure the best possible time. It is good practice to tell them to continue to sprint 5 yards (4.6 m) past the finish line (19).

Descriptive Data

See tables 2.1 and 2.2 for the pro-agility (5-10-5) test descriptive data.

TABLE 2.1 Descriptive Data for the Pro-Agility (5-10-5) Assessment

Group/sport (sex)	Time	Reference
High school soccer (girls)	Mean: 4.91 s ± 0.22 s	33
High school soccer (girls)	<99th percentile: 4.42 s 90th percentile: 4.63 s 75th percentile: 4.74 s 50th percentile: 4.91 s 25th percentile: 5.05 s 10th percentile: 5.26 s >1st percentile: 5.57 s	3
Active 12-15 year old (boys)	Mean: 5.6 s	11
Middle school soccer (girls)	<99th percentile: 4.38 s 90th percentile: 4.71 s 75th percentile: 4.93 s 50th percentile: 5.21 s 25th percentile: 5.39 s 10th percentile: 5.69 s >1st percentile: 6.33 s	3
High school basketball (girls)	Mean: 6.14 s ± 0.32 s	13
High school basketball (boys)	Mean: 5.63 s ± 0.31 s	13
Teenage athletes, general (pooled sexes)	Mean: 5.12-5.17 s ± 0.31-0.36 s	9
High school wrestling (boys)	14 years old: 50th percentile: 5.415 s 15 years old: 50th percentile: 5.347 s 16 years old: 50th percentile: 5.258 s	1

TABLE 2.2   Percentile Values of the Pro-Agility (5-10-5) Test in High School Football Athletes (in Seconds)

Percentile rank	DB	DL	LB, DE, TE	OL	QB	RB	WR
90	4.26	4.47	4.35	4.67	4.33	4.27	4.25
80	4.33	4.57	4.43	4.77	4.40	4.35	4.32
70	4.38	4.65	4.50	4.87	4.45	4.41	4.37
60	4.43	4.71	4.56	4.94	4.51	4.46	4.43
50	4.48	4.79	4.61	5.01	4.56	4.51	4.48
40	4.53	4.87	4.68	5.10	4.61	4.57	4.53
30	4.59	4.97	4.76	5.16	4.67	4.63	4.60
20	4.66	5.11	4.83	5.28	4.74	4.71	4.68
10	4.77	5.29	4.95	5.44	4.86	4.83	4.81
Mean (±SD)							
Freshman	4.61 (0.24)	5.00 (0.43)	4.76 (0.24)	5.18 (0.37)	4.66 (0.24)	4.63 (0.23)	4.62 (0.24)
Sophomore	4.52 (0.22)	4.85 (0.31)	4.66 (0.23)	5.05 (0.31)	4.59 (0.21)	4.53 (0.23)	4.52 (0.22)
Junior	4.46 (0.20)	4.81 (0.34)	4.59 (0.24)	5.02 (0.33)	4.53 (0.20)	4.50 (0.24)	4.46 (0.22)
n	1,307	839	1,189	677	627	1,172	1,462

DB = defensive back, DL = defensive lineman, LB = linebacker, DE = defensive end, TE = tight end, OL = offensive lineman, QB = quarterback, RB = running back, WR = wide receiver. SD = standard deviation, *n* = sample size.

Reprinted by permission from McKay, Miramonti, Gillen, et al. (2020).

Bench Press Strength Assessment

Purpose

This test is designed to measure upper body strength of a student-athlete who has demonstrated proficiency in the proper bench press technique. Although a 1-repetition maximum (1RM) test assesses a student-athlete's *maximal* strength, this carries a higher degree of risk, particularly to inexperienced, untrained individuals. Therefore, a 3RM-5RM assessment, described here, may be more appropriate and safer for younger and less developed student-athletes. If the strength and conditioning professional feels that a 1RM test is warranted for a specific student-athlete, a testing protocol is available (26).

Equipment

- Sturdy bench with a rack or a bench and an adjustable rack
- Barbell
- Weight plates
- Two safety locks for the barbell

Setup

If using an adjustable rack, set it to the appropriate height so that when the weight is racked the student-athlete has slight flexion of the elbows.

Protocol

1. Review and demonstrate proper bench press technique with the student-athletes (see page 105 in chapter 4).

2. A progressive warm-up protocol (sets 1 and 2) is necessary to potentiate the student-athlete to give maximal effort on the test. Allow rest intervals of 3 to 5 minutes between each set for full recovery (table 2.3).

3. For the assessment set (set 3), student-athletes should select a weight they believe they can use to complete 2 or 3 repetitions with proper technique. Athletes should then complete as many repetitions as possible (table 2.3).

4. Use the conversion chart to determine an estimated 1RM and record the number for future programming decisions (table 2.4).

TABLE 2.3   A 3RM-5RM Testing Protocol

Set	Resistance	Reps
1	Student-athletes should select a weight with which they can easily complete 8 to 10 reps with proper technique.	8-10
2	Student-athletes should select a weight with which they can easily complete 5 to 8 reps with proper technique.	5-8
3	Student-athletes should select a weight with which they can complete 2 or 3 reps with proper technique. Student-athletes should complete as many reps as possible. Use table 2.4 to determine an estimated 1RM and record the number for future programming decisions.	As many as possible based on the student-athlete's ability.

TABLE 2.4 Estimating 1RM and Training Loads

Max reps (RM)	1	2	3	4	5	6	7	8	9	10	12	15
%1RM	100	95	93	90	87	85	83	80	77	75	67	65
Load (pounds or kilograms)	10	10	9	9	9	9	8	8	8	8	7	7
	20	19	19	18	17	17	17	16	15	15	13	13
	30	29	28	27	26	26	25	24	23	23	20	20
	40	38	37	36	35	34	33	32	31	30	27	26
	50	48	47	45	44	43	42	40	39	38	34	33
	60	57	56	54	52	51	50	48	46	45	40	39
	70	67	65	63	61	60	58	56	54	53	47	46
	80	76	74	72	70	68	66	64	62	60	54	52
	90	86	84	81	78	77	75	72	69	68	60	59
	100	95	93	90	87	85	83	80	77	75	67	65
	110	105	102	99	96	94	91	88	85	83	74	72
	120	114	112	108	104	102	100	96	92	90	80	78
	130	124	121	117	113	111	108	104	100	98	87	85
	140	133	130	126	122	119	116	112	108	105	94	91
	150	143	140	135	131	128	125	120	116	113	101	98
	160	152	149	144	139	136	133	128	123	120	107	104
	170	162	158	153	148	145	141	136	131	128	114	111
	180	171	167	162	157	153	149	144	139	135	121	117
	190	181	177	171	165	162	158	152	146	143	127	124
	200	190	186	180	174	170	166	160	154	150	134	130
	210	200	195	189	183	179	174	168	162	158	141	137
	220	209	205	198	191	187	183	176	169	165	147	143
	230	219	214	207	200	196	191	184	177	173	154	150
	240	228	223	216	209	204	199	192	185	180	161	156
	250	238	233	225	218	213	208	200	193	188	168	163
	260	247	242	234	226	221	216	206	200	195	174	169
	270	257	251	243	235	230	224	216	208	203	181	176
	280	266	260	252	244	238	232	224	216	210	188	182
	290	276	270	261	252	247	241	232	223	218	194	189
	300	285	279	270	261	255	249	240	231	225	201	195

Max reps (RM)	1	2	3	4	5	6	7	8	9	10	12	15
%1RM	100	95	93	90	87	85	83	80	77	75	67	65
	310	295	288	279	270	264	257	248	239	233	208	202
	320	304	298	288	278	272	266	256	246	240	214	208
	330	314	307	297	287	281	274	264	254	248	221	215
	340	323	316	306	296	289	282	272	262	255	228	221
	350	333	326	315	305	298	291	280	270	263	235	228
	360	342	335	324	313	306	299	288	277	270	241	234
	370	352	344	333	322	315	307	296	285	278	248	241
	380	361	353	342	331	323	315	304	293	285	255	247
	390	371	363	351	339	332	324	312	300	293	261	254
	400	380	372	360	348	340	332	320	308	300	268	260
	410	390	381	369	357	349	340	328	316	308	274	267
	420	399	391	378	365	357	349	336	323	315	281	273
	430	409	400	387	374	366	357	344	331	323	288	280
	440	418	409	396	383	374	365	352	339	330	295	286
	450	428	419	405	392	383	374	360	347	338	302	293
	460	437	428	414	400	391	382	368	354	345	308	299
	470	447	437	423	409	400	390	376	362	353	315	306
	480	456	446	432	418	408	398	384	370	360	322	312
	490	466	456	441	426	417	407	392	377	368	328	319
	500	475	465	450	435	425	415	400	385	375	335	325
	510	485	474	459	444	434	423	408	393	383	342	332
	520	494	484	468	452	442	432	416	400	390	348	338
	530	504	493	477	461	451	440	424	408	398	355	345
	540	513	502	486	470	459	448	432	416	405	362	351
	550	523	512	495	479	468	457	440	424	413	369	358
	560	532	521	504	487	476	465	448	431	420	375	364
	570	542	530	513	496	485	473	456	439	428	382	371
	580	551	539	522	505	493	481	464	447	435	389	377
	590	561	549	531	513	502	490	472	454	443	395	384
	600	570	558	540	522	510	498	480	462	450	402	390

Coaching Tips

- If a student-athlete does not have good technique during the two sets, do not continue the assessment.
- Instruct spotters on how to spot the exercise (19).

Descriptive Data

After the estimated 1RM is determined from a 3RM-5RM, consult tables 2.5 through 2.7 for descriptive data for the 1RM bench press.

TABLE 2.5 Percentile Values of the 1RM Bench Press and Back Squat in High School Football Athletes

	1RM BENCH PRESS		1RM BACK SQUAT		1RM BENCH PRESS		1RM BACK SQUAT	
	lb	kg	lb	kg	lb	kg	lb	kg
Percentile rank	HIGH SCHOOL 14-15 YEARS				HIGH SCHOOL 16-18 YEARS			
90	243	110	385	175	275	125	465	211
80	210	95	344	156	250	114	425	193
70	195	89	325	148	235	107	405	184
60	185	84	305	139	225	102	365	166
50	170	77	295	134	215	98	335	152
40	165	75	275	125	205	93	315	143
30	155	70	255	116	195	89	295	134
20	145	66	236	107	175	80	275	125
10	125	57	205	93	160	73	250	114
Mean	179	81	294	134	214	97	348	158
SD	45	20	73	33	44	20	88	40

SD = standard deviation

Data from Hoffman (8).

TABLE 2.6 Percentile Values of the 1RM Back Squat and 1RM Bench Press in High School Baseball Athletes

| Percentile rank | 1RM BACK SQUAT | | 1RM BENCH PRESS | |
	lb	kg	lb	kg
90-100	365-505	165.9-229.5	235-280	106.8-127.3
80-89.9	320-360	145.5-163.6	220-230	100.0-104.5
70-79.9	290-315	131.8-143.2	205-215	93.2-97.7
60-69.9	270-285	122.7-129.5	190-200	86.4-90.9
50-59.9	255-265	115.9-120.5	180-185	81.8-84.1
40-49.9	245-250	111.4-113.6	170-175	77.3-79.5
30-39.9	225-240	102.3-109.1	160-165	72.7-75.0
20-29.9	205-220	93.2-100.0	145-155	65.9-70.5
10-19.9	180-200	81.8-90.9	130-140	59.1-63.6
<10	125-175	56.8-79.5	95-125	43.2-56.8
Mean	241.0	111.1	171.7	76.1
SD	58.0	28.4	37.7	17.4
n	702			

SD = standard deviation, *n* = sample size

Reprinted by permission from Szymanski and Vazquez (2022, p. 36).

TABLE 2.7 Descriptive Data for the 1RM Bench Press

Group/sport (sex)	Time	Reference
High school athletes, general (girls)	Mean: 79.75 lb ± 13.24 lb (36.25 kg ± 6.02 kg) Minimum: 59 lb (27 kg) Maximum: 114.75 lb (52.16 kg)	2
High school students (boys)	Mean: 89.3-94.6 lb ± 5.1-13.4 lb (40.6-43 kg + 2.3-6.1 kg)	21
U16 rugby league players (boys)	Mean: 162.9 lb ± 29.1 lb (74.0 kg ± 13.2 kg)	30
U17 rugby league players (boys)	Mean: 205.7 lb ± 29.5 lb (93.5 kg ± 13.4 kg)	30
U18 rugby league players (boys)	Mean: 228.6 lb ± 33.7 lb (103.9 kg ± 15.3 kg)	30

Multiply kg by 2.2 to yield pounds.

Back Squat Strength Assessment

Purpose

This test is designed to measure the lower body strength of a student-athlete who has demonstrated proficiency in the proper squat technique. Although a 1RM test assesses a student-athlete's *maximal* strength, this carries a higher degree of risk, particularly to inexperienced, untrained individuals. Therefore, a 3RM-5RM assessment, described here, may be more appropriate and safer for younger and less developed student-athletes. If the strength and conditioning professional feels that a 1RM test is warranted for a specific student-athlete, a testing protocol is available (26).

Equipment

- Barbell
- Squat rack with catches and spotting bars that are adjustable to each student-athlete's height
- Weight plates and two safety locks for the barbell
- Flat, solid, and dry surface

Setup

Set the safety crossbars at the appropriate height.

Protocol

1. Review and demonstrate proper back squat technique with the student-athletes (see page 138 in chapter 4).

2. A progressive warm-up protocol (sets 1 and 2) is necessary to potentiate the student-athlete to give maximal effort on the test. Allow rest intervals of 3 to 5 minutes between each set for full recovery (table 2.3).

3. For the assessment set (set 3), student-athletes should select a weight they believe they can use to complete 2 or 3 repetitions with proper technique. Student-athletes should then complete as many repetitions as possible (table 2.3).

4. Use the conversion chart to determine an estimated 1RM and record the number for future programming decisions (table 2.4).

Coaching Tips

- If a student-athlete does not have good technique during the first two sets, do not continue the assessment.
- Instruct spotters on how to spot the exercise (19).

Descriptive Data

After the estimated 1RM is determined from a 3RM-5RM, consult tables 2.5, 2.6, and 2.8 for descriptive data for the 1RM back squat.

TABLE 2.8 Descriptive Data for the 1RM Back Squat

Group/sport (sex)	Time	Reference
High school junior soccer (boys)	Mean: 231-238 lb ± 24-31 lb (105-108 kg ± 11-14 kg)	5
U16 rugby league players (boys)	Mean: 221.3 lb ± 48.3 lb (100.4 kg ± 21.9 kg)	30
U17 rugby league players (boys)	Mean: 269.4 lb ± 41.2 lb (122.2 kg ± 18.7 kg)	30
U18 rugby league players (boys)	Mean: 295.4 lb ± 34.2 lb (134.0 kg ± 15.5 kg)	30

Multiply kg by 2.2 to yield pounds.

Vertical Jump

Purpose
The vertical jump test assesses lower body power and explosiveness.

Equipment
- Masking, duct, or athletic tape
- Permanent marker
- Measuring tape
- Smooth, high wall with no obstructions
- Alternative: a commercially available system (e.g., Vertec)

Setup
1. Adhere tape to a smooth, high wall that is next to a floor that is flat and safe for student-athletes to jump on.

2. Mark the tape in half-inch (1.3 cm) increments to a height that is 40 inches (102 cm) higher than your tallest student-athlete's reach when standing and reaching vertically with their dominant hand.

Protocol
1. Instruct student-athletes on proper testing procedures.

2. The student-athlete should stand with their dominant shoulder next to the wall.

3. Reaching vertically, the student-athlete should touch the tape, and the sport coach should record the number indicated.

4. The student-athlete should use a countermovement (flexing the knees and hips as well as swinging the arms behind the body) and then jump as high as possible, only elevating the dominant hand (closest to the wall) to touch the tape at the highest point (figure 2.7).

5. The sport coach should record the highest point and then subtract the standing point. The difference will be the student-athlete's vertical jump.

6. Student-athletes should be given three attempts, and the scores should be recorded to the nearest half inch or full centimeter.

Coaching Tips
- Instruct the student-athletes on the test protocol in advance of testing, and allow them to practice.
- Be sure student-athletes have proficient jumping mechanics (countermovement and landing mechanics).
- Position the sport coach who is recording the results far enough away from the wall so that where the student's hand touches during the test is easily visible.

Descriptive Data
See tables 2.9 and 2.10 and figure 2.8 for the vertical jump descriptive data.

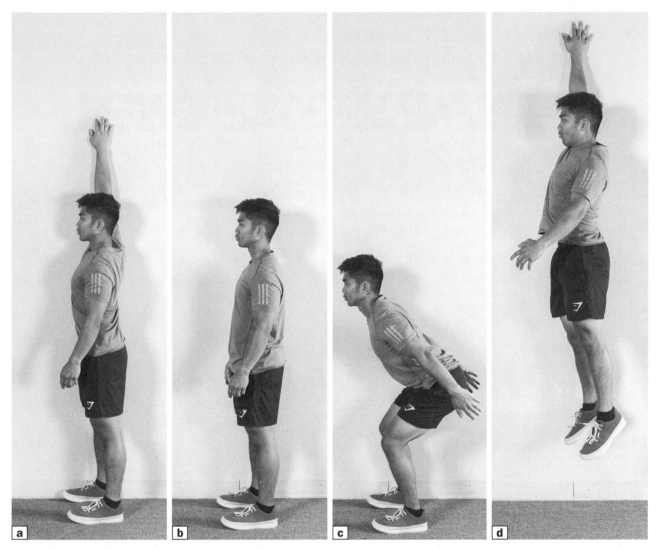

FIGURE 2.7 Vertical jump test: *(a)* measurement of standing height, *(b)* beginning position, *(c)* counter-movement, and *(d)* maximum jump (reach).

TABLE 2.9 Descriptive Data for the Vertical Jump

Group/sport (sex)	HEIGHT[a]		Reference
	in.	cm	
High school volleyball (girls)	18.5 ± 3.3	47.0 ± 8.4[b]	25
Junior national volleyball (boys)	21.5 ± 0.9	54.6 ± 2.3[b]	13
Junior national volleyball (girls)	18.0 ± 0.6	45.7 ± 1.5[b]	13
High school baseball (boys)	21.0 ± 3.1	53.3 ± 7.9[b]	28
High school soccer (girls)	15.6 ± 1.9	39.6 ± 4.8	33
National junior soccer (boys)	17.3 ± 1.9	43.9 ± 4.8	22
National junior soccer (girls)	11.2 ± 0.8	28.4 ± 2.0	22
U17 soccer (girls)	11.4 ± 0.8	29.0 ± 2.0	4
High school rugby league (boys)	16.3 ± 2.1	41.4 ± 5.3	29
U16 rugby league (boys)	18.0 ± 2.0	45.7 ± 5.1	30
U17 rugby league (boys)	19.3 ± 2.3	49.0 ± 5.8	30
U18 rugby league (boys)	19.9 ± 2.2	50.5 ± 5.6	30

[a]Mean ± standard deviation.

[b]Jumps performed with arm swing.

TABLE 2.10   Percentile Values of the Vertical Jump in High School Football Athletes (in Inches)

Percentile rank	DB	DL	LB, DE, TE	OL	QB	RB	WR
90	31.0	28.0	29.2	25.5	30.0	31.0	31.0
80	29.0	26.0	27.5	24.0	28.0	29.0	29.0
70	28.0	24.8	26.5	22.5	27.0	28.0	27.5
60	27.0	23.5	25.0	21.0	26.0	27.0	26.5
50	26.0	22.5	24.5	20.0	25.0	26.0	26.0
40	25.0	21.5	23.5	19.5	24.5	25.0	25.0
30	24.0	20.5	22.5	18.5	23.0	24.0	24.0
20	23.0	19.5	21.5	18.0	22.5	23.0	23.0
10	22.0	17.5	20.0	16.5	21.0	21.5	22.0
Mean (±SD)							
Freshman	23.7 (3.1)	20.9 (3.7)	22.7 (3.3)	19.7 (3.5)	23.9 (3.3)	24.5 (3.1)	24.4 (3.1)
Sophomore	26.1 (3.2)	22.2 (3.9)	24.4 (3.3)	20.4 (3.5)	24.9 (3.4)	26.2 (3.7)	26.0 (3.4)
Junior	27.1 (3.8)	23.4 (4.3)	25.4 (3.7)	21.2 (4.0)	26.5 (4.0)	26.7 (3.9)	26.8 (3.6)
n	1,308	847	1,196	670	625	1,161	1,455

DB = defensive back, DL = defensive lineman, LB = linebacker, DE = defensive end, TE = tight end, OL = offensive lineman, QB = quarterback, RB = running back, WR = wide receiver. SD = standard deviation, *n* = sample size.

Multiply inches by 2.54 to yield cm.

Reprinted by permission from McKay, Miramonti, Gillen, et al. (2020).

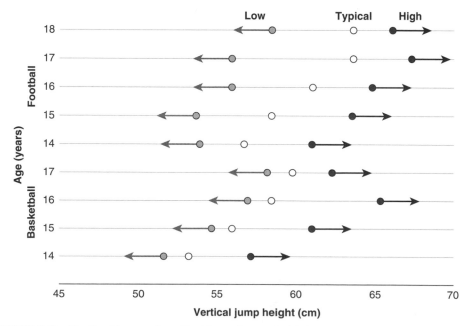

FIGURE 2.8   Vertical jump classifications for male high school American football and basketball players: high—70th percentile; typical—50th percentile; low—30th percentile (divide cm by 2.54 to yield inches).

Reprinted by permission from Fukuda (2019, p. 138).

Standing Long Jump

Purpose
The standing long jump (also called the broad jump) assesses leg power and explosiveness.

Equipment
- Flat, nonslip surface that is suitable for athletic activity
- Masking or duct tape
- Measuring tape
- Alternative: A commercial long jump mat that is properly secured to the floor

Setup
1. Place a 3-foot (0.9 m) long piece of tape on the floor for a starting point.
2. Alternative: Set up the commercial long jump mat on a flat, nonslip floor.

Protocol
1. The student-athlete should stand closely behind the tape without touching it.
2. The student-athlete should use a countermovement and then jump forward as far as possible (figure 2.9).
3. For the jump to count and be scored, the student-athlete must stick the landing and remain on their feet.
4. After a successful jump, the measurement is taken from the back of the student-athlete's rearmost heel to the starting line.
5. The best of three trials is recorded to the nearest half inch or full centimeter.

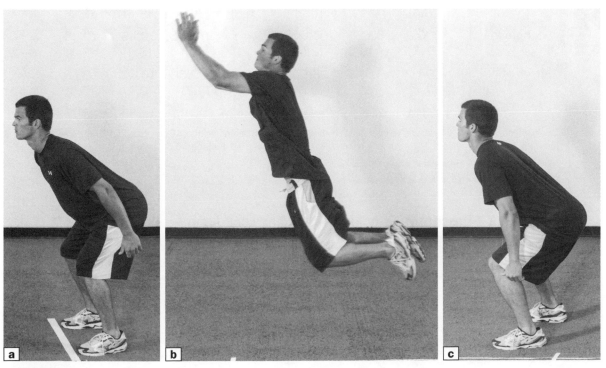

FIGURE 2.9 Standing long jump test: *(a)* beginning position, *(b)* countermovement, and *(c)* maximum jump (distance).

Coaching Tips

- Position your distance judge several feet down the jumping area from the starting line for more accurate judging.
- Be sure to teach proper form for the countermovement, jump, and landing mechanics before the test (19).

Descriptive Data

See tables 2.11 and 2.12 and figures 2.10 and 2.11 for the standing long jump descriptive data.

TABLE 2.11 Percentile Values of the Standing Long Jump in High School Football Athletes (in Inches)

Percentile rank	DB	DL	LB, DE, TE	OL	QB	RB	WR
90	112.0	104.0	108.0	94.0	109.0	111.0	112.0
80	109.0	99.0	104.0	90.0	105.0	107.0	109.0
70	107.0	95.0	101.0	88.0	102.0	105.0	106.0
60	104.0	92.0	98.0	85.0	100.0	103.0	104.0
50	102.0	90.0	96.0	83.0	98.0	100.0	102.0
40	100.0	87.0	94.0	81.0	96.0	98.0	100.0
30	98.0	85.0	91.0	78.0	93.0	96.0	97.0
20	95.0	81.0	88.8	75.0	91.0	93.0	95.0
10	91.0	75.0	85.0	70.0	87.0	89.0	90.0
Mean (±SD)							
Freshman	95.5 (8.4)	83.7 (11.2)	90.5 (8.2)	77.6 (10.8)	93.4 (7.9)	95.8 (8.4)	95.9 (8.2)
Sophomore	100.0 (7.7)	88.9 (10.2)	95.0 (8.5)	81.4 (9.2)	97.5 (8.0)	100.3 (8.4)	100.6 (7.6)
Junior	104.2 (7.6)	91.7 (10.7)	98.5 (8.8)	84.0 (8.9)	100.3 (8.7)	101.2 (9.9)	103.6 (8.0)
n	1,311	836	1,198	676	626	1,169	1,475

DB = defensive back, DL = defensive lineman, LB = linebacker, DE = defensive end, TE = tight end, OL = offensive lineman, QB = quarterback, RB = running back, WR = wide receiver. SD = standard deviation, n = sample size.

Multiply inches by 2.54 to yield cm.

Reprinted by permission from McKay, Miramonti, Gillen, et al. (2020).

TABLE 2.12 Descriptive Data for the Standing Long Jump

Category	BOYS		GIRLS	
	in.	cm	in.	cm
Excellent	79	201	65	165
Above average	73	185	61	155
Average	69	175	57	145
Below average	65	165	53	135

Reprinted by permission from Hoffman (2006, p. 58).

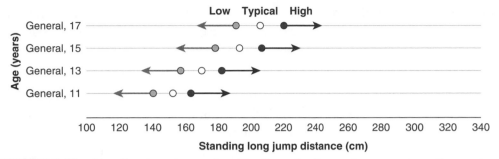

FIGURE 2.10 Standing long jump classifications for the male general youth population: high—70th percentile; typical—50th percentile; low—30th percentile (divide cm by 2.54 to yield inches).

Reprinted by permission from Fukuda (2019, p. 143).

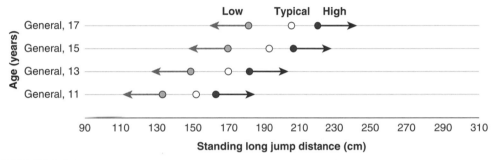

FIGURE 2.11 Standing long jump classifications for the female general youth population: high—70th percentile; typical—50th percentile; low—30th percentile (divide cm by 2.54 to yield inches).

Reprinted by permission from Fukuda (2019, p. 142).

Conclusion

Strength and conditioning professionals have become more common in high school athletics; however, many strength and conditioning practitioners at the high school level are not certified, and strength and conditioning services may not be equally administered to all athletes. As the physiological and psychological benefits of strength and conditioning become more apparent to leadership at the high school level, more scholastic programs are working to incorporate NSCA-certified staff to appropriately train athletes. Schools can implement NSCA-certified strength and conditioning professionals in an extracurricular or a curricular framework.

The purpose of this chapter was to identify and outline instructional frameworks that professionals can use to embed strength and conditioning into the curricular day and to discuss various strength and conditioning assessments that will yield data that will support the program. This chapter featured resources for the school-based strength and conditioning professional regarding prevalent school-day class frameworks, lesson plan considerations, and assessment considerations. As illustrated in this chapter, the administrative responsibilities and professional opportunities differ slightly between a curricular strength and conditioning professional and an extracurricular strength and conditioning professional; however, including curricular strength and conditioning professionals in the curriculum offers many benefits, including the following:

- Maximize student exposure to strength and conditioning
- Increase training consistency and frequency, especially for in-season athletes
- Physical education paradigm shift from general physical activity to data-based performance measurables for all students
- Opportunity for vertical curriculum alignment in K-12 HPE to support a long-term athletic development model
- Opportunity to become better ingrained into school culture
- Obtain professional support and development from the school district
- Opportunity to become a vital member of the HPE faculty
- Better working hours and job security

3

Strength and Conditioning–Related Resources for Teachers and Professionals

Patrick Mediate, MEd, CSCS,*D
Mike Nitka, MS, CSCS,*D, RSCC*E, FNSCA*E

This chapter presents high school teachers and strength and conditioning professionals with resources from experts in the field that will increase the quality of their programs safely and effectively.

The information provided will give insight regarding the design and transition of new and existing facilities through thoughtful planning. The implementation of the NSCA's standards and guidelines along with proper placement of equipment and use of technology are highlighted in understandable language for all experience levels.

Information Sources and Resources

The understanding of policy and procedural guidelines makes for safe and effective decisions in physical education (PE) and athletic programs. Sources for effective communication and technology platforms along with resistance training and equipment providers allow for thoughtful purchases. Through numerous publications and position statements, NSCA resources for standards and guidelines are provided for assistance in following best practices when designing and maintaining a facility.

Risks and liability concerns that are associated with large-group training can be lessened through precautions that protect teachers and strength and conditioning professionals from events that occur. A proactive review of important safety and exit strategies for the facility can keep everyone safe.

To prevent injuries, it may be helpful to design a unit plan to address maintenance guidelines for substitute teachers and off-campus staff. These tools help establish the foundation for a safe and effective strength and conditioning program for years to come.

Organizations

Organizations available to the teacher and the strength and conditioning professional are an important part of professional growth. They allow the professional to keep abreast of current trends and research in the field. It is important to not only read the discipline's literature but also to make the effort to attend the conferences and clinics that these organizations provide. Such organizations offer many opportunities for learning, whether through presentations or with colleagues after hours. Here are a few notable organizations to explore:

- NSCA: www.nsca.com
- SHAPE America: www.shapeamerica.org
- American College of Sports Medicine: www.acsm.org
- National Athletic Trainers Association: www.nata.org
- USA Powerlifting: www.usapowerlifting.com
- USA Weightlifting: www.teamusa.org/USA-Weightlifting

Books

Numerous books in the field of strength and conditioning exist for study and self-improvement, and notable researchers and practitioners have made great efforts to share their experiences and philosophies. It is advisable to take advantage of the NSCA's recommendations applicable to the teacher and strength and conditioning professional, such as *Essentials of Strength Training and Conditioning* (3), *Exercise Technique Manual for Resistance Training* (6), *Weight Training: Steps to Success* (1), and *Designing Resistance Training Programs* (2). Books are peer reviewed and edited. The only caveat with depending solely on books is that unlike articles and research in journals and newsletters put out by the organizations mentioned in this chapter, the most current information may have already been improved upon by the time the book goes to print.

Businesses

Various businesses dedicated to the field of strength and conditioning offer products that give the strength and conditioning professional many choices of equipment to fill their needs in the weight room. Websites, catalogs, and expert advice from professionals well versed in products can help outfit fitness centers with the proper equipment. Some companies produce their own equipment, and others offer selections from many. Researching options available to compare cost and quality is necessary to acquire the best choices.

Community Services

YMCA, YWCA, Boys and Girls Clubs of America, religious groups, municipal recreation centers, and after-school intramurals are available community services familiar to student-athletes, who may have grown up playing pickup and league games at local fields and courts through the various institutions in town. These outlets are based on kids playing games for fun. This concept of playing for enjoyment is the basis for all sport yet is not always apparent with secondary school team sport coaches. Although the equipment and facilities at these venues may be different than what is at school, kids know their purpose. The recreational facilities at these sites may be well funded but not necessarily administered or supervised by individuals as qualified as the high school PE teacher and strength and conditioning professional. Caution student-athletes against overtraining at the local gym. Advice from well-meaning local personal trainers may not reflect the school's training philosophy and could result in an overuse injury.

Descriptions, Uses, and Guidelines for Purchasing Common Exercise Equipment

This section outlines best practices on obtaining the proper equipment desired by staff for an effective program. The relationships established with vendors and experts in the field can enable good decisions regarding quality equipment at a practical cost that serves the needs of the program.

Successful student-athletes are training in traditional weight rooms, using basic equipment. Before the advent of large commercial facilities, resistance training was often performed in local gyms, garages, and basements.

Purchasing athletic equipment is generally done through the school's athletic and PE budgets a year in advance. Choose wisely and plan ahead, because the funds often have to be shared with other department staff. Demonstrate how specific equipment will benefit the entire department in some way.

If funding allows for the design of a new facility, it will be necessary to research basic equipment that most participants will use regularly. Design the current resistance training program according to the available equipment. As a strength and conditioning program evolves and student-athletes begin exhibiting gains, a more efficient weight room will help move their sport performance to a higher level. New equipment can pique interest and be a great motivator if the necessities are present. What works for a school's program may be different from the gym downtown.

Athletic directors (ADs), department heads, athletic trainers, and head coaches can use purchase order requests for equipment needs. Staff can request catalogs and communicate with equipment manufacturers for equipment options and cost. Companies that specialize in weight rooms and fitness centers have the expertise to offer recommendations for what equipment to purchase for any budget. Doing business with local companies offers the benefit of being able to see and test future purchases before they are ordered. Take a few assistants and student-athletes along to test and comment. Staying local helps foster long-lasting relationships for future purchases with trusted people. Their equipment has to be good, but their service must be better.

Resistance Training Machines

Resistance training machines can be found with individual stations or an all-in-one combined universal design. Purchases depend on facility space, layout, and training philosophy. Machines come in the form of cable or pulley, plate loaded, hydraulic piston, air compression, cam devices, and band assisted (see figure 3.1).

Machines can be an integral and nonthreatening part of the facility for untrained and inexperienced student-athletes and for secondary movement training modalities. They can also be used by the athletic training staff for rehabilitation purposes. Input from athletic trainers can be instrumental when selecting equipment for the facility. These machines are great for individual exercise and circuit training. Pulleys used for lat pulls and seated rows can augment free-weight workouts. However, pulling movements can be easily performed with bands, while back and reverse hyperextensions need only a partner or inflatable gym ball to be effective.

If the goal of a workout is to train individual muscles, a machine will do the job. Its role in athletics is limited, however. The individual station on a typical plate-loaded machine is designed to isolate a muscle in a seated position. This body position is not a functional way to train athletic movements. Machines isolate muscles, whereas free-weight movement patterns integrate them in a more balanced way. Isolating a muscle can also create an imbalance, with opposing groups leading to performance injuries.

The reality is that there is no machine specific to each individual. These machines are often designed for the general public to perform in a seated position. Because most sports are not played sitting down, the carryover to sport applications is limited when using machines. Machine-based circuit training can, however, lend itself well to both the PE classroom and athletics.

Machines must be commercial grade. Be wary of accepting home equipment from private-sector donors. The expense of moving such equipment and the upkeep it will need may not be worth the time and effort. Breakdowns equal

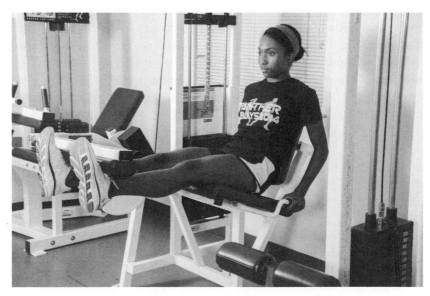

FIGURE 3.1 Example of a selectorized resistance training machine.

workout time lost. As such, the school system should consider purchasing a service contract from the equipment supplier. The suppliers are hired by the school district and are prepared to service and replace parts on a regular basis. Machines of any type are expensive. Look carefully at the budget and decide what can be better served by free weights.

Free Weights and Related Equipment

Purchasing free weights can be a simple task. Free-weight training and competition sets are common. Long bars range from 6 to 7 feet (1.8-2.1 m) with ball bearing sleeves and collars or locks that secure the plates during the exercise. They are designed to allow for efficient rotation of the bar, especially during Olympic lifts.

The bars used for resistance training come in a variety of lengths and configurations depending on their application (see figure 3.2a). Olympic, trap, hex, safety squat, close grip bench, EZ-curl (see figure 3.2b), Swiss, cambered, and fat bars are often useful for movement variations. Always purchase quality bars for smooth action, durability, and collars/locks that will withstand constant floor contact and not fall off.

Rubber bumper plates or polyurethane materials can be used with different results and bounce; rubber will bounce more from a drop, whereas the composite material will land with less movement (see figure 3.3). Determine if the facility has an area to drop the weights after an Olympic clean or snatch.

Individual free-weight plates start at 2.5 pounds (1.1 kg) and usually increase to 45 pounds (20 kg). This range in weight addresses most PE classes and sport team needs.

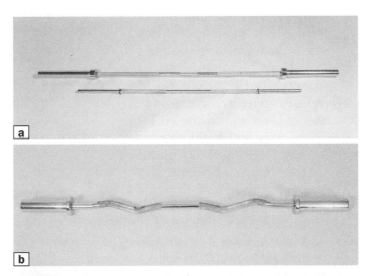

FIGURE 3.2   Examples of bars used for resistance training: *(a)* Olympic (top) and standard (bottom) bars and *(b)* EZ-curl bar.

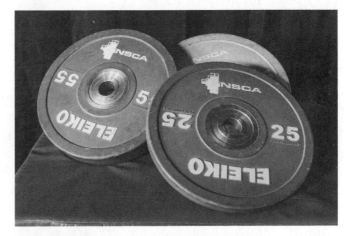

FIGURE 3.3   Example of bumper plates.

The Olympic lifts and their variations serve as the basis for most resistance training programs. Typically, a designated area such as a wooden platform, a rubber mat, or an inlaid floor outlines the plate location for Olympic lifting (see figure 3.4).

Weighted Implements

Weighted implements that complement bar work come in a variety of forms. Dumbbells, medicine balls, kettlebells, sandbags, weighted vests, ropes, chains, individual plates, and landmines are often used for variations in a resistance training program. These types of unconventional weighted equipment are necessary tools for a well-rounded PE curriculum and athletic program. Keeping the workout interesting, challenging, and fresh is a good way to pique interest and improve participation. These implements do not rely on a fixed axis or a bar. Many high school athletes use these weighted implements in combination with barbells and dumbbells to perform complex movements (see figure 3.5).

Conditioning Equipment

Conditioning equipment comes in many forms and allows the strength and conditioning professional to effectively teach to different learning styles and exercise regimens. Dot drill mats, jump ropes, resistance bands, ladders, minihurdles, heavy ropes, plyometric jump boxes, sleds and towing apparatus for pushing and pulling, oversized tires, strong man hammers,

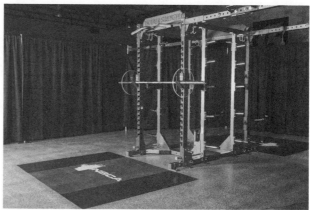

FIGURE 3.4   Example of an Olympic platform in front of a power rack.

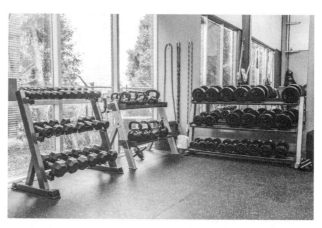

FIGURE 3.5   Examples of kettlebells and various types of dumbbells.

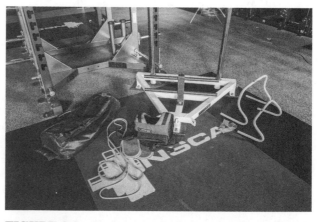

FIGURE 3.6   Examples of various conditioning equipment.

sandbags, abdominal or core training equipment, parachutes, and balance boards could have a big impact on programming (see figure 3.6).

Bodyweight exercise equipment is also an important element for all gyms. Here are a few basic stations that foster competition and improve strength.

1. Pull-up station
2. Dip station (see figure 3.7)
3. Back hyperextension station
4. Reverse hyperextension station

The inclusion of jumping and the use of plyometric boxes are an important part of many complex training programs. The composition of the plyometric box is an important factor to consider (see figure 3.8). Wooden boxes are durable and maintain a stable base but can increase the risk of injury because they provide a less forgiving surface. In contrast, materials such as foam and plastic are lighter and allow for a softer landing but are less stable and lend to students piling them higher. High school students' competitive instincts lead to a different type of injury: falling from high places!

Aerobic Machines

Treadmills, ellipticals, stair climbers, stationary bikes (see figure 3.9), rowing machines, and an array of other apparatus that raise heart rate have a large footprint. Aerobic machines enable students to warm up or provide an adaptive variation for students with limitations due to injury or condition. Despite their value, aerobic machines require a routine maintenance schedule and close monitoring to ensure target heart rates and cardio goals are being met.

The use of aerobic machines offers a limited role in sport applications, where they are primarily used for warm-up, cooldown, or testing. While these pieces are usually expensive, they do serve a role in classroom settings, where student-athletes can monitor their progress with instant feedback on heart rate, distance traveled, and intensity. High schools often desire to mimic big gym facilities designed for the general public. The

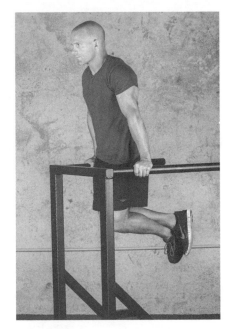

FIGURE 3.7 Example of a bodyweight exercise station.

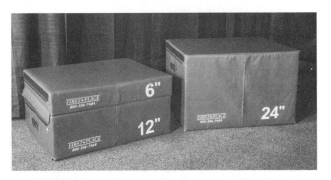

FIGURE 3.8 Examples of various heights of plyometric boxes.

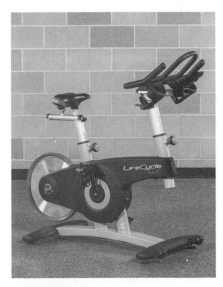

FIGURE 3.9 Example of an aerobic machine.

addition of too many large-footprint aerobic machines such as treadmills and ellipticals may not be necessary if most sport teams' main aerobic activity is field based. PE classes often use the aerobic section of a fitness facility more than a team.

Standards and Guidelines

Lawsuits against resistance training instructors and strength and conditioning professionals usually involve injuries caused by inappropriate supervision in one or more of the following areas (8, 9):

- Failure to meet the accepted professional standards in the field
- Failure to take the medical history of participants before allowing them to participate in a strength and conditioning program
- Failure to wear the proper footwear and clothing while training
- Failure to warn the participants of inherent risks of participation
- Failure to calculate the proper percentage of resistance used
- Failure to inspect and evaluate using risk management protocols
- Failure to maintain the facility and its equipment
- Failure to hire an adequate number of qualified staff members
- Failure to actively supervise

Being in charge of, or assisting with, a strength and conditioning program for high school PE teachers and sport coaches involves having qualified staff. A qualified staff member should possess competencies in one or all of the following: exercise science, administration, management, teaching, and coaching.

Most high school fitness centers and weight rooms are used by PE classes, sport teams, and staff. The safety and success of all those involved is a big responsibility and involves several decisions, such as which staff member will have the final say on who uses the facility before or after school. It is important to have a way of knowing when a class or team will be there. Have a schedule printed out and posted or have an electronic copy that can be shared with all involved. Without a schedule anybody with a key to the weight room can bring a class or team in and train, posing threats of overcrowding and scheduling conflicts.

In addition to traditional keys, some schools issue a faculty scan card to keep a record of who was in last to aid with security. Keys or cards should only be given out to those teachers and strength and conditioning professionals who use the room daily. A sport coach from outside the building may be expected to return their key to the AD when their season is over to prevent unwanted personal use. Usage of the facility should be addressed in the policies and procedures manual.

PE teachers, strength and conditioning professionals, and sport coaches must be aware of local, state, and national laws and regulations. It is challenging and requires substantial experience and expertise to effectively address all regulations, but it is necessary to prevent potential injury and related claims and lawsuits. Involve the risk management team to assist with developing safety guidelines.

Budgets, equipment, facilities, and qualified staff are often limited or lacking in various school systems. In school districts where these issues are identified, an imbalance exists between the student-athlete's expectation of a safe and effective program and the school's ability to provide it. This may lead to future risk management issues and should be addressed. It is important for teachers, strength and conditioning professionals, and administrators to understand that the standard of care for the student-athlete is a shared duty between the school and the teacher or strength and conditioning professional.

NSCA *Strength and Conditioning Professional Standards and Guidelines* (9) (see the appendix; page 345) reflects the profession's best practices and identifies nine common areas of liability exposure. This document will help a high school PE teacher, strength and conditioning professional, sport coach, principal, AD, and school board develop a policies and procedures manual specific to their school's needs. The original document has been updated several times, which ultimately improved the standard of care offered. It is hoped that PE teachers, sport coaches, and strength and conditioning professionals will mutually benefit and enhance the quality of instruction provided to their programs.

The areas of liability concern that teachers and strength and conditioning professionals are responsible for include the following (9):

1. Preparticipation screening and clearance
2. Personnel qualifications
3. Program supervision and instruction
4. Facility and equipment setup, inspection, maintenance, repair, and signage
5. Emergency planning and response
6. Records and record keeping
7. Equal opportunity and access
8. Participation in strength and conditioning activities by children
9. Supplements, ergogenic aids, and drugs

A committee from the NSCA was tasked to review and modify those areas of liability concern where needed to create an evaluation tool that could be used by all high school PE teachers and strength and conditioning professionals responsible for operating a safe facility. The end product was free downloadable criteria called the NSCA Strength of America Award (see www.nsca.com/membership/awards/special-recognition/strength-of-america-award). This project was put in place to help high school PE teachers and strength and conditioning professionals evaluate their program and compare it to the NSCA standards and guidelines that identify areas of liability concern. While weight room management style will determine the method of delivery, the Strength of America Award will assist staff in monitoring operational details that are part of any management style.

A responsibility that all teachers and strength and conditioning professionals have is to critique their programs regularly. The Strength of America committee has developed a checklist to evaluate and identify excellence in high school strength and conditioning programs. It uses the following criteria:

- Supervision: 35 possible points
- Education: 15 possible points
- Program: 22 possible points
- Facility: 33 possible points

A minimum of 90 points is required to be recognized for the award. While it may be a humbling experience for teachers and strength and conditioning professionals to critique their own program, the great ones are constantly looking for ways to improve.

Another high school strength and conditioning program evaluation tool from the NSCA is called Why Your High School Needs a Qualified Strength and Conditioning Professional (7). This free packet can be downloaded and contains a site evaluation worksheet that references the NSCA standards and guidelines document targeted at ADs and administrators to help them evaluate their program and create awareness of performance and liability concerns. Both the Strength of America Award and the NSCA's program evaluation tool have been successful in identifying weaknesses and strengths in high school strength and conditioning programs across the country.

Weight Room Facility

With student-athlete safety and welfare a priority, developing a policy and procedures manual provides a blueprint for implementing safe and effective programs and services. Policies are the facility's rules and regulations that reflect the goals and objectives of the program. Procedures describe how policies are met and carried out by every teacher, sport coach, and staff member using the weight room. It is necessary to examine program goals and objectives with administrators and staff. Additionally, specific policies and procedures should include elements that protect the program and its employees from a risk of litigation; issues such as guidelines for supervision and instruction, facility administration, and emergency action planning and response should be included. The goal of this section is to identify areas of risk exposure and means of increasing safety, as well as to guide the strength and conditioning professional in providing and enhancing the quality of services and programs (8). When developing a manual, the following questions may be a helpful guide.

- What are the current policies and procedures for operating the weight room?
- Are the current policies and procedures based on current best practices?
- Did administrators review and approve them?
- Do all the staff members understand and follow the policy and procedure manual?
- Are the policies and procedures in compliance with the NSCA standards and guidelines (9) that are being used in the profession?
- When was the last time the policies and procedures manual was reviewed and updated by the staff and approved and accepted by the administration?

If no such policies and procedures manual exists, now may be the time to develop one. It is a wise investment of time to put the policies and procedures down on paper so that when administrators, parent groups, sport coaches, student-athletes, and others ask why things are done a certain way, they can refer to the policies and procedures manual.

Using the nine areas of liability concern, explain to all staff that a policies and procedures manual will show others what and how the performance culture will be developed and improved by clarifying various progression goals for each class and team that would participate in the strength and conditioning program. When all who use the weight room understand the daily operational policies and procedures of a strength and conditioning program, it will help direct all involved to achieve the program's goals and objectives.

So how does a PE teacher or strength and conditioning professional begin to develop a policies and procedures manual? Begin by writing the strength and conditioning mission statement.

Classes or sport coaches should never come into the weight room and follow a non-evidence-based training program. There may be discussions and debates about programming, but the teacher or strength and conditioning professional should explain what the literature says will work best for the high school population. Sharing that expertise will inform all staff and sport coaches that the profession of strength and conditioning, and the operation of a high school weight room, have standards and guidelines to follow, and it will make the next step of writing a weight room mission statement a bit easier.

A weight room mission statement should be written based on the accepted standards and guidelines. When drafting this mission statement, invite all who will be affected by its adoption to provide input because they may offer a perspective that had not been discussed earlier.

A well-written mission statement provides the PE teacher, strength and conditioning professional, and all student-athletes and staff using the facility with direction and focus. The NSCA provides guidelines for drafting a mission statement (8):

- Short and sharply focused
- Clear and easy to understand
- Defines why the group exists
- Does not prescribe a means
- Broad in scope
- Provides direction for upholding a code of ethics
- Addresses and matches the school's scope of practice
- Inspires commitment

Using the criteria above, a sample mission statement could read like this: *To provide all student-athletes the opportunity by which they can train year-round under the supervision of a qualified professional, following an age-appropriate, evidenced-based program throughout their high school career in a safe and clean environment that may contribute to minimizing serious injury during training and competition. The ultimate goal of our program will be to improve athletic performance.*

Liability Concepts and Guidelines

Depending on school system policies, strength and conditioning professionals should take time to review their personal insurance plan and its coverage in a high school weight room setting. Most schools have full coverage for liability while school is in session or coaching is in season. If not, strength and conditioning professionals must be proactive to protect themselves by contacting their insurance agent about what the job entails. ADs and human resource staff can assist with the coverage provided by the school system. Strength and conditioning professionals should ask their school's HR staff the following questions to understand the insurance coverage:

1. What will the school district's policy cover if there is an injury to students or myself during my PE class?
2. Do I need separate contracts for before- and after-school strength and conditioning sessions?
3. Am I covered when using all inside facilities (e.g., the various gyms, swimming pool, hallways, stairwells)?
4. Am I covered when using all outdoor facilities on campus?
5. Am I covered when taking student-athletes to or meeting them at off-campus facilities during contests or camps?

Organizations such as the NSCA offer coverage for their certified members to help cover some of these issues.

Many school districts are asking the following question during the interview process: "Are you qualified to be a strength and conditioning coach?" In many states sport coaches must first take and pass a rules test before they are allowed to coach a sport, yet there is no organization that says a PE teacher, strength and conditioning professional, or sport coach must know and follow certain rules before they can teach or coach in the weight room.

These rules are referred to as either standards or guidelines. A standard is a rule that must be followed each day in the weight room, and a guideline is a measurement that should identify an area in the program that could be improved on in the near future. Keep a record detailing how staff is working to improve a weakness if approached by the administration or risk management team.

Nine areas of liability concern have been identified and are being used by the legal system to hold strength and conditioning professionals accountable for their actions. In each of the nine areas of liability concern, legal teams refer to the standard or guideline subcategories. These are examined by lawyers when a PE teacher, strength and conditioning professional, or sport coach was accused of negligence when supervising a student-athlete on the day of an incident. The NSCA *Strength and Conditioning Professional Standards and Guidelines* document has been modified for this chapter for a high school PE teacher, sport coach, or strength and conditioning professional (9).

Area of Liability Concern 1: Preparticipation Screening and Clearance

- Modified Standard 1.1: Student-athletes are not allowed to participate until they have a current physical on file.
- Modified Guideline 1.1: Identify who in the school or on staff is responsible for making sure participants have a physical on file before they participate. (The school health office most often is responsible for checking.)

Area of Liability Concern 2: Personnel Qualifications

- Modified Guideline 2.1: The people designing programs and supervising the student-athletes should have a BS in one or more of the scientific foundations.
- Modified Guideline 2.2: Each practitioner must have and maintain professional certifications such as first aid and CPR with continuing education requirements.
- Modified Guideline 2.3: The teaching and coaching staff should be assigned to supervise only areas in which they have expertise.

Area of Liability Concern 3: Qualified Program Supervision and Instruction

"Qualified" has been defined by the NSCA as being certified by the NSCA or another accredited agency to do the job. This qualified person will have and maintain certifications in standard first aid, CPR, and AED. A qualified strength and conditioning professional should have a degree in one of the scientific foundations, have several years of experience in the practical application for the age group with whom they plan to work, and be aware of and well versed on proper equipment layout and spacing for safe and effective training.

- Modified Standard 3.1: At least one qualified supervisor (BS in one of the scientific foundations and a Certified Strength and Conditioning Specialist) must be in the weight room when student-athletes are present.
- Modified Standard 3.2: The supervisors should be in-serviced on how to spot the various exercises, and records of the last in-service should be readily available.
- Modified Guideline 3.1a: The administration should limit class or team size in the facility to a ratio of one student-athlete per 100 square feet.
- Modified Guideline 3.1b: The facility should be staffed with one qualified teacher or strength and conditioning professional per 15 high school student-athletes during class and before and after school.
- Modified Guideline 3.1c: The room should be adequately equipped so that no more than three student-athletes are at each training station.

Area of Liability Concern 4: Facility and Equipment Setup, Inspection, Maintenance, Repair, and Signage

- Modified Standard 4.1: Assembly records should be kept on all pieces of equipment.
- Modified Standard 4.2: Maintenance records should be kept on all pieces of equipment.
- Modified Standard 4.3: Inspection records should be kept on all pieces of equipment.
- Modified Standard 4.4a: If a piece of equipment is broken, a "Do not use" sign should be placed on it for all to see.
- Modified Standard 4.4b: If an accident occurred on a piece of equipment, a "Do not use" sign should be placed on it until an administrator inspects it and the technician responsible for repairs approves its return to use.
- Modified Guideline 4.1: Identify who designed the facility's floor plan regarding equipment placement.
- Modified Guideline 4.2: Ensure that all teachers, sport coaches, and strength and conditioning professionals read the manuals on how to use each piece of equipment before bringing in a class or team.
- Modified Guideline 4.3: Give an in-service to all student-athletes and coaches on how to disinfect the equipment and document the day this in-service was held.

Area of Liability Concern 5: Emergency Planning and Response

- Modified Standard 5.1: Identify who is responsible for seeing that all staff are currently trained and certified in first aid and CPR.
- Modified Standard 5.2: Ensure that a written emergency response plan has been approved by the administration and is posted at several strategic areas within the weight room.
- Modified Guideline 5.1: Components of this plan must include access to a doctor or medical facility and appropriate, necessary, on-site, and accessible emergency care equipment.

Area of Liability Concern 6: Records and Record Keeping
- Modified Guideline 6.1: Keep various operational records, operating manuals, warranties, cleaning maintenance, and repair schedules.

Area of Liability Concern 7: Equal Opportunity and Access
- Modified Standard 7.1: Staff must know and follow the laws on equal opportunity access and non-discrimination.
- Modified Guideline 7.1: A procedure must be in place to report discriminatory violations to the administration.

Area of Liability Concern 8: Participation in Strength and Conditioning Activities by Children
- Modified Guideline 8.1: Children under 7 should not be permitted to engage in strength and conditioning activities designed for adults.
- Modified Guideline 8.2: A policy should be in place defining what modified strength and conditioning activities children between 7 and 14 may participate in.
- Modified Guideline 8.3: A policy should be in place allowing children 14 and older to participate in strength and conditioning activities that are designed for adults with acceptable progressions.

Areas of Liability Concern 9: Supplements, Ergogenic Aids, and Drug Use
- Modified Standard 9.1: Be aware of the school rules that discuss bringing and using supplements to school and be aware of what supplements individual state athletic associations allow student-athletes to use.

These nine areas of liability concern with each standard and guideline may be unfamiliar to many, but prosecuting attorneys know these nine areas well and will not take ignorance as an excuse. It is critical to be aware of and follow the rules.

Facility Design

While it may be a great opportunity to be a part of and assist in building a new weight room from the ground up, most high school weight rooms are redesigned to fit into preexisting spaces (see figure 3.10).

The following suggestions provide guidance on how to build a new facility or retrofit an existing one with the space and equipment that fits the program's current and future needs.

Strength and conditioning professionals may be con-

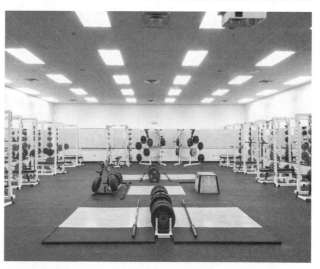

FIGURE 3.10 Example of the layout of a high school weight room.

sulted and asked to share ideas for the new facility and should be prepared to answer the following questions:

- How many student-athletes will be using the facility hourly, daily, and seasonally?
- What are the training goals for the teachers, student-athletes, sport coaches, strength and conditioning professionals, and administration?
- What will the training experience of the student-athletes be?
- Who will manage the scheduling of the facility?
- What equipment will need to be repaired, modified, or purchased to fit the anticipated needs?

Study future enrollment projections and stress to the committee that the group should allow enough space for the program to grow into the future. Not having enough space will have a large impact on the training environment and scheduling (4).

Communities often fund the building of new schools if they include a multipurpose recreation facility that can be used by student-athletes during the day and shared by the community during the evenings. From concept to completion, new facilities take a long time and a lot of planning. Members of a committee usually consist of the architect, the winning contractor, equipment companies, lawyers, the strength and conditioning professional, and other key decision makers. A model that has been used in new facility design includes the following four phases (4):

1. Predesign
    a. Conduct a needs analysis.
    b. Conduct a feasibility study.
    c. Create the master plan.
    d. Hire the architect.
2. Design
    a. Finalize the design committee.
    b. Create the blueprint.
3. Construction
    a. This includes the time from breaking ground to opening the doors.
    b. Lawyers are needed here to keep the project on track.
4. Preoperation
    a. Finish the interior decorations.
    b. Identify what certifications are acceptable to the district administration and hire a qualified staff.
    c. Have a policies and procedures manual for the new staff.

More realistically, strength and conditioning professionals will be asked to update the strength and conditioning program, which may call for a modification of the existing space. Whether it is the strength and conditioning professional's first day or 43rd year on the job, they are reviewing the seemingly never-ending process of modifying their current facility by considering if they can tear down walls or move racks and benches for a more efficient and safer flow of traffic throughout the room.

Remember the line from the movie *Field of Dreams*, "If you build it, they will come"? Improving facilities will attract the attention of more sport coaches, who will begin to request and use the strength and conditioning professional's services. As more students and teams want to train with the strength and conditioning professional, these daily numbers can quickly outgrow the current facility.

Many details need careful attention before the project begins. The more research the strength and conditioning professional and the committee can do, the fewer delays will be experienced. It is important to have qualified and knowledgeable practitioners involved in the process from beginning to end. Too many voices, however, may slow progress. Input from the individuals using the facility the most and working in it will be an important step in the final outcome that addresses the program's goals.

Prior to arranging the equipment in a strength and conditioning facility, the type of facility desired for a new or preexisting site must be considered. Both options require serious planning before any equipment can be purchased. Special attention needs to be paid to the location of the site and easy access for the delivery of equipment and for supervision, environmental factors, mechanicals, and the physical dimensions of the site. Important factors are described in the following section (4).

- *Location:* In many schools the classrooms were originally designed to only hold desks and students. If repurposing a classroom, make sure that it is on the ground floor or has a load-bearing capability of at least 100 pounds per square foot. Ask the custodial staff who might have that information. If possible, the new weight room should be as far away as possible from offices or classrooms because both students and staff in these areas may be distracted by the hourly flow of student-athlete traffic coming to the weight room and going back to the locker room.

- *Supervision location:* Where will the main desk be placed? Walk through the room and select a spot that has as clear a sight line as possible of the entire weight room. If finding that spot is difficult, strategically place mirrors on the wall to assist supervision of the entire room with a few glances. Ideally, this main desk or supervisor's spot would also be used for student-athletes to check in and pick up their program. This spot should be the heart of the weight room where all the assorted necessities to run the weight room can be found. Strength and conditioning professionals should not use this area for staff meetings to discuss practice planning while the class or team is training unsupervised. After an incident, a lawyer will ask, "Where were you when the incident happened, and what were you doing?"

- *ADA access:* The person in charge of the building and grounds can find the Americans with Disabilities Act (ADA) compliance guidelines, which will assist in the design of the facility. Students with special needs in the school district would benefit by having an opportunity to train with the strength and conditioning professional. If students with special needs are in wheelchairs or riding scooters, are the aisles wide enough for them to easily maneuver around the room? Giving these students this option allows them to feel included, and their parents will support the program.

- *Double doors:* Many renovation projects will not add the double door to their room design because of the additional expense. Explain to administrators that double doors will not require equipment to be disassembled and reassembled in order for it to fit through the doors. Also educate the administrative team that double doors are appreciated by the fire department when there is an emergency, and the double doors will allow EMTs to enter and exit with their equipment more easily. Fight hard to get at least one double door in your room.

- *Ceiling height:* Ceiling height should be able to accommodate all jumping activities safely inside the weight room. The recommended ceiling height of 12 to 14 feet (3.7-4.3 m) should allow this. If the current ceiling is low, there may be room above the existing drop ceiling. Take a look above and see if some of that space can be reclaimed by removing the tiles. Bring in an administrator when the basketball team is performing overhead barbell presses and show them that ceiling tiles may be broken in the near future. Ask them for permission to remove some tiles over the jumping or pressing areas.

- *Flooring:* If an abandoned classroom is being converted to a weight room, the floor will probably be tile. Most renovations will place rubber flooring over the existing tile. Rubber flooring comes in various thicknesses, so the thickness of the flooring should depend on what type of exercises will be performed off of the floor. On the plus side, rubber floors are easy to sweep, vacuum, and mop when needed; a negative is that they have a strong rubber smell. Another increasingly popular option is indoor turf. When space is available, sections of turf (10-20 yds [9-18 m]) are installed in the weight room where speed and agility drills can be performed. The last floor covering option is antifungal carpeting. Machines can be placed on top of the carpeting or in a separate area where student-athletes will sit on the carpeting and take a test, watch an instructional video, or work on improving their flexibility. A bit of goodwill can be earned if the cheerleaders, dance team, or other groups are allowed to use the turf or carpeted areas when classes or teams are not training.

- *Lighting:* Many weight rooms are placed in the basement of the school, and some of the basement rooms will have no windows, resulting in a dungeon-like space. Unfortunately, lighting selection is costly but critical for waking up students in early-morning classes. It is suggested that there be a reading of between 50 and 100 lumens measured at the floor. Visit the science department and ask to borrow a light meter or ask a science teacher if their class would like to visit the weight room and take sample readings for an experiment.

- *Temperature:* The temperature will vary between 68 and 78 degrees Fahrenheit (20-26 °C). This range depends on the time of year. Many suggest that 72 degrees Fahrenheit (22 °C) is optimal. A room that is too hot or too cold may affect training in a negative way. Classes and teams will speak up if they would like it warmer or colder.

- *Relative humidity:* This should not exceed 60 percent. Monitoring the humidity will help prevent bacterial growth, avoid the spread of infections and disease, and minimize the rusting of the equipment.

- *Circulation:* The air in a weight room should be exchanged anywhere from 8 to 12 times per hour, which will help prevent odors caused by stagnant air. The custodial staff may be able to identify how many air exchanges the room has per hour by looking at their computer program. If the HVAC system does not currently meet the recommended number of air exchanges, large fans can assist with circulating the air in the room. When necessary, have 2 to 4 fans per every 1,200 square feet of the room to meet the suggested number of air exchanges per hour.

• *Sound system:* Consider meeting with the chairpeople of the music and theater departments when purchasing a sound system; they have probably worked with more sound systems, so asking for their input may save some time and result in a lead on where to purchase this equipment. A quality sound system may be conducive to improving the training environment. While considered non-essential by some staff, music may help motivate student-athletes. The sound should be less than 90 decibels so the student-athletes can hear instruction and cues throughout the room without the strength and conditioning professional having to yell. Ask the science department if they can lend one of their sound meters or would like to visit the weight room and perform an experiment on noise.

• *Electrical service:* Ask the school electrician to explain the existing code for outlet spacing along the ceiling or floor. Have a floor plan ready showing where machines, sound systems, video monitors, and other items requiring electricity will be located. The electrician will identify where the 110-volt outlets should be placed and where the 220-volt outlets should be placed. Ground fault circuits are an additional expense but will be necessary to ensure safety of the student-athletes and protect the machines in case of a lightning strike.

• *Mirrors:* Mirrors in a weight room have always been a topic of debate. They can be placed strategically to create an illusion of additional space, or they can be used as a coaching tool that provides visual feedback when placed at the right height. To avoid broken mirrors, place them at least 6 inches (15 cm) away from dumbbell racks or other equipment and at least 20 inches (51 cm) off the floor.

• *Water:* Drinking fountains or water bottle fillers should be placed away from the free-weight training area and should not interrupt the traffic flow of a class or team. Originally placed outside a classroom in the hall, they are now often fitted inside the weight room next to the entrance where student-athletes can be monitored.

• *Landline phone placement:* Even though most people will have a cell phone, a reliable landline phone mounted on the wall where it is ADA accessible and where all student-athletes and staff will have access to it is still a good idea as long as everybody has been shown how to get the school operator or an outside line when needed.

• *Storage space:* Storage space is often included in the initial design plan but is then eliminated as unexpected expansion costs become an issue and something has to be cut to stay on budget. Ask the architect to find other areas to cut costs in an effort to keep a reasonable amount of storage space.

• *Security cameras:* Cameras have become more common in weight rooms because they are a good way to help monitor activity during a class or training session. Security video has been used to answer questions about injury claims, bullying, damage, and misuse of equipment. As a courtesy, make sure that the student-athletes and staff are notified with posted signs that cameras are monitoring the facility 24-7 (4).

Facility Layout and Equipment Spacing

The process of designing a facility layout sometimes involves trying to get the proverbial 10 pounds of stuff into a 5-pound bag. Organize the floor plan by drawing a square or rectangle and sketching in where the doors and windows are. Next, identify the location of the supervisor's desk. Then find a designated warm-up space. Now add all the cardio equipment. Where will the free weights be placed? Remember to follow the guideline of having at least 3 to 4 feet (0.9-1.2 m) between equipment (see figure 3.11) and between the ends of bars resting on benches or racks and an aisle space wide enough to accommodate a stretcher in and out in case of an emergency. The guidelines for laying out a facility and providing proper spacing include the following (4):

- *Traffic flow:* It can be a challenge to place equipment with the proper spacing while designing a safe weight room floor plan that flows well. Planning the traffic pattern in a room is just as important as planning the workout. Planned traffic patterns allow for a safe and more efficient way to move from one area to the next and complete workout sessions in the time allotted. For example, an area for stretching, warming up, and cooling down could be placed near the entrance so that when a class comes in, they are not walking through the entire room to warm up, and it will be their last stop as they work on their flexibility before they leave the room.

- *Machine area:* If there is a machine circuit resistance training area, it can be set up in a classic push–pull format. Resistance training on machines helps develop confidence in the untrained and inexperienced student-athletes. If the budget permits, purchase enough equipment (15 pieces for a class of 30) so that when one student-athlete is training, another is recovering and completing their workout card. Ask the local equipment dealer for notification of when a gym is upgrading their circuit line and make them an offer on the used equipment. Student-athletes typically stay motivated during circuit training because they are

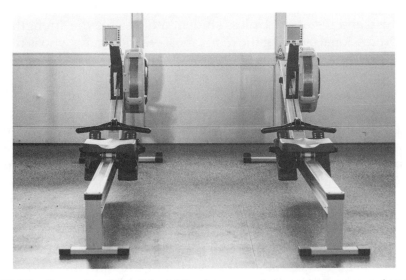

FIGURE 3.11   Example of the 3-foot (.9 m) space minimum between equipment.

either lifting or recovering and recording the repetitions completed. Motivation can be improved even more by having a timing device on the wall showing the student-athletes how to monitor tempo and keeping track of the time left in the set.

- *Free-weight area:* Strategically placing equipment (tall against the wall) offers a better opportunity to observe the entire room without the line of sight being obstructed. It is also a good idea to place power racks facing a mirrored wall to provide feedback to student-athletes. Mirrors, while not essential, can provide the necessary feedback, which can be used as a teaching tool to improve technique.

- *Olympic lifting area:* In the past, this has been a separate 8 foot by 8 foot (2.4 m by 2.4 m) wooden platform with a squat rack placed on top of it; however, equipment companies are promoting a designated space built into the rubber floor in front of a squat rack. This new surface still allows the student-athlete to shuffle the feet as needed to complete the various Olympic lifts and opens up the floor by not having a platform take up that space.

- *Aerobic area:* This is where the cardiorespiratory equipment is grouped together. This equipment usually consists of stationary bikes, stair climbers, elliptical machines, treadmills, rowers, and upper body ergometers. If the class size is 30, consider purchasing five different pieces so the student-athletes will have the opportunity to learn how to use five different machines. Have the class rotate to a new piece of equipment every other class.

Maintenance and Cleaning

One of the most important factors in the safety of the facility is its ability to stay open. If there is any instance of infection or sickness attributed to its maintenance and cleaning, trust will be lost, and the program will suffer. This section outlines some of the procedural actions that should be followed for a facility to function effectively.

Who will be responsible for cleaning the weight room? Is there a weight room fairy who visits nightly to return all equipment to its proper place and to vacuum, dust, and disinfect? Unless student-athletes see the strength and conditioning professional cleaning the room, most will not know who is responsible for its upkeep. The policies and procedures manual should include a schedule of how all who use the facility are expected to help with its maintenance. Get the student-athletes to understand that this is their weight room, and therefore they have a responsibility to keep it clean. While they may ask why they have to clean up initially, they will develop a sense of pride in the room, and it will become second nature to them. Host an in-service each semester for new faculty or coaching staff who will be using the weight room and share the directions for what is to be done before their class leaves.

The custodial department is invaluable. They are probably given an area of the school to clean each night and only have so many minutes to get it done. Negotiate a deal with them. Tell them that the strength and conditioning professional and student-athletes will keep the room clean if they will provide the supplies as needed. Ask that a custodian stop in every evening to empty the trash, leave more paper towels, and refill the disinfectant bottles. Establishing a good relationship with custodial staff is very important. They will take care of the facility as if it were their own if they feel they are part of the program. Something as simple as a T-shirt with the weight room logo on it goes a long way.

A facility is a reflection of the strength and conditioning professional and will affect all of the athletic program's culture. If it looks clean and organized when student-athletes enter, it must be clean and organized when they leave. This takes time and relies on the consistent expectations of the PE department and sport coaches. When the facility is clean and orderly, it sets a standard for all other staff. The ultimate responsibility of maintaining a clean and safe environment falls on the strength and conditioning professional or sport coach in charge at the moment. A good practice is to have participants wipe down exercise equipment immediately after using it. It is also important to develop a system through which all teams sanitize the bars, pads, and all equipment used for that workout before they leave the room. Make each team and their strength and conditioning professional or sport coach aware of these procedures in advance and hold others accountable if the procedures are not followed after their class or team trains.

Some surfaces have a greater chance of developing bacterial growth and could close down a facility when left unchecked. Using an approved germicide can prevent the spread of transmissible diseases. Sanitizing each piece of equipment after each exercise is an easy way to make student-athletes take responsibility for their room. All floors should be mopped regularly for the removal of dust and grime that could cause foot slippage (4).

The upkeep of equipment is important. Maintenance on the equipment should be checked for broken or damaged parts. It is cheaper to maintain than to replace a piece of equipment. If a piece of equipment is broken, it should be removed from the floor, or it should have a "Do not use" sign attached to it. It is a good idea to have a stocked toolbox to adjust, tighten, and make minor repairs (4).

If your budget allows, get to know which companies will visit and inspect all resistance training machines and other weight room equipment. Usually, it is a branch of the company where the equipment was purchased. These technicians are trained to spot, repair, and replace equipment with the proper parts and material. They are contracted and will perform general and specific tasks brought to their attention. Keep records in case there is an equipment failure that could prevent full implementation of the daily program (9).

Assign these tasks to develop a sense of ownership in the room and keep a record of who did the work and on what day and time. A cleaning and maintenance schedule should be made that specifies what equipment is to be cleaned and inspected daily, weekly, or monthly. (See the checklists at the end of the chapter.) Maintenance materials should be kept in storage or a closet, cleaning materials should be kept at a central site where all will have access as needed, and the toolbox should be put away out of sight. Supervisors are responsible for checking and recommending what cleaning supplies will be needed for the weight room several months in advance. Budgets are planned far ahead, and these cleaning items need to be purchased through the school's general fund. Make an effort to keep records of the amount of cleaning materials used during the previous year to make sure enough is ordered.

Risk Analysis Checklist

PE teachers and strength and conditioning professionals must be aware of their legal liability each day they open the doors to the weight room. While the risk of injury cannot be totally eliminated, it can be anticipated and effectively managed using risk management strategies (9). Risk management is the use of strategies that decrease and control the risk of liability exposure. Some districts have someone with the title of risk manager who could tour the facility, looking for areas that may be classified as an area of liability.

"Liability" and other legal terms are nothing to be afraid of. It is important to understand the responsibilities of the strength and conditioning professional or sport coach and to understand the definitions of the following terms in risk management and how they affect day-to-day interactions with student-athletes (8).

- *Informed consent:* The process by which a procedure or event is described to a participant
- *Liability:* A legal responsibility, duty, or obligation
- *Standard of care:* What a reasonable and prudent person would do under similar circumstances
- *Negligence:* Failure to act as a reasonable and prudent person would under similar circumstances
- *Assumption of risk:* Knowing that an inherent risk exists with participation in an activity and voluntarily deciding to participate anyway

It is advisable to meet with the administration, each sport coach, and their teams prior to their season to review all the rules, regulations, and workouts. Scheduling one team at a time may be ideal because there will be less chaos and more focus, but it is difficult to fit all the sessions in when a group would like to train. Usually, scheduling the in-season teams first and then filling in the schedule with the off-season teams works well.

Take attendance of the entire team and coaching staff. All sport coaches should participate in the review session before they can be part of team supervision in the weight room. This will help promote a safe weight room culture, minimize serious accidents, and keep things in order. Make sure the room is checked and all participants have exited when the door is locked.

Regular staff in-services may help prevent future litigation against the strength and conditional professional for not addressing the above content before the workouts begin. It is also advisable that each teacher and strength and conditioning professional do a quick walk-through of the facility prior to the beginning of their classes or before a team enters the weight room.

A sample mental walk-through could go something like this: A strength and conditioning professional or sport coach is about to bring a class or team into the weight room. They open the door, turn on the lights, and begin to perform a quick scan for the following:

1. Is there anything observable that may cause someone harm?
2. If a hazard was observed, decide who may be harmed, and how.
3. After evaluating the risks, decide on what precautions to take, and take them.
4. Record the finding and make a record of it in the log.
5. What action could be taken so this will not happen again?
6. If a staff member or team constantly ignores requests to keep the room in order, consider reporting the finding to the proper administrator.
7. What is the school's chain of command for complaints?

Review the assessment as soon as time permits and take the necessary action (8).

Sample Emergency Action Plans or Procedures

An emergency action plan (EAP) is a written document that details the proper procedures for reacting to various scenarios and emergencies. Have a written response plan for environmental situations as well as both life-threatening and non-life-threatening situations. The development of this document usually includes input from the PE and athletic department, strength and conditioning professionals, medical personnel, and sport coaches. This emergency response plan is specific to each high school and weight room facility and must be approved by the administration for liability concerns, reviewed with staff and student-athletes before the beginning of a semester or season, and clearly posted at several sites in the weight room (8).

Strength and conditioning professionals who are new to the school can ask any of the following people if the school has an EAP in place:

- Any member in the PE department
- Department administrator
- School nurse
- AD

Look for a date on the document. When was the plan last revised? If there is no date it would be a wise idea to thoroughly review and make necessary revisions, then meet with whichever administrator is responsible for weight room risk management and ask that they review and sign off on it before it is put in place.

The following are usually included or are described in an EAP (8):

- Current EMS activation procedure
- Names and phone numbers of people to contact
- Address of the facility
- Locations of the telephones
- Locations of the nearest exits and entrances
- Designated personnel to care for injuries
- Ambulance access
- Location of emergency supplies and first aid kit
- Plan of action in case of fire, tornado, life-threatening injury, non-life-threatening injury, crime, terrorism, and any other incident that your district suggests you plan for

The following four aspects of an EAP warrant additional detail:

- *Emergency personnel:* As a potential first responder, the strength and conditioning professional should acquire and maintain a professional certification including standard first aid, CPR, and AED. A supervisor is usually given up to six months to acquire the necessary certifications after being hired. Until then they should not be allowed to supervise a class or team alone (8).

- *Emergency communication:* The ability to immediately communicate is crucial for the quick delivery of care. While most people have cell phones, it is possible the cell service would not work when needed. A suggestion is to have access to a landline that has an operator during the school day or an extension code that will allow the caller to get an outside line before or after school hours when an operator is not available (8).

- *Emergency equipment:* Maintaining professional certifications means that the strength and conditional professional has been trained on, is certified in, and has practiced how to respond to emergencies using basic lifesaving equipment until professional emergency personnel arrive on the scene. The basic equipment should be readily available in an emergency situation. Know where the nearest AED and first aid kit are located. Ask the school nurse to inspect them on a regular basis and keep the kit stocked with the necessary supplies. Having the nurse's assistance would be a valuable addition (8).

- *Rules within the emergency team:* Each building in the district usually asks for volunteers to be on an emergency response team. These volunteers have been trained and are certified in basic first aid and CPR. In the case of an emergency the first person on the scene will be in charge until more qualified personnel arrive. In-services are great opportunities to plan and practice what will work at the school. Discuss various strategies for handling situations that have occurred in the school over the past year or have happened nationally to date (8).

A plan is only as good as the practice sessions that help prepare for it. It is suggested that this plan is practiced on a quarterly basis with all staff who are teaching or training student-athletes in this facility during this quarter (8).

Recommendations for Communication

Communication recommendations with student-athletes, parents, administrators, sport coaches, and strength and conditioning professionals are plentiful. While social media platforms such as Instagram, Facebook, and Twitter have their pitfalls, they are the accepted ways we communicate with one another on a daily basis. All of these pose some concerns. Misuse can have dramatic repercussions for student-athletes and their teams. Reputations, scholarships, and careers have been destroyed by a simple text message sent in haste.

School systems have their own rules and guidelines for proper social media use. These recommendations should be explored before using any social media to contact students. Student-athletes should also be aware of their actions and responsibilities. Teachers and sport coaches should have scheduled in-services on acceptable and proper use of social media so they can explain the repercussions of poor choices such as bullying and inappropriate comments. Although it is difficult to monitor each player's conversations, it is a sport coach's responsibility to address these concerns and make a very clear statement about this type of behavior on the team platform.

Communication while in the school building is paramount if a sport coach, strength and conditioning professional, teacher, administrator, nurse, or security officer needs to be contacted. The use of walkie talkies, cell phones, wall intercoms, and direct lines inside and outside the building is necessary. Distinguish which form of communication the school or facility recognizes and test it periodically to make sure it works.

Athletic departments and schools have websites. Many schools and teams have their tech and media departments design communication platforms to get messages for specific sports and are very helpful in getting information to parents and players quickly. This can be as easy as developing your own free website available through most carriers such as Gmail or going a step further by purchasing services through various commercial apps such as sportsYou, Drivn, or GroupMe.

Unplanned meetings in the community can occur, so it is important that staff are prepared to discuss various topics with parents and other community members.

Options for Incorporating Technology

Technology applications such as apps, computer programs, websites, Google Classroom, and various measurement devices all enable teachers to become better organized and to serve their program well. Ethical, motivational, and student-athlete learning modalities that foster honest feedback are also addressed.

Apps

PE has been ahead of other disciplines when it comes to analysis, feedback, and measurement tools. Heart rate monitors, pedometers, Apple Watch, Fitbit, Fitness-Gram, and accelerometers are programs or devices that use digital technology to gather student-athlete data. With this ability, there may be ethical implications with student-athlete data being uploaded into an external platform of a private company. This is not a simple issue and should be contemplated for its inherent nature and ramifications.

Technology is very easy for students to master because student-athletes have grown up with a high degree of exposure to computers and technology-driven devices from an early age. Technology may incorporate a basic stopwatch or expensive tools to measure bar speed through a cell phone to record movement patterns. This equipment can be a great motivator yet may lose its luster as time goes on.

With the advent of computers of diminishing size, communication is often via cell phones and text messages. Teams and staff can also communicate through various apps available to record exercises, supply data, and record video. Apps can also monitor attendance and time spent on the site. Taking advantage of this technology allows student-athletes, sport coaches, and strength and conditioning professionals access to a constant form of communication to gauge progress and adherence.

It is important to prepare a budget and foresee needs that may allow for more efficiency when it comes to technology. Technology can be elusive, but it is often second nature to the student-athlete. Many communication and technical programs such as graphs, workout forms, and attendance procedures are beneficial to managers and tech-savvy players on the team or student-athletes in class.

Privacy issues and the inability of some student-athletes to access computers or internet services outside of school are concerning. The use of technology can also diminish their ability to perform mathematical computations without the use of the device.

The goal of technology is to augment, not replace, classroom instruction and learning. The resources student-athletes and schools have may present limitations. PE teachers may also have a variety of philosophies on the use of technology in PE.

Google School

Google School (also called Google Classroom) is an efficient way to create and share lesson plans with student-athletes and staff. It allows for constant interaction between editors on the same page in real time. The ability to do a presentation in a PowerPoint format can be a useful tool.

A sample unit plan can include lessons in the order the teacher wants to pursue, such as the following:

1. Purpose
2. Elements to be included
3. What to expect each week
4. Lesson 1:
   a. The athletic position
   b. Visualization of bar movement in straight lines
   c. Spotting

Templates for Designing Strength and Conditioning Programs

The setup of a unit plan (long-term goals) and daily lesson plans (short-term goals) is essential. A lesson plan is a good way to be organized for an efficient classroom and sport instructional period. Daily, weekly, and monthly programs can be presented in many creative formats.

A simple template for PE teachers is based on comfort level with the activity. Many PE teachers and sport coaches do not have expertise in strength and conditioning. Classroom PE teachers are free to develop their own method of delivering a sound strength and conditioning program. There is no particular set rule to its inception, other than simplicity is the rule of thumb.

For sport coaches and strength and conditioning professionals, a simple template allows for instruction and supervision of a large group. Workouts can be separated into daily, weekly, monthly, seasonal, and annual plans. If a school system and coaching staff are fortunate enough to have a member who is proficient and current in the field of strength and conditioning, they are usually aligned with the NSCA or a very select few other organizations in some capacity.

Teams use a more involved management presentation. This is usually posted in various locations in the workout facility in weekly or monthly formats. The program incorporates a well-thought-out periodization program designed to produce results.

Computer programs are commercially available with websites that can help make programs more organized and easier to use. Here are a few suggestions:

- NSCA's Program Design Essentials (www.nsca.com/education/tools-and-resources/program-design-essentials/)
- TeamBuildr (www.teambuildr.com)
- Excel Templates for Coaches (www.exceltrainingdesigns.com/)

The high school strength and conditioning program should have a goal in mind. These goals should be presented through research-based progressions that lead to success and consider the student-athlete's participation in multiple sports. High school student-athletes who specialize in one sport have opportunities to advance strength gains beyond those moving from sport to sport through a yearly program.

A high school may be fortunate enough to have a designated strength and conditioning professional on staff and an AD who can aid in the administration of a required program to all teams regardless of the sport. This concept can limit the introduction of workouts that are counterproductive to the student-athlete.

Strength and conditioning professionals have the ability and responsibility to present their programs in an organized fashion through media available in the school's system. This presentation can be posted either electronically or visually in the room. With numerous teams having access to the facility, it is important to differentiate between PE and sport-specific workouts and further separate off-season and in-season workouts for each sport team.

Guidelines for Substitute Teachers

Most substitute teachers are not qualified to deliver proper supervision, care, or expertise for a class that involves resistance training. Although most PE departments would feel uncomfortable having a substitute teach a class in the fitness facility, some activities may be safe for a class of high school student-athletes familiar with the safety protocols in the facility.

School policy will often dictate what substitutes can and cannot do; however, program administrators have the obligation to set the rules that day. This may involve having a substitute teacher change places with a full-time teacher or limiting access to the weight room entirely. The department often has a list of substitute teachers who are qualified in specific areas stated on the teaching license.

In the event a substitute teacher lands in the facility, the regular PE teacher should have clear and explicit lesson plans outlined. For instance:

1. The use of free weights by student-athletes when a substitute teacher is supervising is not allowed.

2. The use of the following equipment in a PE or strength and conditioning class may be acceptable if the administration feels the substitute teacher is qualified:
   a. Aerobic equipment following safe protocol
   b. Pin-loaded circuit machines
   c. Medicine ball training with a partner (5)
   d. All jump ropes and resistance band routines
   e. Mats for stretching

3. Have the class watch a training video or read a fitness article from a referenced source and complete a quiz on the subject.

A PE teacher's classes have been trained to follow proper weight room etiquette and are aware of the rules and regulations. Lesson plans are specific to expectations and rules for class that day even if it only specifies aerobic and stretching options. Having a substitute "teach the class" may not be a wise decision for a variety of reasons. The safety of the student-athletes must be a priority. Here are examples of what PE teachers might say regarding substitute teachers:

- If I know of an upcoming absence, I try to work with the department and help to select a qualified substitute such as another PE teacher or sport coach.

- Unless a substitute teacher is qualified and experienced in a strength and conditioning setting, keep them out for liability reasons.

- Ever since a student dropped a weight plate on his foot under the supervision of a non-qualified substitute teacher, only a PE teacher can substitute teach in the weight room in our district.

Knowing these policies in advance could help PE teachers prepare a substitute teaching plan while they are out of class. Scouting all the subs hired in the system may be a good approach as to whether they could substitute for a resistance training class. If one has been identified, notify the appropriate secretaries of substitutes that are qualified.

Conclusion

Evidence-based information should be the basis and foundation for successful strength and conditioning instruction. The suggestions in this chapter and identifying standards and guidelines help keep a facility running safely, efficiently, and productively.

Checklist for Cleaning Floors, Walls, and Ceilings

Floors

- ☐ Check for large cracks and standing dirt or grime.
- ☐ Check for splintering on platforms.
- ☐ Check any bolts or screws that go into the floor.
- ☐ Ensure that no glue is protruding from the floor.
- ☐ Ensure that the flooring is sturdy and locked in place.
- ☐ Check carpet for mold, mildew, and tears.

Walls

- ☐ Check walls for dirt buildup.
- ☐ Replace mirrors if cracked as soon as possible.
- ☐ Clean mirrors of smudges at least once weekly.
- ☐ Clean windows of smudges at least once weekly.
- ☐ Dust windowsills and any shelving weekly.
- ☐ Mirrors should be at least 20 inches (51 cm) off the floor.

Ceilings

- ☐ Ensure that all lights work properly.
- ☐ Check for dust and cobweb buildup.
- ☐ Ensure that nothing attached to the ceiling is loose.
- ☐ Replace ceiling tiles when needed.
- ☐ Ceilings should be at least 12 feet (3.7 m) high to ensure clearance.

Reprinted by permission from Haff and Triplett (2016, p. 636).

NSCA's Safety Checklist for Exercise Facility and Equipment Maintenance

Exercise Facility

Floor

- ☐ Inspected and cleaned daily
- ☐ Wooden flooring free of splinters, holes, protruding nails, and loose screws
- ☐ Tile flooring resistant to slipping; no moisture or chalk accumulation
- ☐ Rubber flooring free of cuts, slits, and large gaps between pieces
- ☐ Interlocking mats secure and arranged with no protruding tabs
- ☐ Nonabsorbent carpet free of tears; wear areas protected by throw mats
- ☐ Area swept and vacuumed or mopped on a regular basis
- ☐ Flooring glued or fastened down properly

Walls

- ☐ Wall surfaces cleaned two or three times a week (or more often if needed)
- ☐ Walls in high-activity areas free of protruding appliances, equipment, or wall hangings
- ☐ Mirrors and shelves securely fixed to walls
- ☐ Mirrors and windows cleaned regularly (especially in high-activity areas, such as around drinking fountains and in doorways)
- ☐ Mirrors placed a minimum of 20 inches (51 cm) off the floor in all areas
- ☐ Mirrors not cracked or distorted (replace immediately if damaged)

Ceiling

- ☐ All ceiling fixtures and attachments dusted regularly
- ☐ Ceiling tile kept clean
- ☐ Damaged or missing ceiling tile replaced as needed
- ☐ Open ceilings with exposed pipes and ducts cleaned as needed

Exercise Equipment

Stretching and Bodyweight Exercise Area

- ☐ Mat area free of weight benches and equipment
- ☐ Mats and bench upholstery free of cracks and tears
- ☐ No large gaps between stretching mats
- ☐ Area swept and disinfected daily
- ☐ Equipment properly stored after use
- ☐ Elastic cords secured to base with safety knot and checked for wear
- ☐ Surfaces that contact skin treated with antifungal and antibacterial agents daily
- ☐ Nonslip material on the top surface and bottom or base of plyometric boxes
- ☐ Ceiling height sufficient for overhead exercises (12 feet [3.7 m] minimum) and free of low-hanging apparatus (beams, pipes, lighting, signs, and so on)

> *continued*

NSCA's Safety Checklist for Exercise Facility and Equipment Maintenance   > *continued*

Resistance Training Machine Area

- ☐ Easy access to each station (a minimum of 2 feet [61 cm] between machines; 3 feet [91 cm] is optimal)
- ☐ Area free of loose bolts, screws, cables, and chains
- ☐ Proper selectorized pins used
- ☐ Securing straps functional
- ☐ Parts and surfaces properly lubricated and cleaned
- ☐ Protective padding free of cracks and tears
- ☐ Surfaces that contact skin treated with antifungal and antibacterial agents daily
- ☐ No protruding screws or parts that need tightening or removal
- ☐ Belts, chains, and cables aligned with machine parts
- ☐ No worn parts (frayed cable, loose chains, worn bolts, cracked joints, and so on)

Resistance Training Free-Weight Area

- ☐ Easy access to each bench or area (a minimum of 2 feet [61 cm] between benches; 3 feet [91 cm] is optimal)
- ☐ Olympic bars properly spaced (3 feet [91 cm]) between ends
- ☐ All equipment returned after use to avoid obstruction of pathway
- ☐ Safety equipment (belts, collars, safety bars) used and returned
- ☐ Protective padding free of cracks and tears
- ☐ Surfaces that contact skin treated with antifungal and antibacterial agents daily
- ☐ Securing bolts and apparatus parts (collars, curl bars) tightly fastened
- ☐ Nonslip mats on squat rack floor area
- ☐ Olympic bars turn properly and are properly lubricated and tightened
- ☐ Benches, weight racks, standards, and the like secured to the floor or wall
- ☐ Nonfunctional or broken equipment removed from area or locked out of service
- ☐ Ceiling height sufficient for overhead exercises (12 feet [3.7 m] minimum) and free of low-hanging apparatus (beams, pipes, lighting, signs, and so on)

Weightlifting Area

- ☐ Olympic bars properly spaced (3 feet [91 cm]) between ends
- ☐ All equipment returned after use to avoid obstruction of lifting area
- ☐ Olympic bars turn properly and are properly lubricated and tightened
- ☐ Bent Olympic bars replaced; knurling clear of debris
- ☐ Collars functioning
- ☐ Sufficient chalk available
- ☐ Wrist straps, belts, and knee wraps available, functioning, and stored properly
- ☐ Benches, chairs, and boxes kept at a distance from lifting area
- ☐ No gaps, cuts, slits, or splinters in mats

☐ Area properly swept and mopped to remove splinters and chalk

☐ Ceiling height sufficient for overhead exercises (12 feet [3.7 m] minimum) and free of low-hanging apparatus (beams, pipes, lighting, signs, and so on)

Aerobic Exercise Area

☐ Easy access to each station (a minimum of 2 feet [61 cm] between machines; 3 feet [91 cm] is optimal)

☐ Bolts and screws tight

☐ Functioning parts easily adjustable

☐ Parts and surfaces properly lubricated and cleaned

☐ Foot and body straps secure and not ripped

☐ Measurement devices for tension, time, and revolutions per minute properly functioning

☐ Surfaces that contact skin treated with antifungal and antibacterial agents daily

Frequency of Maintenance and Cleaning Tasks

Daily

☐ Inspect all flooring for damage or wear.

☐ Clean (sweep, vacuum, or mop and disinfect) all flooring.

☐ Clean and disinfect upholstery.

☐ Clean and disinfect the drinking fountain.

☐ Inspect fixed equipment's connection with the floor.

☐ Clean and disinfect equipment surfaces that contact skin.

☐ Clean mirrors.

☐ Clean windows.

☐ Inspect mirrors for damage.

☐ Inspect all equipment for damage; wear; loose or protruding belts, screws, cables, or chains; insecure or nonfunctioning foot and body straps; improper functioning or improper use of attachments, pins, or other devices.

☐ Clean and lubricate moving parts of equipment.

☐ Inspect all protective padding for cracks and tears.

☐ Inspect nonslip material and mats for proper placement, damage, and wear.

☐ Remove trash and garbage.

☐ Clean light covers, fans, air vents, clocks, and speakers.

☐ Ensure that equipment is returned and stored properly after use.

Two or Three Times per Week

☐ Clean and lubricate aerobic machines and the guide rods on selectorized resistance training machines.

Once per Week

☐ Clean (dust) ceiling fixtures and attachments.

☐ Clean ceiling tile.

> continued

NSCA's Safety Checklist for Exercise Facility and Equipment Maintenance > *continued*

As Needed

☐ Replace light bulbs.

☐ Clean walls.

☐ Replace damaged or missing ceiling tiles.

☐ Clean open ceilings with exposed pipes or ducts.

☐ Remove (or place sign on) broken equipment.

☐ Fill chalk boxes.

☐ Clean bar knurling.

☐ Clean rust from floor, plates, bars, and equipment with a rust-removing solution.

Reprinted by permission from Haff and Triplett (2016, pp. 637-639).

Resistance Training Exercises

Scott Sahli, MEd, CSCS,*D, NSCA-CPT,*D, RSCC*E,
USAW National Coach

Developing strength makes a difference in the career and future life of a high school student-athlete. A stronger student-athlete can perform fundamental movements better and can thus be a more effective student-athlete. By using proper movement and regularly doing the exercises that make them stronger, student-athletes will become more flexible and more powerful and will thicken and strengthen their bones, ligaments, tendons, and muscles. Doing the exercises that get them stronger will develop body armor, helping protect them against the effects of collisions, bumps, and bruises, and is therefore a factor in reducing injuries. Being strong will allow the student-athlete to do many strenuous tasks in life more efficiently. This chapter will serve as a guideline for a high school teacher or strength and conditioning professional to teach safe and effective exercise techniques. This includes making the exercise essentials clear, emphasizing important terms, and helping the student-athlete to know and understand the underlying keys to exercise technique.

Exercise Essentials

In order to conduct a successful program that teaches safe and effective exercise technique, it is important to follow some essential principles.

1. There must be designated areas in the weight room for specific exercises—for example, platforms or a designated space for power exercises and deadlifts; racks for squats, presses, and so on; and areas for the bench press and for assistance exercises. It is also important that the area where the exercises are being taught and conducted is clear of all other equipment to make it a safe environment.

I would like to express my gratitude to Roger Earle and Mike Nitka for their invaluable guidance, insight, suggestions, and expertise. Thank you to Scott Caulfield and Doug Berringer for their inspiration.

2. It is of the utmost importance to have and to use the proper tools and implements in order to execute the exercises properly. There must be bars of different weights that are appropriate for student-athletes of varying age, size, experience, and strength (e.g., a 15 lb bar, a 25 lb bar, a 15 kg or 35 lb bar, and a 20 kg or 45 lb bar) (see figure 3.2 on page 67). Machines should also be able to be adjusted to accommodate student-athletes of vastly different sizes.

3. Safety is the highest priority. This includes paying attention to and being aware of what is around the student-athlete, using the proper implements and loads, keeping the different areas clean and accessible, always using collars when weights are on a bar, using competent spotters and spotting techniques when appropriate, and using a weightlifting belt when needed. It is important to stay off and away from platforms or designated areas when they are being used for the power exercises by another student-athlete.

4. The most important step of the functional part of doing exercises is learning and becoming competent with the proper fundamental movements. Proper movement must be a priority before emphasizing strength. The student-athlete should first learn how to do the proper movements and technique with no weight or with empty bars. Everyone progresses at a different rate, so it may be difficult for the strength and conditioning professional to know whether a weight is too heavy. If, in the eyes of the strength and conditioning professional, a student-athlete is unable to perform the movements easily, correctly, and competently, that student-athlete should be guided to go with lighter weight or a lighter bar. The student-athlete should learn and then practice the exercises correctly and with manageable weight before beginning a progressive overload process. It is important to have an appropriate and periodized program designed by an NSCA-certified professional.

5. Teachers and strength and conditioning professionals expect their student-athletes to stay motivated and eager to learn, to work hard, and constantly to give their best and they, too, should be motivated to improve their programs and constantly learn by reading and by attending clinics and conferences in person or online. An ideal goal of all strength and conditioning professionals is to become a Certified Strength and Conditioning Specialist (CSCS) as part of their pursuit to improve their knowledge and art of the craft of strength. They should never assume that a student-athlete will always use proper technique. Their job is to be in perpetual motion: constantly teaching, correcting, and adjusting technique and equipment if necessary. In the weight room, the strength and conditioning professional should never remain seated but instead should always be actively coaching.

Key Fundamentals to Exercise Technique

There are several keys to exercising properly beyond using the proper equipment. These include using a proper handgrip and grip width, setting a proper body position to begin each exercise, using proper breathing patterns, using weight belts in the correct situations, and following proper spotting guidelines appropriately.

Using the proper width for hands during an exercise increases the likelihood of success because it puts the arms and hands into an anatomically more advantageous and safer position.

Helpful Terms

Collars: Devices put on the bars to secure the weight plates so they do not slide off; also called clips, fasteners, clamps, or locks (figure 4.1).

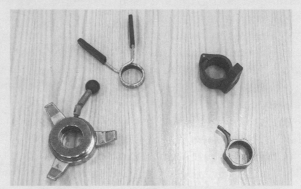

FIGURE 4.1 Examples of various types of collars (locks).

Concentric movement: The phase of the movement that is overcoming gravity or resistance as the muscle is being shortened or contracted.

Eccentric movement: The phase of the movement during which resistance force is greater than contraction force and the muscle lengthens.

Isometric movement: An action that occurs when a muscle generates a force against a resistance but does not overcome it, so that no movement takes place.

Lordotic curve: The normal inward curve of the lower back (figure 4.2).

Multijoint exercise: An exercise that involves movement at two or more primary joints.

Neutral spine: The position or alignment of the torso in which the three curves of the spine (cervical, thoracic, and lumbar) are in their natural, balanced position; when viewed from the side, these curves form an S.

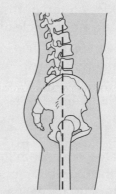

FIGURE 4.2 Lordotic curve of the vertebral column.

Power exercises: Exercises (clean, snatch, and clean and jerk, and their various versions) that help student-athletes develop tremendous amounts of power (force × velocity).

Platform: A designated area in the weight room (commonly 8 feet by 8 feet [about 3 m by 3 m]) where the exercises that develop the most power, such as the clean and its progressions or the snatch and its progressions, are performed for safety reasons. Other exercises can be performed on a platform, too (e.g., the deadlift; even though the deadlift is not a power exercise, a platform is the most appropriate place to do this exercise).

Power lifting: A sport composed of three competitive exercises (back squat, bench press, and deadlift) that can develop tremendous amounts of strength—the ability to resist force or move objects—but not a lot of power. Strength is a fundamental element of developing power.

Single-joint exercise: An exercise that involves movement at only one primary joint.

Triple-joint extension: A position achieved while pulling on a bar by simultaneously extending the hips, knees, and ankles to achieve maximum power.

Weightlifting: A sport involving the Olympic lifts (snatch and clean and jerk) that generate tremendous amounts of power. Power is a prerequisite for many athletic activities, sports, and fundamental movements.

Hand Grips

Different hand grips are used for different exercises because they are not only more comfortable, but they also anatomically put the student-athlete in a much better position to be successful in the exercise. Using the proper hand grip is also safer for the student-athlete. See figure 4.3 for examples of hand grips.

1. *Pronated grip:* This is an overhand grip with the knuckles on top of the bar, as in doing a power clean.

2. *Supinated grip:* This is an underhand grip with the knuckles facing downward and the palms up, as in performing a biceps curl.

3. *Closed grip:* This can be a pronated or a supinated grip

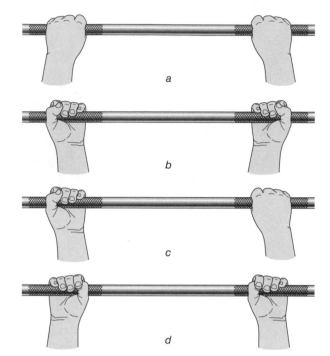

FIGURE 4.3 Types of hand grips: *(a)* pronated, *(b)* supinated, *(c)* alternated, and *(d)* hook (posterior view).

with the thumb wrapped around the bar the opposite way as the fingers so that the student-athlete has better control of the bar and a stronger grip.

4. *Open grip or false grip:* This is a grip with the thumb grabbing the bar on the same side and in the same way as the fingers. (In most exercises this is considered unsafe.) Although often used while doing the front squat and sometimes during the back squat, this grip is not considered as safe as a closed grip because it is much easier for the bar to slip out of the student-athlete's grasp.

5. *Neutral grip:* In this grip, the palm of the hand is facing toward the body, as in holding a hammer. It is often used with kettlebells, dumbbells, and machines that are pulling stations.

6. *Alternated grip:* In this grip, one hand is pronated in a closed grip and the other hand is supinated in a closed grip. This is often used with some deadlifts and spotting techniques.

7. *Hook grip:* This is a pronated grip in which the thumb is wrapped around the bar in the opposite direction as the fingers, and the fingers grasp the thumb. This grip is used for the Olympic lifts because it is a stronger grip and assists in lifting heavy weight rapidly. The reason that this grip is important to teach is that the hands are often considered the weakest part of the body used when pulling weights. A hook grip helps strengthen that weakness.

Grip Width

Using the proper width for hands during an exercise increases the likelihood of success with the exercise because it puts the arms and hands into an anatomically more advantageous and safer position (figure 4.4).

1. *Common grip width:* In this grip, the hands are outside the legs and near the width of the shoulders, but equidistant from the ends of the bar. It is often used for the bench press, standing front press, power clean, deadlift, and Romanian deadlift.

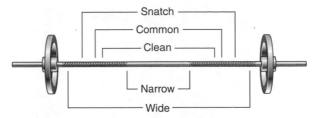

FIGURE 4.4   Common grip widths.

2. *Wide grip:* This grip is wider than a common grip and is outside the shoulders. It is often used when squatting.

3. *Narrow grip:* This grip is usually inside the width of the shoulders and is commonly used for assistance exercises. Depending on the exercise it could be pronated closed grips or supinated closed grips.

4. *Clean grip:* This grip is about one half to one full fist width wider than the shoulders; it is a pronated hook grip.

5. *Snatch grip:* This grip is wider to enable the bar to be snatched, or lifted, over the head in one movement. A wider grip allows this to happen more easily. This width can be determined by having the student-athlete stand up tall and grasp the bar with a pronated hook grip and with the arms hanging down in front. The student-athlete pulls the bar into the hip crease and then lifts up a thigh to hip crease height. While keeping the bar in the hip crease the student-athlete moves the hands out until the arms are extended. The student-athlete then lifts the bar above the head, making sure it clears the top of the head.

Body Position Sets the Foundation for Proper Execution of the Exercise

No matter what exercise is being done, the body needs to be in a strong and stable position to execute it properly, regardless of whether using a machine or free weights. The body is the foundation upon which the exercise is executed. A proper foundation alignment ensures that the proper muscles and joints are stressed appropriately. The objective of the exercise is to eventually complete the movement through the full range of motion in order to promote flexibility and proper muscle, ligament, tendon, and joint development.

Exercises executed while standing require that the feet be arranged so that the heels are below the outside of the hips and the toes are pointed slightly out. Weight should be distributed evenly on the whole foot, and the knees should be slightly flexed with an erect neutral spine (slightly lordotic).

Exercises done on a machine often require the student-athlete to make several adjustments. Numerous kinds of machines are used to exercise different parts of the body. Most of them require the student-athlete to move or adjust back pads, chest pads, head pads, and foot platforms; to fasten or adjust belts; and often to adjust arm, leg, or ankle rollers for the proper individual fit. Often these machines have figures that show the proper alignment of the body to the cams or levers so that the student-athlete can effectively and safely move through the proper range of motion during the exercise. It is important for the strength and conditioning professional to teach and demonstrate to the student-athletes how to use and properly adjust each machine to get maximum benefit in the proper way, and then to continually monitor the correct alignment daily (2, 18, 19).

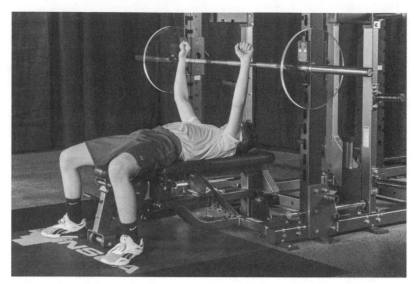

FIGURE 4.5   Five-point body contact.

Seated or supine (lying face up) exercises require five points of body contact with the bench or machine for a safe, proper, and effective position for developing strength (figure 4.5):

1. The buttocks are placed firmly on the bench or seat.
2. The shoulders and upper back are distributed evenly and firmly on the bench or back pad.
3. The head is placed firmly on the bench or head pad.
4. The right foot is flat and firmly on the floor.
5. The left foot is flat and firmly on the floor.

Keeping to these five points of contact is crucial to successful execution of the exercises and helps ensure stability and spinal support.

Movements done on a platform or designated area will often necessitate the use of a **hip hinge** movement to allow the proper execution of exercises in which pulling movements are done (9). A hip hinge is a movement that is used to give a stable position for the body to pull weight and properly protect joints and the spine. In this movement, the student-athlete

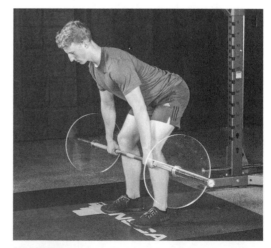

FIGURE 4.6   End of hip hinge movement.

approaches and grasps the bar with a pronated hook grip with the spine in a neutral position, the hips extended back behind the heels and slightly higher than the knees, the chest spread, and the shoulders and chest above the hips, with the shoulders and head slightly in front of the bar. The head is neutral, the knees are slightly flexed, the feet are flat and about hip-width apart with the toes pointing out 5 to 10 or more degrees, and the shoulders and chest are slightly in front of the bar (figure 4.6).

Effective Breathing Patterns

All muscle movements have three parts: eccentric, isometric, and concentric. Often the most difficult part of the exercise movement is the transition from somewhere in the isometric or transfer stage to somewhere in the concentric portion of the movement. This is referred to as the **sticking point**, which is a very individual spot for each person, depending upon the person's strengths and weaknesses while lifting and where there is the least mechanical advantage (22, 23). A general guideline is that for most exercises—especially exercises that are not power exercises or squats—the student-athlete should inhale on the eccentric or lengthening part of the exercise and exhale through the sticking point and the concentric part of the exercise. More trained and experienced student-athletes who are doing power exercises on platforms or squats in a squat rack might find breath-holding techniques useful when performing structural exercises (exercises that load and stress the vertebral column, such as squats or heavy pulls) with heavy loads.

The **Valsalva maneuver** is one such technique that helps keep proper vertebral support and alignment (1, 11, 12, 13). The Valsalva maneuver helps the student-athlete maintain a **neutral spine** with a normal lordotic curve and erect upper body position. The maneuver is done by taking a deep breath and exhaling against a closed glottis while simultaneously contracting the abdomen and rib cage muscles. This creates rigid compartments of fluid (called the *fluid ball*) in the lower torso and air in the upper torso. It thereby increases the rigidity of the entire torso to aid in supporting the vertebral column, which in turn reduces the associated compressive forces on the disks during lifting. Potential negative side effects include dizziness, high blood pressure, and blacking out. The breath-holding phase should be only 2 seconds at most. This maneuver must be done quickly and not extended (11, 17). Inexperienced student-athletes should not intentionally use it.

Weight Belts

The NSCA recommends that a weight belt be worn for exercises that place stress on the lower back and during sets that use near-maximal or maximal loads (2, 12, 15, 16). Wearing a weight belt all the time will keep the lower back and abdominal muscles from being trained appropriately. Untrained and inexperienced student-athletes should train with lighter weight until they are able to demonstrate competence with the movements before going heavy.

Spotting Guidelines

A spotter is a person who not only encourages and assists student-athletes but also helps prevent injury if the student-athlete needs help completing the exercise. Spotters must be taught how to spot properly. They should be tall enough, experienced enough, and strong enough so they can effectively help the student-athlete when necessary. The number of spotters needed is largely determined by the load being lifted, the experience and ability of the student-athlete and the spotters, and the physical strength of the spotters. Heavier loads increase the likelihood and severity of an injury. Once the load exceeds a spotter's ability to protect the student-athlete (and the spotter) effectively, another spotter must become involved. On the other hand, a single spotter is preferred if the load can be handled easily, because two or more spotters would have to coordinate their actions with those of the student-athlete. As the number of spotters increases, so does the chance of an error in timing or technique. Therefore it is a set of skills that should be taught and practiced using lighter weights.

Spotting is a very important responsibility to keep student-athletes safe, and is a must for any of the following situations:

1. Any exercise that is being done with weight resting on the front of the shoulders—for example, the front squat.

2. Any exercise that is done above the head, face, or throat—for example, the shoulder press, bench press, incline bench press, incline dumbbell press, or lying triceps extension.

3. Any exercise that involves a bar on the back of the shoulders or the trapezius, such as the back squat.

4. Olympic lifts that go over the head, or their variants (snatch, clean and jerk, power jerk, power snatch, push press), should not be spotted. Having a spotter on a platform to spot an Olympic lift would endanger both the spotter and the student-athlete because of the position of the bar and the speed at which it is lifted. Instead, it is safer for student-athletes to simply dump the bar in front of them with the clean, or in front or behind them in the snatch. Student-athletes need to learn early in their instruction of the platform exercises how to "miss" a repetition properly and safely.

5. Any exercise that is done with very heavy weight (one with which the student-athlete expects to get only 1 to 3 repetitions) will necessitate two or three spotters.

Spotting Guidelines for the Front Squat and the Back Squat

Depending on the amount of weight being lifted while squatting, a spotter or spotters should be required. The spotters should be experienced, strong enough, and tall enough to actually spot correctly. If not, either those spotters should not be used, or the weight should not be lifted. A spotter's first job is to make sure the bar has collars on each side of the bar and that the safety bars are at the right height for the student-athlete doing the lifting.

If one spotter is used for lighter weight, the spotter should be behind the student-athlete, squatting with the hands in a neutral handshake position under the student-athlete's armpits. This enables the spotter to assist the student-athlete up. The spotter's body should be close to, though not touching, the student-athlete's torso. Spotters should descend by flexing at the knees and hips along with the student-athlete while keeping their own torso upright and strong and rise up as the squatter rises by extending the knees and hips. If the student-athlete needs assistance, the spotter grabs the student-athlete under the armpits and helps him or her rise to the standards in the uprights. For safety reasons, spotters never pull a squatter back into themselves but only help the student-athlete to rise up if possible. If the student-athlete is unable to complete the repetition, the spotter helps the student-athlete place the bar on the safety bars smoothly and in a controlled manner.

When two spotters are used, one should be on each side of the bar with one of them designated as the head spotter. Both spotters will take a stance similar to the student-athlete's: chest spread, upright neutral spine, knees slightly flexed, and head neutral. Both hands should be placed under the bar; the hands do not touch the bar unless the student-athlete wants help lifting the bar off the supports, however. When the student-athlete is standing up and has control of the bar, the two spotters slowly let go of the bar at the same time. The spotters keep their hands close to and under the bar during the whole exercise and for all the repetitions. The spotters follow the bar down by flexing their knees and hips and follow it up by extending them. At the end of the exercise, or at the student-athlete's signal, or if the spotters see signs of trouble, the student-athlete and the spotters communicate, and the spotters grab the bar at the same time and guide or help the student-athlete safely back up to the supports. If the student-athlete is struggling or is not in a safe, strong position to complete the exercise properly, the head spotter says "down" and slowly and safely helps the student-athlete lower the bar to the safety bars. Sometimes the role of the spotters is simply to encourage the student-athlete lifting the weight.

When three spotters are used (which is highly recommended when a new maximum is being attempted), there should be one spotter on each side of the bar and one spotter behind the student-athlete who has his or her hands open, palms facing inward toward the student-athlete's body, and under—but not touching—the student-athlete's armpits. The spotter in the back is the head spotter in this situation. If the student-athlete needs assistance to complete the exercise, all three spotters will simultaneously lift up together on the command of "up." If the student-athlete seems unable to complete the exercise safely, the head spotter says "down," and helps the student-athlete guide the bar down to the safety bars in a controlled manner.

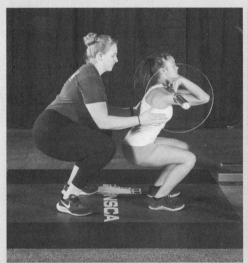

Front squat with one spotter.

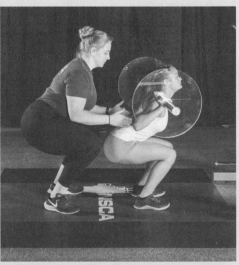

Back squat with one spotter.

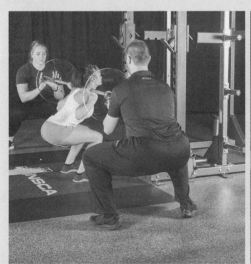

Back squat with two spotters.

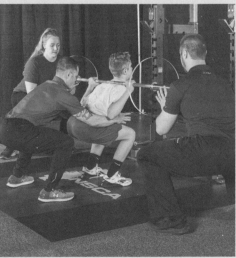

Back squat with three spotters.

Top-Down and Bottom-Up Technique Instruction Approaches

Both the clean and the snatch can be taught with two different instructional approaches: the bottom-up and the top-down techniques. The bottom-up technique teaches the lifting progression from the floor, where the exercise actually begins. This technique works very well and has significant merit (18).

Although the weight is ultimately lifted from the floor when doing the exercise, learning the exercise "backward" or from the top down has proven to be an effective and beneficial method. The guidelines in this chapter will follow the top-down approach (4, 7, 8, 9, 20). The bottom-up method is the exact opposite of the top-down approach.

Exercise Finder

Upper Body Exercises

Bench Press

Exercise Type

Multijoint

Primary Muscles Trained

Chest, shoulders, triceps (pectoralis major, triceps brachii, anterior deltoids)

Beginning Position

• The student-athlete sits on the bench and tightens the upper back by retracting and depressing the scapula; this is the solid foundation from which to push the weight up.

• Lying down on the bench in a supinated five points of body contact position, the student-athlete drives the feet so that the upper back is pushed upward until the eyes are underneath the bar and the upper back is tight and providing a strong base.

• The student-athlete's back will have a slightly lordotic curve, which is normal. There is no need to hyperextend the lumbar area.

• The eyes should be focused on a spot above the bar and the shoulders because that is where the bar is going to be pushed to.

• Using a pronated closed grip, the student-athlete places the bar in the heel of the hands and grabs the bar with the hands hip-width apart while keeping the wrists stiff and locked. While the bar is being lifted, the student-athlete should attempt to squeeze the bar while pushing it up (22).

• The student-athlete should make eye contact and verbal contact with the spotter for assistance in moving the bar from the supports to the ready position directly above the chest and shoulders (22).

Movement Phases

1. The student-athlete lowers the bar to the sternum on the chest near the nipples with the elbows somewhat close to the body and the arms parallel to one another. The elbows should not be out so they are straight in line with the shoulders; rather the elbows should be somewhere between 70 to 80 degrees of abduction (22).

2. Five points of contact should be maintained throughout the exercise.

3. The student-athlete presses the bar upward, without arching or raising the buttocks, until the elbows are fully extended (23). The student-athlete drives the weight from the base of the upper back and pushes the feet into the floor. In a controlled manner, the student-athlete returns the bar to the chest and repeats until all repetitions are complete.

4. When finished, the student-athlete signals the spotter and continues holding on to the bar until it is racked and in the uprights.

Breathing Guidelines

Inhale before lowering the bar to the chest on each repetition, and exhale when the weight is raised and the repetition is finished.

Spotting Guidelines

The spotter stands very close to the student-athlete's head on the bench. The spotter must be experienced and strong enough to spot the amount of weight being lifted, should stand in a strong upright position with the knees slightly flexed and the feet hip-width apart, and should grab the bar with an alternated closed grip between the student-athlete's hands. The spotter and the student-athlete should make eye contact and communicate verbally and lift the weight from the supports on the designated signal of "ready, 1, 2, 3" (lifting up on 3). When the student-athlete has control of the bar, the spotter should gently release the grip from the bar but keep the hands very close to the bar for all the repetitions. As the weight is lowered, the spotter should flex the knees and follow the bar down while staying in a strong upright position. As the weight is raised, the spotter should follow the bar up by extending the knees and hips. As the repetitions are completed, the spotter should again be prepared to grab the bar and help the student-athlete return it to the supports. If the student-athlete is struggling, the spotter can assist the student-athlete with a forced repetition or grab the bar and help the student-athlete return it to the supports.

If the weight is very heavy, as during a maximum or testing attempt, two or three spotters should be used. If two spotters are available, one should be at one end of the bar and the other should assist the student-athlete in lifting the bar from the uprights and then walk around to the open end of the bar. Both spotters should have hands open, under, and close to the bar. If three spotters are available, as for a max-out or very heavy exercise, one spotter should stand behind the supports by the student-athlete's head and the other two should be at opposite ends of the bar. The spotters on the ends should have their hands under the bar in a supinated position and the one behind the supports and bar should have an alternated grip. The spotters should have their bodies in a strong upright position with the knees slightly flexed and the hands under the bar, and they should follow the bar down and back up. The spotter by the student-athlete's head is the one in charge.

Exercise Modifications and Variations

This exercise can also be completed with a narrow grip—a pronated closed grip with the hands inside the shoulders. A spotter should grab the bar outside the student-athlete's hands. A lighter weight should be used than with a regular bench press. Another option is to do the bench press with two dumbbells, using a pronated closed grip. In this case the spotter will assist by spotting at the two wrists and not at or under the elbow.

Coaching Tip

Have the student-athlete push the body away from the weight as they press the bar up; this activates the upper back more. While pushing the bar away, the student-athlete should act as though trying to bend the bar at the same time as also squeezing it.

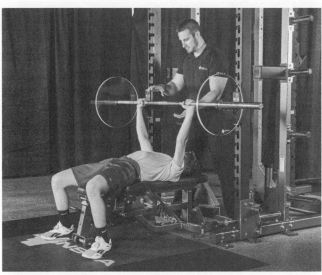

Beginning position (after lift-off) showing one spotter.

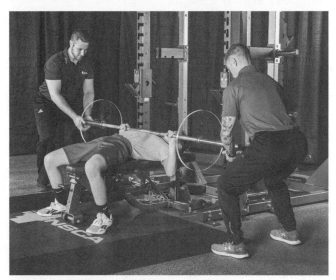

Bottom position showing two spotters.

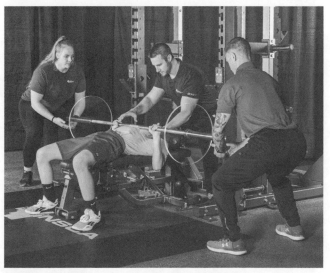

Bottom position showing three spotters.

Bent-Over Row

Exercise Type

Multijoint

Primary Muscles Trained

Upper back, shoulders (latissimus dorsi, teres major, middle trapezius, rhomboids, posterior deltoids)

Beginning Position

- The feet should be hip-width to shoulder-width apart, with the hips back in a hinge position and the body weight on the whole foot.
- Flex the knees a little, with the back and the head in a neutral position (straight, or slightly lordotic); the gaze should be down and slightly forward.
- The chest should be spread, and the hips should be close to level, with the back and shoulders very slightly elevated.
- The arms should be hanging down, extended, with the elbows out and a pronated closed grip just outside the shoulders.

Movement Phases

1. Keep a neutral (normal, slightly lordotic) spine with the trunk fixed, tight, and firm. Flex the knees slightly.

2. Pull the bar up by bending the elbows up and touch the bar near the sternum.

3. Pull smoothly. Lower the bar back down with control until the arms are once again extended with the elbows out. Repeat until the set is completed.

Breathing Guidelines

Exhale while pulling the weight toward the sternum and inhale while lowering the weight.

Coaching Tip

The student-athlete should flex the knees, with a spread chest and flat back, and "blow" the weight up.

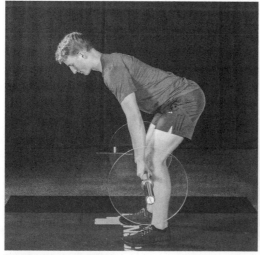

Beginning position

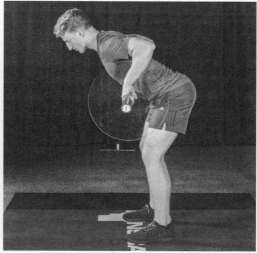

End position

Biceps Curl

Exercise Type
Single-joint

Primary Muscles Trained
Biceps (biceps brachii, brachioradialis, brachialis)

Beginning Position
- Grip the bar with a shoulder-width supinated closed grip.
- Extend the arms down, with the elbows and arms touching the trunk.
- Have the feet shoulder-width apart, with the weight on the whole foot and the knees slightly relaxed or flexed, and the toes slightly turned out.
- Stand up straight with a neutral spine and neutral head, and gaze forward.

Movement Phases
1. Keep an upright neutral spine but a rigid torso.
2. Flexing the elbows, very smoothly pull the bar up until it is near the upper chest and the anterior deltoids.
3. Lower the bar smoothly by extending the arms fully while keeping the torso upright. Repeat until the set is completed.

Breathing Guidelines
Exhale while raising the weight and inhale while lowering it.

Exercise Modifications and Variations
The biceps curl has many variations. This same exercise can be done using dumbbells while standing. The student-athlete can raise both dumbbells at once or with one arm at a time. This exercise can also be done at a padded curling

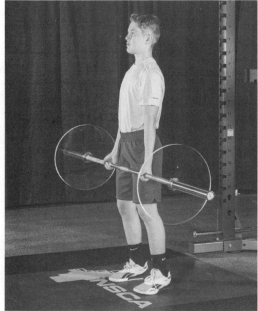

Beginning position   **End position**

station. The student-athlete sits on the seat facing the pad, rests the back of the arms and elbows on the pad, holds the bar in a supinated closed grip position, and curls the weight up toward the face until the mechanical advantage is lost, at which time the student-athlete lowers it. There are also many different machines that are designed to exercise the biceps. In this case it is important to follow the drawings and directions on the machine. Another popular version of this exercise is the hammer curl, in which the student-athlete holds the dumbbells with a neutral grip, as in holding a hammer, and curls from that position, alternating arms.

Coaching Tip

The strength and conditioning professional should help the student-athlete avoid cheating from swinging the body or bouncing the weight off the hips to gain a mechanical advantage. The student-athlete should concentrate on the biceps doing the work.

Lat Pulldown

Exercise Type

Multijoint

Primary Muscles Trained

Upper and middle back, back of shoulders (latissimus dorsi, rhomboids, middle trapezius, teres major, posterior deltoids)

Beginning Position

• To find the proper position to use the machine, the student-athlete should sit down on the seat facing the machine, adjust the pads, and place the knees or the thighs under the pads so they are secure and the feet are flat on the floor.

• Once the machine has been properly adjusted, the student-athlete should set the proper weight and then stand up, extend the arms up, grab the bar with a grip a little wider than hip-width using a closed pronated grip, and then return to the proper beginning position.

• The chest should be spread a little and the trunk leaned slightly backward.

Movement Phases

1. Pull the bar downward to the sternum or upper chest area.

2. Extend the arms slowly back to the beginning position and repeat for the necessary repetitions.

3. When finished, slowly stand up while keeping hold of the bar, and return to the beginning position.

Breathing Guidelines

Inhale while pulling the bar down and exhale while returning the bar to the beginning position.

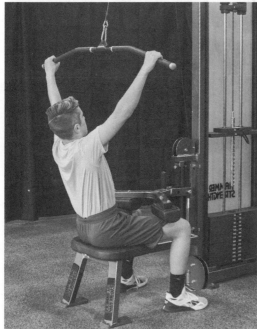
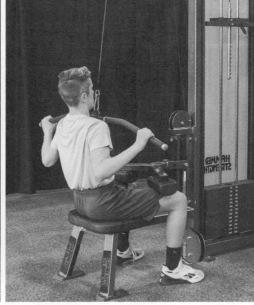

Beginning position   **End position**

Exercise Modifications and Variations

A number of different types of bars and attachments can be used for this exercise. The bar can also be gripped at different widths. Signs and directions are posted on the machines.

Coaching Tips

- Lift the weight smoothly and with control.
- Concentrate on using the back muscles and maintain a neutral spine throughout the exercise.
- "Blow" the weight up the weight stack.

Seated Barbell Shoulder Press

Exercise Type

Multijoint

Primary Muscles Trained

Front and middle shoulders and triceps (anterior and medial deltoids, triceps brachii)

Beginning Position

• Sit on a sturdy bench that is made for a seated shoulder press, with the body in a five points of contact position. This is best done in a power rack or with a sturdy bench and supports.

• Grip the bar between shoulder-width and one-fist-width out from the shoulders with a pronated, closed grip. The bar should be placed in the heel of the hand.

• A spotter should be available and in communication with the student-athlete. Using a signal of *ready, 1, 2, 3* (lifting up on *3*), lift off the standards and locate it directly above the shoulders. When steady and ready, the spotter lets go of the bar.

Movement Phases

1. Slowly lower the bar in front of the body and around the face by flexing the elbows and keeping the forearms parallel and in sync with one another to the shoulders (anterior deltoids).

2. Maintaining five points of contact, press the bar up and around the face and overhead, keeping the wrists stiff until the elbows are extended and pointing out. Repeat until the set is completed.

3. When the repetitions are completed, work with the spotter helping to rack the bar. Do not let go of the bar until it is completely racked.

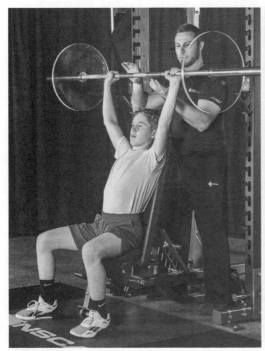

Beginning position

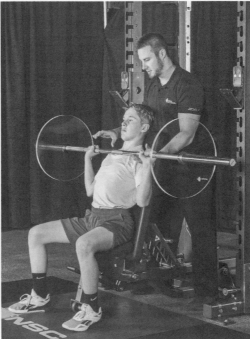

Bottom position

Breathing Guidelines

Inhale while lowering the weight and exhale while raising it.

Spotting Guidelines

It is imperative to have a spotter for this exercise. If the spotter is not tall enough, up high enough, experienced enough, and strong enough to spot properly, this exercise should not be done. All these factors are important and necessary. The spotter and the student-athlete should make sure that their communication is clear before they begin the exercise. The spotter stands behind the vertical or incline bench with a strong and stable hip-width stance, knees slightly flexed and toes slightly out. Before the exercise is begun, the spotter grabs the bar with a closed alternated grip while it is still in the rack. At the student-athlete's signal the spotter assists in moving the bar off the supports and helps locate the bar over the student-athlete's head with the student-athlete's arms fully extended. The spotter does not touch the bar but keeps an alternated grip very close to the bar as it is lowered while simultaneously keeping a strong upright torso. The spotter follows the bar back up while keeping an alternated grip that is not touching the bar. As the bar is raised, the spotter extends the hips, knees, and torso. At the signal, the spotter grabs the bar together with the student-athlete and they rack it into the supports, never letting go of the bar until it is safely in the racks.

Exercise Modifications and Variations

This exercise can also be done with dumbbells. In this variation, the student-athlete lifts the dumbbells up to the shoulders and then sits down in the five points of contact position before the exercise begins. The spotter's role is the same, except that the spotter's hands are close to the student-athlete's wrist and forearms in order to grab them if assistance is needed. Another modification is to do a shoulder press on a machine. In this modification, the student-athlete adjusts the seat and back of the machine to properly fit the body and then sits down firmly in the five points of contact position before performing the exercise.

Coaching Tips

- Push the weight up overhead, behind the ears (but not behind the head), not out and away.
- "Blow" the weight up.

Triceps Pushdown

Exercise Type
Single-Joint

Primary Muscles Trained
Triceps (triceps brachii)

Beginning Position
- Place the pin in the weight to be lifted.
- Have the body close enough to the bar so the head and torso do not touch it, but so that it can easily be grabbed with the hands while the elbows stay down and very close to the body, and the bar can still be grabbed and moved up and down with control.
- Stand with the torso upright and the knees slightly flexed with a hip-width stance.
- Grab the bar with a narrow pronated closed grip that is 6 to 10 inches (15-25 cm) apart.
- Pull the bar down so that the elbows are flexed at about 90 degrees and the upper arms are alongside the torso. Each repetition begins from this position.

Movement Phases
1. Keeping the upper body upright and somewhat rigid, push down on the bar until the elbows are fully extended. Always keep the elbows close to the body.
2. Keep the hands pronated (palms facing rear) when the arms reach full extension at the bottom.

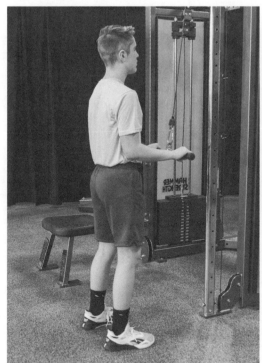
Beginning position

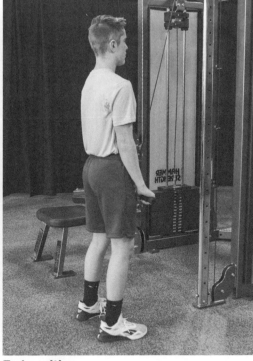
End position

3. Do not change the position of the upper arms.

4. In a controlled manner, allow the elbows to flex back to the beginning position and repeat until the set is complete.

5. When finished, lower the weight in a controlled manner back to its resting position on the stack.

Breathing Guidelines

Exhale while pushing the bar down and inhale while returning the bar to the beginning position.

Coaching Tip

In the starting and stopping positions, the student-athlete should keep the torso upright and the elbows close to the body.

Lower Body Exercises

Deadlift

Exercise Type
Multijoint

Primary Muscles Trained
Glutes, hips, thighs, hamstrings (gluteus maximus, rectus femoris, vastus medialis, vastus intermedius, vastus lateralis, semimembranosus, semitendinosus, biceps femoris)

Beginning Position
• Walk up to and touch the bar with the shins. The bar will then be right above the middle of the foot.

• The feet are flat and hip-width apart or a little narrower, with the toes out between 10 and 30 degrees.

• Lower toward the bar by doing a little hip hinge and slightly flexing the knees. Grab the knees while lowering and hinging the hips and extend the arms by pushing on them and simultaneously spreading the chest. This is called the *lock position* as it prepares and "locks in" the torso correctly (19). The student-athlete is now prepared to lower down to grab the bar.

• At this point the hips should be higher than the knees and the chest higher than the hips. The head is in front of the bar and the shoulders are slightly in front of the bar or right above it.

• Lower down to the bar by simultaneously flexing the knees and hip-hinging a little deeper and further back.

• The bar is above the middle of the foot.

• The head is neutral, the gaze forward and slightly down.

• The chest is spread, the back is neutral, and the torso is rigid.

• The head and shoulders are slightly in front of the bar and above the height of the hips.

• The hips are above the height of the knees.

• Grab the bar with a common width grip, with hands outside the knees. Place the bar in the part of the hand where the fingers meet the palm, using a pronated closed grip. This grip is also better preparation for pulling for the clean and snatch. Another option is the alternated grip.

Movement Phases
1. Begin the movement up by squeezing the glutes.

2. Extend the hips and knees while simultaneously raising the chest at the same constant rate and angle. (Important: The hips should *not* come up first, because that would cause forward movement.)

3. The arms remain extended and the elbows out.

4. As the bar comes off the floor, move the knees back until the shins are vertical and out of the path of the bar. Keep the bar tight to the body with the chest spread, the spine neutral, and the torso rigid. *Never* allow any part of the back to round; it must be kept *flat* and tight.

5. Keep the shoulders over and slightly in front of the bar until the bar passes by the knees and is halfway up the thighs, at which point the hips are extended and the legs are driven until the torso, legs, and hips are in full extension.

6. Fully extend—but do not hyperextend—the knees (22).

7. Now begin to lower the bar to the floor with control in exactly the opposite way it was lifted up. Keep the chest spread, the torso rigid, and the back flat while simultaneously flexing the hips and knees until the weight is on the floor. Alternatively, once the bar is raised it can just be dropped. Dropping it eliminates the eccentric component, however.

Breathing Guidelines

Take a deep breath before lifting the bar off the floor. Exhale when the repetition has been completed.

Exercise Modifications and Variations

The deadlift can also be done with an alternated grip; this often works very well with very heavy loads. It can also be done with a wide sumo stance and with a closed alternated grip inside of the legs.

Coaching Tips

• Use a weight belt when loads are very heavy, or when testing or maxing out.

• Keep the back flat or neutral by simultaneously spreading the chest and hip-hinging back. Hip hinge tip: Spread the chest, relax the knees, put each index finger on the same side hip crease, and just push the hips back. Keep the chest up, the back flat, and the shoulders forward. It is very important *not* to have the hips come up before the shoulders. The angle needs to remain constant, with the chest up, the legs driving, the knees and hips extended. As the bar is being lifted, imagine pushing the floor away.

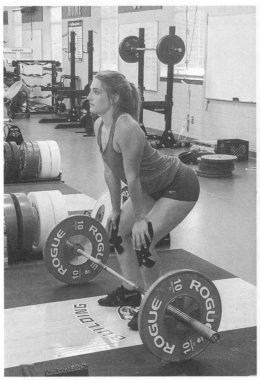

Lock position

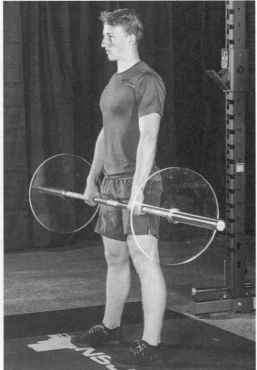

Beginning position

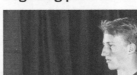

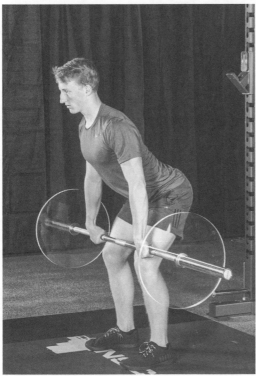

Middle of upward movement

End position

Forward Lunge With Dumbbells

Exercise Type
Multijoint

Primary Muscles Trained
Glutes, thighs, hamstrings, psoas (gluteus maximus, vastus lateralis, vastus intermedius, vastus medialis, rectus femoris, biceps femoris, semitendinosus, semimembranosus, iliopsoas)

Beginning Position
- Learn and practice the exercise with no weight first, then progress to using resistance.
- Pick up a dumbbell of the same weight in each hand with a pronated closed grip.
- The feet are parallel and hip-width apart with toes pointing forward.
- Stand up straight and tall in an area that allows enough room for a couple of steps forward and back with the arms extended down the sides of the body and the elbows and the knuckles facing outward.

Movement Phases
1. Keep the chest spread and the gaze forward.
2. Take a large step forward with one leg while keeping the torso rigid, tall, and perpendicular to the floor
3. Keep the arms extended and the elbows outward.
4. Flex the knees, hips, and ankles until the foot of the lead leg comes in contact with the floor while the rear knee comes close to the floor but does not come in contact with it.
5. The lead knee should be above the lead foot, with body weight equally balanced between both feet, which are hip-width apart. (*Note*: The exercise is more effective if done with a positive shin angle of the front leg in the lunged position. The torso should then match the angle of the shin.)
6. Keep the chest spread and the torso tall to keep from leaning forward.
7. Begin movement backward by powerfully extending the knees and hips.
8. Keep the chest spread, gaze forward, and the torso rigid and upright.
9. Bring the lead leg back until it is parallel with the other leg and foot and the body is upright.
10. Alternate feet and continue this process until all repetitions are completed.

Breathing Guidelines
Inhale as the body goes forward and the weight and the body are lowered toward the floor. Exhale as the body is driven backward to the beginning position.

Coaching Tips
- Spread the chest.
- Stay tall.
- Keep the knees above the toes.

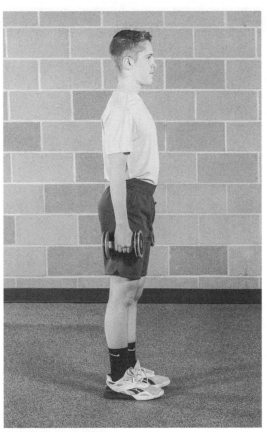

Beginning position

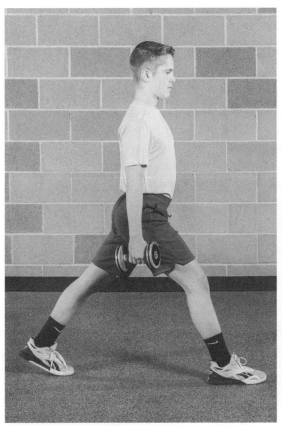

Middle of forward step

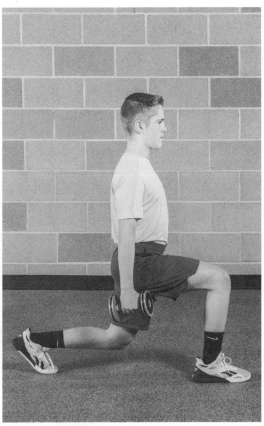

Lunged position

Good Morning

Exercise Type

Multijoint

Primary Muscles Trained

Glutes, hamstrings, muscles parallel to the spine (gluteus maximus, erector spinae, biceps femoris, semimembranosus, semitendinosus)

Beginning Position

• Place hands on the bar a little wider than hip-width using a pronated closed grip.

• Using a shallow squat stance to get under the bar, lift the elbows up and back and then place the bar at the base of the neck on the upper back and back of the shoulders.

• Spread the chest and keep the torso rigid and strong, the head neutral, the gaze slightly upward, and the feet about hip-width apart and the toes pointing slightly out.

• Stand up by extending the knees.

• Step back and away two or three steps from the uprights for clearance.

Movement Phases

1. Keeping the torso strong and rigid and the back slightly lordotic, begin a hip hinge.

2. Hip hinge by pushing the hips backward and slightly down while flexing the knees slightly.

3. Keep the back flat and slightly lordotic with the chest spread and the gaze slightly up. (Never allow the back to round.)

4. The feet remain flat as the chest and torso descend toward the floor but remain above and parallel to the floor.

5. After descending, raise the chest and torso back up by extending the hips forward and slightly extending the knees, although they will still be flexed a little. The back must not round and must remain neutral or slightly lordotic.

6. Continue until all the repetitions are completed. Then walk back into the uprights or rack and in a controlled manner set the bar on the uprights.

Breathing Guidelines

Inhale while lowering the weight and exhale while raising it.

Coaching Tips

• Push the hips back, spread the chest, and look slightly upward. If the knees do not flex on the descent, the back will round.

• Push the hips back at the same time as the knees flex.

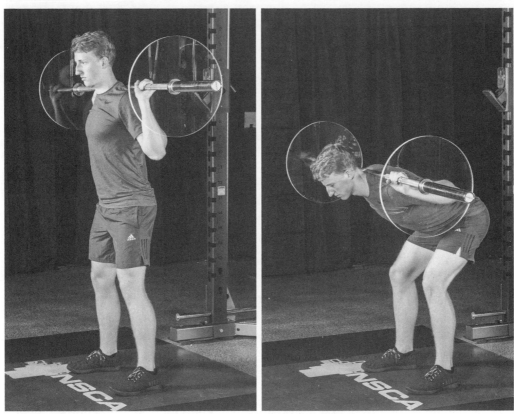

Beginning position

Bottom position

Leg Press

Exercise Type

Multijoint

Primary Muscles Trained

Glutes, thighs, hamstrings (gluteus maximus, rectus femoris, vastus intermedius, vastus lateralis, semimembranosus, semitendinosus, biceps femoris)

Beginning Position

- If the machine being used allows for it, follow the five points of contact guidelines. Sit in the machine with the head, shoulders, and hips placed firmly on the pads provided.
- Place the other two points of contact—the right foot and the left foot—hip-width apart, with the toes slightly out on the foot support provided.
- Stay in the proper position, grab the handles provided, and extend the legs out. Unlatch the lock mechanism of the machine and begin the movement.

Movement Phases

1. In a controlled manner, bring the legs and knees back toward the body to lower the weight.
2. Stay in a five points of contact position and keep the feet and knees aligned.
3. Lower the weight by flexing the knees and hips until they are parallel to the foot support.
4. Keep the whole foot in contact with the foot support the entire time.
5. Push the foot support up and away by extending the legs and keeping the knees and hips aligned.
6. At the end of the repetitions, return to the beginning position and latch the lock mechanism of the machine.

Breathing Guidelines

Inhale as the weight is lowered and exhale as the weight is pushed up.

Coaching Tip

- Maintain the five points of contact with the machine.
- "Blow" the weight up.

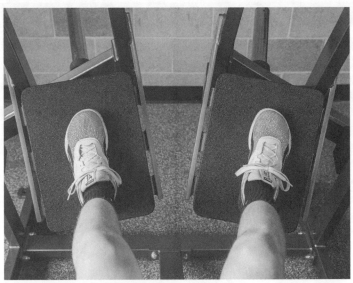

Close-up of foot placement

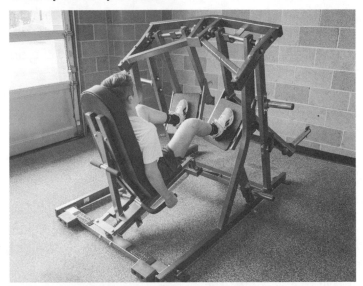

Beginning position

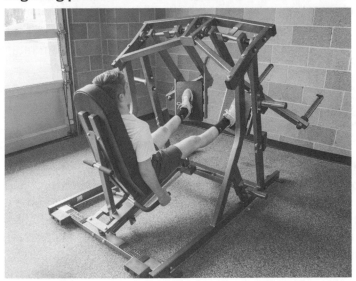

End position

Romanian Deadlift (RDL)

The Romanian deadlift is an important assistance exercise in that it prepares the body for strength movements such as squat progressions, cleans, and snatches. It also prepares the body for everyday life movements such as pushing, pulling, lifting, and carrying.

Exercise Type

Multijoint

Primary Muscles Trained

Glutes, lower back, hamstrings (gluteus maximus, erector spinae, semitendinosus, semimembranosus, biceps femoris)

Beginning Position

- This exercise can be done with either a clean grip or a snatch grip, a pronated closed grip or a pronated hook grip.
- Approach the bar and squat down with a hip hinge movement to grasp the bar (with either a hip-width "clean" grip or an outside-the-shoulders "snatch" grip).
- Keep the knuckles down, the elbows pointed out, and the arms extended but not locked.
- Keep the feet hip-width apart or a little wider and the toes slightly turned out.
- Distribute the weight across the whole foot and equally between both feet.
- Deadlift the bar and stand up with it while keeping it tight to the body.
- Flex the knees slightly, spread the chest, and keep the back neutral, the torso rigid, the head neutral, and the gaze straight ahead.

Movement Phases

1. While keeping the bar close to the body, begin to descend using a hip hinge movement by simultaneously flexing the knees and pushing the hips back, thereby moving the trunk forward.

2. The knees will track over the toes.

3. The shoulders, upper chest, and head should be slightly in front of the bar, which remains close to the body.

4. Lower the bar to the bottom of the kneecap, with the arms remaining extended during the whole exercise.

5. At this point the hips are hinged back, higher than the knees and lower than the shoulders.

6. The back is neutral (slightly lordotic), and the torso is rigid with the scapula and shoulders retracted. The back, chest, shoulders, and head will be above the hips.

7. The arms are extended, with the elbows out and a pronated closed grip.

8. At this point, begin the ascent by extending the knees and hips and raising the bar up and tight to the body. Return to the beginning position, but do not lock out the knees or hips; rather, keep them slightly flexed at the conclusion of the exercise because this keeps them prepared to hip hinge again. Repeat until all repetitions are completed.

Breathing Guidelines

Inhale while lowering the weight and exhale while raising it.

Exercise Modifications and Variations

Another version of this exercise is a straight-leg or stiff-leg deadlift. The exercise is done the same way as the RDL, except that the knees are straighter, the back more rigid (less flexed), and the descent deeper and much closer to the floor by lowering the bar until the plates touch the floor. This exercise can also be done with dumbbells.

Coaching Tip

If the student-athlete is having trouble with the hip hinge or the back is rounding, have the student-athlete try this: Stand up straight, spread the chest, flex the knees, and put the index finger of each hand on the hip crease of the same side. Keeping the back neutral, have the student-athlete push the hips back with the fingers while also slightly flexing the knees.

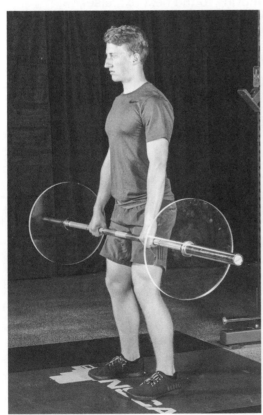

Beginning position

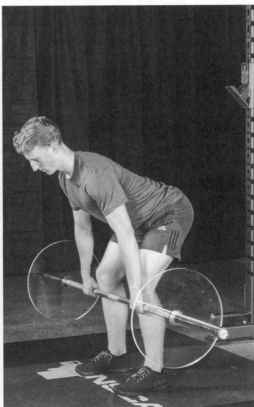

Bottom position

Squat Progressions

Squats are one of the very best ways to improve strength. Pushing, jumping, running, stopping, and lifting are very important athletic activities. All these activities are improved by doing the squat (17). Squatting also helps improve stability and strength not only within the knee but in the entire body (5). Squat strength is also important for the total body exercises to be effective.

Although squatting is a simple exercise, it is not necessarily easy for everyone to do properly. Squat progressions prepare the student-athlete to be able to do both the front and back squats effectively and correctly.

An example of a squat progression is a sequence of bodyweight squat, anchored squat, goblet squat, front squat, and back squat—either the high bar or the low bar option (10, 14). Remember, always emphasize proper movement first, without resistance. Following this progression for the squats will make it possible to see where the student-athlete may have shortcomings or flexibility issues.

Movement through the progression will vary greatly depending upon the student-athlete's flexibility. It is important that the student-athlete demonstrate competence in each progression before moving to the next exercise.

Exercise Type

Multijoint

Primary Muscles Trained for the Squat Progressions

Glutes, thighs, hamstrings (gluteus maximus, rectus femoris, vastus medialis, vastus intermedius, vastus lateralis, semimembranosus, semitendinosus, biceps femoris)

Bodyweight Squat

The bodyweight squat allows the strength and conditioning professional to assess the student-athlete's flexibility, balance, strength, and posture. This, in turn, helps to determine the appropriate next step in the progression that will ultimately enable the student-athlete to successfully do a weighted front or back squat.

Beginning Position

- Stand independently without an implement and without holding on to anything. There is no spotter.

- Have the feet hip- to shoulder-width apart (wider than what is seen in the photos) and the toes pointed out 10 degrees or a little more (more than what is seen in the photos), with the body weight distributed evenly on the whole foot.

- Stand upright with the chest spread and a neutral spine.

- The head is neutral, and the gaze is straight ahead at about eye height or a little above.

- The arms may be extended ahead and held out parallel to the floor (as shown in the photo) or with the elbows flexed and the hands just above the shoulders with the thumbs pointed down to the shoulders (like when doing a front squat).

Movement Phases

1. Begin the descent by flexing both the knees and the hips at the same time and at the same rate. This is a critical component for success.

2. While descending by flexing the knees over the toes, keep the trunk upright and the spine neutral (slightly lordotic).

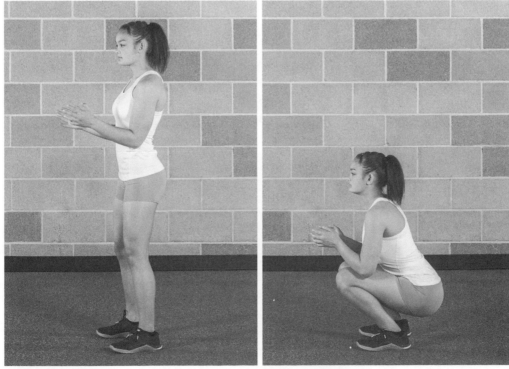

Beginning position   **Bottom position**

3. The ultimate objective of a great squat is to squat to a depth that puts the hip crease below the knee. Going to this depth generates more strength and muscle and develops protection for the knee. Attempt to descend to a depth at which the hip crease is below that of the knee as seen in the second photo. The hips drop between the legs and the heels.

4. While still on the whole foot, begin the ascent up from the bodyweight squat with a concentrated drive from the heel, extending the hips and legs simultaneously until a standing position is reached. Repeat until the set is completed.

Breathing Guidelines

Inhale while descending and exhale while ascending.

Coaching Tips

- Hinge the hips and the knees at the same time.
- Drive the hips and the legs up at the same time by extending them.
- Spread the chest.
- It is very important not to allow the knees to come inward (valgus); keep the knees over the toes.

Note: Not all student-athletes will be able to do this squat correctly nor descend to the depth shown in the second photo. If flexibility is not very good or there is not good postural control, it is important to learn and do the anchored squat, which will be next in the progression. It may also be necessary to change the desired descent level temporarily to where the top of the thigh is parallel to the floor. Everyone is different.

Anchored Squat

The bodyweight squat offers a very quick assessment and understanding of the student-athlete's abilities and body control during a squat. The anchored squat allows the student-athlete to grab hold of something to anchor them into a solid, sturdy position in which they can assist themselves slightly with their arms if necessary. A student-athlete who has mastered the bodyweight squat can next progress to the anchored squat to learn how it feels to flex the knees and the hips at the same time and how it feels to drop the hips between the legs and the heels and slightly behind the heels. Even the most experienced squatters learn from this. If the bodyweight squat did not go well, the anchored squat will be one of the keys to developing flexibility and proper body control for the squat (14).

Beginning Position

• Stand within 3 or 4 inches (8-10 cm) of a solid, upright pole or the upright part of a power rack (closer than what is seen in the photo) to anchor to a sturdy, solid position.

• The feet will be hip- to shoulder-width apart (slightly wider than what is seen in the photos), with the toes turned out 10 to 30 degrees and the weight distributed evenly over both feet. The legs are parallel and the knees track over the feet.

• The chest is spread, the torso is upright, and the spine is neutral.

• The head is neutral and the gaze is straight ahead or slightly up.

• Grab the upright loosely with both hands a little above waist height.

Movement Phases

1. Standing erect and holding on to the upright, begin descending by flexing the knees and hips simultaneously and at the same rate. Keep the trunk upright, spread the chest, and retract and depress the shoulder blades. If the hips go back first it means that they are flexing first rather than the knees and hips flexing at the same time. This simultaneous flexing is the purpose of this exercise.

2. Keep the weight distributed evenly over the feet while descending to a depth where the hip flexors are slightly below the knees. It is important to drop the hips straight down between the legs and heels, and a little behind the heels. If it is not possible to achieve that depth yet, that will become a target for practicing this exercise, and in the meantime should change the immediate goal to that of lowering the top of the thigh to be parallel to the floor.

3. Begin the ascent by driving through the feet (a little more toward the heels), with the hips and knees simultaneously extending until upright. It is fine to control the balance somewhat by gripping the upright. Continue until all repetitions are complete.

Breathing Guidelines

Inhale while descending and exhale while ascending.

Coaching Tips

• The hips and knees need to flex and extend at the same time for this to be done correctly. If the hips flex first, it is as though the student-athlete were sitting back into a chair, which is incorrect.

- Give a coaching cue of "drop straight down." (This seems to make the student-athlete flex the knees and the hips at the same time.) The upright the student-athlete is standing directly in front of and holding on to the anchor will help keep the back upright because it keeps the student-athlete from leaning forward very far. If the hips go back first, the chest will bump into the bar and prevent a proper descent. *Note*: This prepares the student-athlete for front squats and high bar back squats. A low bar back squat is used by powerlifters who want to have the torso lean more forward.

If the student-athlete demonstrates competence in the anchored squat, the next step in the progression is the goblet squat. The rate at which student-athletes go through the progression depends upon the individual. Some may go through it in one or two days and others may take 2 or 3 weeks to progress through the first three exercises of the progression. These progressive exercises may need to be revisited periodically to fix technique issues.

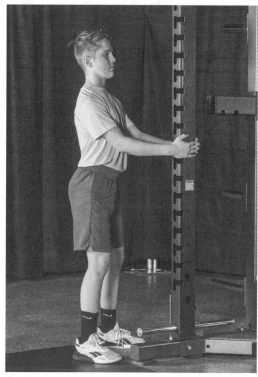
Beginning position

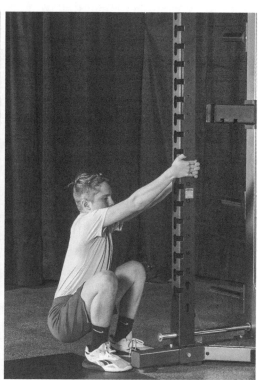
End position

Goblet Squat

A goblet squat is a squat with a kettlebell or a dumbbell being held like a big cup filled with liquid. The objective is to squat while holding it and not spill any fluid, which indicates that the student-athlete is doing a smooth and balanced multijoint squat (3).

Exercise Type

Multijoint

Primary Muscles Trained

Glutes, thighs, hamstrings (gluteus maximus, rectus femoris, vastus medialis, vastus intermedius, vastus lateralis, semimembranosus, semitendinosus, biceps femoris)

Beginning Position

• The student-athlete picks up and holds a light- to medium-weight kettlebell by the horns with the horns at the top of the kettlebell. (A dumbbell will also work and is shown in the photos.)

• The feet are hip- to shoulder-width apart, with the toes pointed out 10 to 30 degrees and the weight distributed evenly over both feet. The legs are parallel.

• The chest is spread and the torso is upright, with the spine neutral.

• The head is neutral and the gaze is straight ahead or slightly up.

• The goblet is held in front of the student-athlete against the body, with the hands on the horns at the top, elbows flexed and facing down, and the bell on the bottom.

• The elbows are held such that during descent they will be on the inside of (or directly over) the legs.

Movement Phases

1. The student-athlete begins to descend, holding the goblet in front and against the body while standing in an upright position with a spread chest and neutral spine.

2. To descend, the student-athlete flexes both the hips and knees simultaneously and does a controlled squat right between the legs to the point where the hip crease is below the knees. If the student-athlete is unable to squat below parallel, squatting to parallel might become the temporary immediate goal.

3. The knees continue to track over the feet (the toes of which are turned slightly outward), which allows the hips to drop between the legs.

4. Keep the torso-to-floor ratio the same throughout the whole descent.

5. Upon reaching the bottom of the squat, drive the legs and hips through the feet (toward the heel) to extension while keeping the torso upright with a neutral spine.

6. Stand up, keeping the chest spread and the torso erect until upright, but knees not locked.

7. Repeat for the designated number of repetitions.

This exercise prepares the student-athlete by improving hip and trunk mobility, balance, better understanding of concentric drive, and preparing to handle weight.

Breathing Guidelines

Inhale while lowering the weight and exhale while raising it.

Coaching Tips

- Keep the goblet tight to the body.
- Sit and rise tall.
- Hip and knee drive at the same time; do not let hips rise first.

Once this exercise is done with competence, the student-athlete is ready to do a front squat.

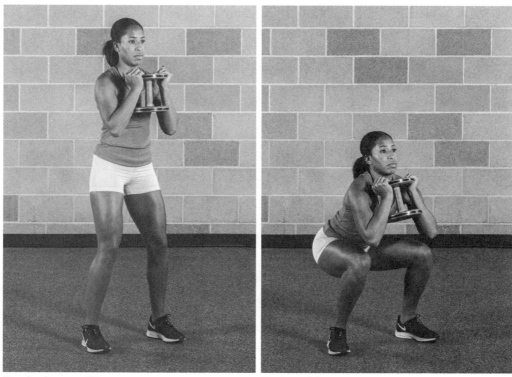

Beginning position   **End position**

Front Squat

A successful and competent front squat is a prerequisite for doing a correct deep squat clean (3).

Exercise Type

Multijoint

Primary Muscles Trained

Glutes, thighs, hamstrings (gluteus maximus, rectus femoris, vastus medialis, vastus intermedius, vastus lateralis, semimembranosus, semitendinosus, biceps femoris)

Before Beginning

• To set the proper height for the bar, stand with the shoulder next to the end of the bar in the rack. The bar should be set at a height matching the middle of the medial deltoid on the shoulder.

• Set the safety bars 1 to 2 inches (3-5 cm) below the height of the bar on the shoulders during the deepest part of the squat. The safety bar should be at a height that will not impede the exercise but close enough to keep the student-athlete safe.

• Put collars on the bar to secure the weights.

Beginning Position

• Begin with an empty bar or with a light weight that is appropriate for learning the movement properly.

• Grasp the bar with the hands about hip-width apart or within a fist-width of the shoulders. Use a pronated and closed grip.

• Dip under the bar with both legs parallel in a square stance.

• Place the bar on the anterior deltoids by flexing the elbows and pushing them forward and up so they are parallel with the floor. The bar should not be on the clavicle or the throat.

• Keep the chest spread, the spine and the head neutral, and the gaze straight ahead or raised slightly (3).

Movement Phases

1. Communicate with the spotter and lift the bar off the supports on the count of *ready, 1, 2, 3* (stand up with the bar on *3*). Be sure to remain upright and straight and under control. Then take a step or two back.

2. Place the feet hip- to shoulder-width apart (wider than what is seen in the second or third photos) and the toes out 10 to 30 degrees (more than what is seen in the photos), with the weight distributed evenly between both feet.

3. Keeping the chest spread, the spine neutral, the torso tight, and the elbows up, begin to descend by flexing the knees and hips at the same time.

4. Squat down between the legs with the hip crease below the knees. If unable to squat to this depth, have a temporary goal of squatting parallel to the floor or go back to one of the previous squat progressions to work on flexibility.

5. Begin the ascent by squeezing the glutes, driving and extending the hips and knees at the same time while pushing through the feet (more toward the heel). While driving the legs up the knees remain above the toes.

6. Continue until all repetitions are completed. Stand completely upright, but with the knees not locked.

7. When finished, walk into the rack with the spotter's help and guidance. At the instruction "down," lower safely to the supports.

Breathing Guidelines

Inhale before descending in the front squat. It is usual to hold the breath throughout the squat. Many will begin to exhale a little on the ascent and exhale the rest of the air at the completion of the exercise. Most student-athletes do the Valsalva maneuver naturally. *Note*: The Valsalva maneuver should never be held for more than 2 seconds; doing so could be dangerous by raising blood pressure and creating dizziness. It is important to keep the bar off the carotid artery and the clavicle. For more detail, refer to the Effective Breathing Patterns section earlier in the chapter that explains the Valsalva maneuver.

Spotting Guidelines

See the sidebar on Spotting Guidelines for the Front Squat and the Back Squat earlier in this chapter.

Coaching Tips

• Weight belts are recommended for loads that are considered heavy for the particular student-athlete. (Refer to the Key Fundamentals to Exercise Technique section.)

• Keep the elbows up and parallel to keep the back from rounding. Sit tall with the chest up in front.

Note: Student-athletes who find it difficult to rack the bar properly on the front of the shoulders should continue to do goblet squats while at the same time working on increasing wrist flexibility.

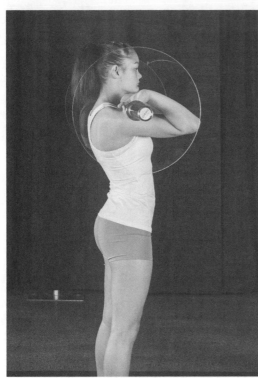

Close-up of the arm position with the bar racked at the shoulders

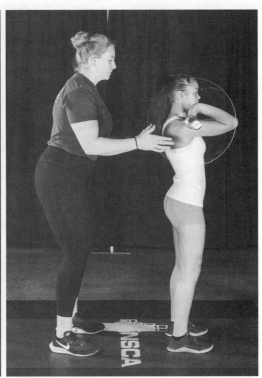

Beginning position

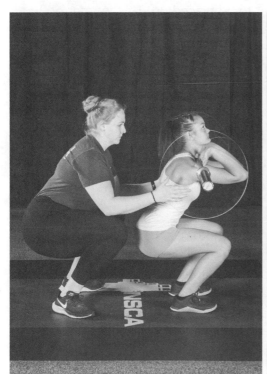

Normal parallel front squat bottom position showing one spotter

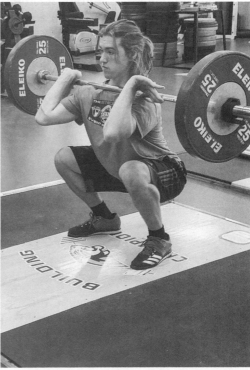

Advanced deep front squat bottom position (shown for body position only)

Back Squat

A back squat can be done with either a high bar or a low bar (10).

Exercise Type

Multijoint

Primary Muscles Trained

Glutes, thighs, hamstrings (gluteus medius, rectus femoris, vastus medialis, vastus intermedius, vastus lateralis, semimembranosus, semitendinosus, biceps femoris)

Before Beginning

• Set the height of the bar by locating the uprights at the height of the middle of the medial deltoid (on the shoulder) and make sure the safety bars in the rack are set to the proper height.

• Put collars on the bar to secure the weights.

Beginning Position

• Grasp the bar with the hands about hip-width apart or within fist-width of the shoulders. Use a pronated and closed grip.

• Dip under the bar, resting it on the upper trapezius and the posterior deltoids at the base of the neck, with the legs parallel in a square stance.

• Lift the elbows up, in, and back. This will create a shelf on the upper trapezius and the posterior deltoids for the bar to be placed on. This is referred to as a *high bar squat*. *Note*: Do not place the bar on the vertebral bone(s). Make sure it is on the muscle instead.

• Keep the chest spread, the spine neutral, and the head neutral and up, with the gaze straight ahead or raised slightly.

• Pull down slightly on the bar.

Movement Phases

1. Communicate with the spotter and lift the bar off the supports on the count of *ready, 1, 2, 3* (stand up with the bar on *3*). Be sure to remain upright and straight and under control. Then take a step or two back.

2. Place the feet shoulder-width apart, the toes turned out 10 to 30 degrees (more than what is seen in the second or third photos), and the weight distributed evenly over both feet.

3. Keeping the chest spread, the spine neutral, the torso tight, and the elbows up, begin to descend by flexing the knees and hips at the same time.

4. At the start of the descent, the forearms and elbows should be parallel with the torso and the shins. They should all be in alignment if the form is correct.

5. Pull downward somewhat on the bar as it rests on the posterior deltoids and the upper trapezius.

6. Retract and depress the shoulder blades.

7. The knees track over the toes.

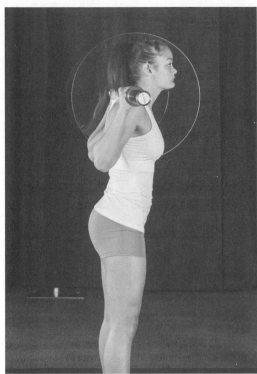

Close-up of the bar racked on the upper back at the base of the neck

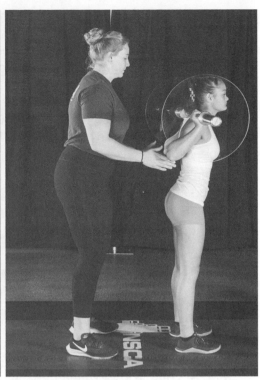

Beginning position

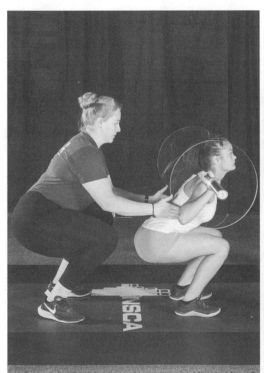

Normal parallel back squat bottom position showing one spotter

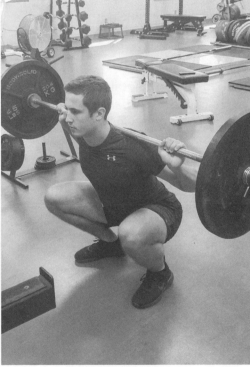

Advanced deep back squat bottom position (shown for body position only)

8. Squat down between the legs and heels until the hip crease is parallel with the knees, keeping the chest spread and the back and the head neutral the whole time. Often a parallel squat is the lowest depth that can be safely attained by those who are untrained and inexperienced and those with longer limb length or flexibility issues. This is normal and acceptable for many. An advanced back squat involves squatting below parallel as seen in the last photo in the series. If reaching a depth below parallel is difficult but attainable over time, the student-athlete may want to make a short-term goal of squatting parallel to the floor or go back to one of the previous squats in the progression to improve flexibility.

9. Begin the ascent by squeezing the glutes, driving and extending the hips and legs at the same time while also pushing through the feet (more toward the heel) and the middle of the foot.

10. Continue until the required repetitions are completed. Stand completely upright, but with the knees not locked.

11. When finished, walk into the rack with the spotter's help and guidance. At the instruction "down," lower safely to the supports. Keep control of the bar until it is set firmly in the rack supports (14, 21, 23).

Breathing Guidelines

See the comments provided in the Breathing Guidelines section of the front squat, and for more detail, refer to the Effective Breathing Patterns section earlier in the chapter that explains the Valsalva maneuver.

Spotting Guidelines

See the sidebar on Spotting Guidelines for the Front Squat and the Back Squat earlier in this chapter.

Exercise Variation

The back squat can also be done with the bar located lower down on the back. This is called a *low bar squat* and is common for competitive powerlifters. In this variation, the bar is located lower on the back across the middle of the trapezius and across the posterior deltoids (10).

Coaching Tips

• A belt should be used with loads that are very heavy or during testing or maxing out.

• Sit tall and drive the hips and the legs. The instruction "chest up first" will help make the student-athlete be sure to keep the hips and knees extended at the same time. If they are not extended at the same time, the buttocks will raise too fast and the chest will lower, and the weight will be transferred forward and to the front part of the foot, causing the student-athlete to lose strength, proper position, and control. This leads to injuries.

Standing Calf Raise

The standing calf raise can be performed using a selectorized or a plate-loaded machine. Those machines are less common in a weight room, so a simple step or raised surface can be used. (*Note:* The exercise is described as if the student-athlete is using a machine, but the photos show the exercise being performed using a step.)

Exercise Type

Single joint

Primary Muscles Trained

Calves (gastrocnemius, soleus)

Beginning Position

- Adjust the pads and the footpad if needed.
- Set the pin in the weight rack at the appropriate weight.
- Get underneath the pads in a position in which everything is balanced. Stand upright with the legs extended and parallel, with a firm torso.
- Grip the handles located by the shoulder pads.
- Step onto the footpad with the feet hip-width apart. The knees should not be locked but slightly flexed.

Movement Phases

1. Keep the balls of the feet on the footpad edge. Lower the heels to a slight stretch position, but one that causes no discomfort.

2. Push straight up as high as possible on the toes while keeping the legs and knees extended. Do this in a controlled manner.

3. In a controlled fashion, lower the heels back to the beginning position. Repeat until the set is complete.

Breathing Guidelines

Exhale while rising up on the balls of the feet and inhale while lowering the heels.

Exercise Modification

Another effective calf exercise, which targets the soleus more, is the seated calf raise. This exercise is done sitting on a seat, usually facing a weight or rack, and placing the thighs and knees under a pad that will need to be adjusted to the appropriate position. Place the ball of the foot on a support under the weight or lever and lower the heels. It may be necessary to rise up high on the balls of the feet in order to enable the machine to work and to unhook or free a lever. Then lower the heels to a position where there is no discomfort and push up again to the balls of the feet. Repeat until the set is completed. Then raise up the weight and hook the lever to the beginning position again.

Coaching Tips

- Keep the legs parallel to each other with the knees extended but not locked.
- Use a weight that helps and challenges but that does not hurt or cause discomfort other than fatigue.

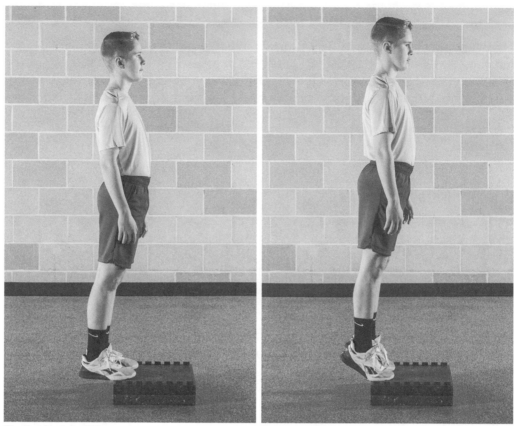

Beginning position   **End position**

Total Body Exercises

It is very important to use the proper implements when learning how to perform power-based total body exercises. Light bars, steel rods, or dowels should be available as tools here. It is important to do the movements with a weight that is light enough to allow the repetitions to be performed without strain, so the proper neural patterns can be developed. It is important that the instructors are CSCS- or USAW-certified and experienced in teaching these exercises and progressions. Resistance should be increased in the exercises based upon technical competence and strength levels. All parts of the progressions of these exercises require the use of the hip hinge movement. The ability to do the power clean and the power snatch with technical competence is greatly enhanced by learning and practicing the following progressions regularly.

Power Clean Progressions

Sports and athletic movements require pushing, pulling, accelerating, stopping, jumping, landing, and power that is initiated at floor level. The power clean is a ground-based exercise that develops tremendous amounts of power, uses the whole kinetic chain, and improves athleticism. The power clean and the squat clean are important because they develop movements that create tremendous amounts of power, which translates directly to sports activities and movements (6, 20).

The student-athlete must be competent in the front squat before beginning to train for the power clean, because the skill to catch the bar with a properly executed front squat is important in order to complete the exercise successfully. Competence in each of these progressions should be demonstrated before moving on to the next. The term *power clean* means that the bar will be caught with the hips above parallel. An advanced student-athlete's goal is to catch the weight with the hips below parallel, in what is known as a *squat clean*.

The power clean progressions are these: muscle clean, clean from the power position, clean from high knee or hang clean, power clean from the floor, clean from the floor. These are done in a top-down progression (4, 6, 7, 9, 18, 20).

Exercise Type

Multijoint

Primary Muscles Trained for the Power Clean Progressions

Glutes, back, thighs, hamstrings, calves (gluteus maximus, trapezius, deltoids, rectus femoris, vastus intermedius, vastus medialis, vastus lateralis, semitendinosus, semimembranosus, biceps femoris, soleus, gastrocnemius)

Muscle Clean

Beginning Position

• Stand upright holding on to a bar. Place the bar high on the thighs, where pockets would be, with the hands about hip-width or one fist wider and a pronated hook grip.

• Have the feet hip-width to a little wider apart, with the legs parallel, the toes out slightly, and the weight distributed evenly over the whole foot.

• Keep the arms extended, with the elbows rotated out and the knuckles facing down.

• Keep the knees slightly flexed.

• Keep the torso upright and the back and the head neutral with the gaze straight forward.

Movement Phases

1. It is important to keep the bar close to the body.

2. Slightly extend the knees and the hips and pull the bar up close to the body by shrugging the shoulders up while simultaneously pulling the elbows up to about parallel with the shoulders and above the hands. Keep the bar tight. Move to a scarecrow position (not seen in the photos).

3. Now turn the bar over by rotating the hands under the bar and driving the elbows forward and up so that the bar is rotated on top of the anterior deltoids and the upper arms are parallel with the floor. Place the bar on the front of the shoulders, not on the clavicle or on the throat.

4. Lower the bar back to the beginning position and repeat until the set is complete.

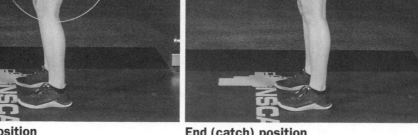

Beginning position   End (catch) position

Power Position Pull and Catch for the Clean

Biomechanically, this is an incredibly powerful position for the body, so it needs to be practiced consistently.

Beginning Position

- Grip the bar in the same way as for the muscle clean, with the arms extended and the elbows rotated outward.

- Have the feet flat and hip-width apart or slightly wider, with the toes turned out 5 to 10 degrees or a little more.

- Flex the knees slightly, with the hips hinged back just enough so that the shoulders are above but just a little in front of the bar.

- Rest the bar on the high part of the thighs, where a pocket would be.

- Have the weight on the whole foot but concentrated more on the heels.

- Keep the chest spread, the torso upright, and the back and the head neutral.

- Keep the gaze straight ahead or a little bit up.

Movement Phases

1. Forcefully drive the legs and the hips straight up into extension while simultaneously shrugging the shoulders up violently.

2. When the leg and hip drive are almost complete, immediately pull up on the bar with the shoulders and the elbows until the elbows rise above the hands and are close to shoulder height.

3. Catch the bar on the front of the shoulders (anterior deltoid), with the elbows, hands, and upper arms in the same position as for the muscle clean finish: parallel with the floor.

4. While pulling under the bar, slide the feet a shoe-width wider sideways to be able to catch the bar in a front squat position. Catching in a deep front squat position is preferable. Not everyone can achieve this depth right away, so catching it in a power clean position (legs slightly above parallel) is acceptable. Advanced student-athletes should have a goal of dropping below parallel on the catch. The hips should be the first part of the body to drop under the bar, dropping straight down between the legs and the heels.

5. Once the weight is caught and control of the bar and weight is achieved, extend the hips and legs forcefully and simultaneously while keeping the upper torso upright and rigid and the elbows to return to a standing position.

6. Then extend the arms to reset, and once again flex the knees and do a hip hinge to the beginning position. Repeat until the set is complete.

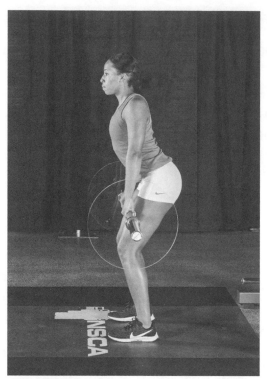

Beginning position

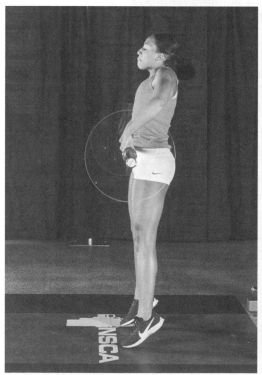

Almost highest bar position

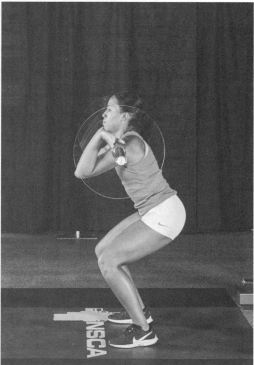

End (catch) position (above parallel)

Hang Clean

This position is an important component of doing the power clean because it prepares the student-athlete to move properly from the transition into the power position.

Movement Phases

1. Get into the high knee position by starting in the power position and lowering the bar against the thighs while the hips hinge further back and down until the bar is directly above the kneecap.

2. Keep the chest spread, the torso rigid, and the back and the head neutral.

3. Push the knees back as the bar is lowered to above the kneecap, so that the shins are vertical, and the weight is on the middle of the foot.

4. Have the head and shoulders in front of the bar, the arms extended, and the scapula and shoulders retracted and depressed.

5. Have the shoulders higher than the hips and the hips above the knees. This is the beginning position for each repetition.

6. Keeping the bar close to the body, begin the ascent with an aggressive pull and a forceful knee and hip extension.

7. As the bar rises up the thighs to the power position, shift the weight to the heel; the knees will go slightly forward as the torso rises, right before full extension.

8. The catch and finish are the same as for the power position catch and finish.

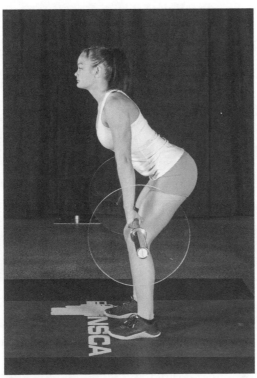

Beginning position

Power Clean

A power clean is a movement in which the weight is pulled and lifted from the floor and is caught with the legs in such a position that the thighs and hips are above a parallel position to the floor. (An advanced and more effective catch would be a deep squat clean catch with the hips below the knees.)

Beginning Position

It can be difficult for untrained and inexperienced student-athletes to lower themselves down to the bar with proper form to do the power clean. This is a challenging position for those with flexibility issues. A process called **lock and load** can help properly teach and develop the proper beginning position for the movement. This could become a normal routine while doing power exercises on the platforms, because it helps ensure that the start of each exercise will be correct and consistent. An incorrect or inconsistent start on a platform exercise greatly raises the probability of technical mistakes and misses. The purpose of this exercise is to improve the likelihood of technical competence and consistency.

Lock Position to Set up the Load (or Beginning) Position Correctly

- Walk up to the bar within 1 inch (3 cm) of the shins.

- Stand with a hip-width or slightly wider stance with the toes turned out slightly or up to 5 to 10 degrees.

- Hip hinge back and grab the knees with the hands. While holding on to the knees, extend the arms and spread the chest to lock the back and torso into a strong, rigid position with the back neutral. As with the lock position of the deadlift (see page 117), this lock position for the power clean locks the body in a good position to correctly move to the load, or beginning, position (19).

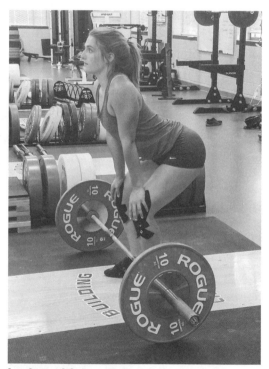

Lock position

Load (or Beginning) Position

- Go down to the bar by simultaneously flexing and lowering the hips and knees to a position in which the bar can be grasped.

- Have the feet hip-width to shoulder-width apart. Point the toes out slightly 5 to 10 degrees or more. The knees should push out against the elbows (arms) and be tracking somewhat over the toes.

- As the body is lowered to the bar, the shins and the knees will come forward and in front of the bar.

- The bar should be above the balls of the feet.

- The grip should be a pronated hook grip about outside of the legs, or a little wider.

• The joints of the shoulders should be directly above the bar, and the top of the shoulders and head should be in front of the bar.

• The shoulders and the head are higher than the hips, and the hips are slightly higher than the knees.

• Keep the chest spread and the back neutral, with the scapula retracted and depressed and the torso rigid.

• Keep the head slightly up and the gaze straight ahead or slightly up.

• Extend the arms, with the elbows rotated out and the knuckles down.

• Concentrate the body weight on the whole foot.

• Just prior to the exercise, very lightly pull up on the bar without moving it up, thus putting a little tension on it.

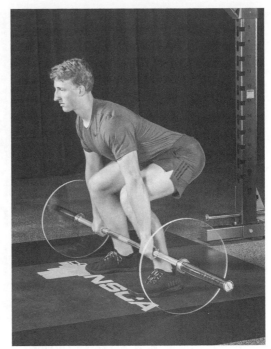
Beginning position

Movement Phases

Phase 1: First Pull from the Power Position

1. Begin ascent by forcefully driving the legs and hips into extension.

2. As the bar begins to rise from the floor, drive the legs until the knees and shins are vertical, with the bar kept tight to the body.

3. Keep the shoulder blades retracted and depressed, with a neutral spine.

4. The rate and angle between the hips and shoulders must remain the same while the bar is pulled up to the top of the kneecaps. Do not raise the hips first.

5. Keep the arms extended with the elbows out.

Transition

1. Continue a powerful knee and hip extension as the bar rises above the knees. It is very important to keep the shoulders in front of and over the bar until about mid-thigh. Keep the bar close to the body.

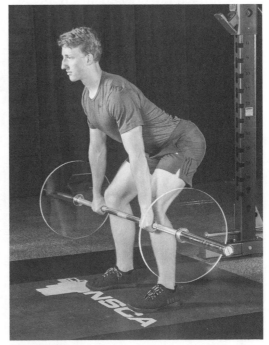
First pull

2. Keep the back neutral and the torso rigid as the bar and the torso rise.

3. Keep the arms extended. The pressure is still on the whole foot but concentrated on the middle of the foot while the bar is being pulled back into the body and nears the power position.

Phase 2: Second Pull from the Power Position

1. As the bar contacts the body at high thigh or high pocket level (the power position), weight distribution on the feet moves more toward the heel, and the knees flex slightly forward, putting the body in the power position.

2. At this point, the torso and the head are above and slightly in front of the bar, the gaze is forward and slightly up, and the bar remains close to the body.

3. The legs and hips drive into full powerful extension straight up while the feet remain in contact with the floor. If the legs and hips keep driving with extension through the whole foot, but a little more toward the heels, the student-athlete can maximize the power that can be produced. The force produced will often cause the upper part of the body and the head to lean back slightly at the top.

4. As the legs and hips are completing full extension with the bar tight to the body, the body will reach maximum height and velocity. (It is common at this point for the student-athlete to go into triple-joint extension or to the ball of the foot as a result of really hard leg and hip drive.)

5. As maximum height and velocity is reached, and the legs and hips are fully extended, the feet and legs will often slightly widen about a shoe width or less to descend under the weight.

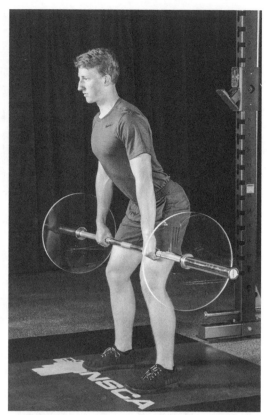

Transition

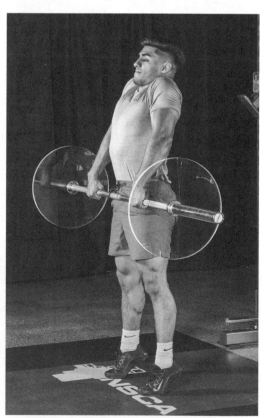

Second pull (showing a different model)

Phase 3: Extension and Catch

1. To help descend under the bar for the catch, pull the body rapidly under the bar by powerfully shrugging the shoulders and trapezius and pulling the elbows up until they are near the height of the shoulders and above the hands.

2. Pull the bar onto the anterior deltoids (front of the shoulders) by rotating the hands and elbows under and around the bar.

3. At the same time, move the feet slightly out and flex the hips and the knees so the body can rest solidly on the whole foot of both feet as the weight is caught.

4. Catching the weight above the line of the thigh when it is parallel with the floor is called a power clean.

5. This catch is completed with the student-athlete sitting tall, with the elbows up and the upper arms up and parallel with the floor, the feet solidly on the floor, and the torso upright (3).

6. Stand up with the weight through the leg and hip extension, safely drop the weight in front of the body to the floor, and repeat until the set is complete. Make sure to start the squat up while sitting tall and driving and extending the knees and hips at the same time. Do not squat up with the hips first, because the load will move forward.

Breathing Guidelines

• Inhale just before lowering to grab the bar immediately prior to the pull. It is usual to hold the breath throughout the pull, the catch, and part of the ascent. Many will begin to exhale a little on the ascent and finish exhaling at the completion of the exercise. Most student-athletes will do this naturally.

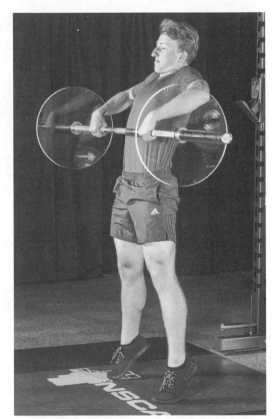

Pulling the elbows up to contribute to the highest bar position

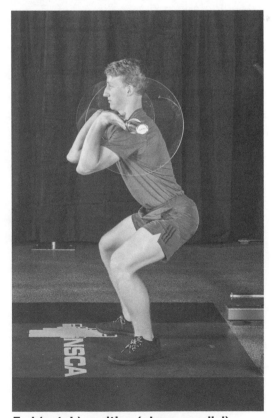

End (catch) position (above parallel)

• The Valsalva maneuver often takes place naturally on the ascent. It is also often done on purpose. *Note*: The Valsalva maneuver should never be held for more than 2 seconds; doing so could be dangerous by raising blood pressure and creating dizziness. It is important to keep the bar off the carotid artery and the clavicle.

Exercise Modification

The most effective version of this exercise is the squat clean, the difference being that the catch is in a low or deep squat position with the hips below parallel. This develops more strength and flexibility and is more athletic.

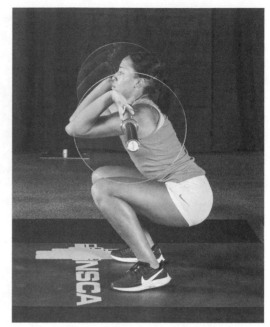

End (catch) position (advanced, deep)

Coaching Tips

• When a heavy weight is being used, it may be advantageous for the student-athlete to use a weight belt. Weight belts should not be used for lifting light weight because that would hinder the development of synergists and the abdominals.

• It is important to continue to drive the legs and the hips to achieve full extension and power.

• When catching the bar, it is very important to keep the elbows up and sit tall and drive the legs; do not let the hips come up first. Remember: chest up first and drive the legs.

• Keep the bar tight.

Power Snatch Progressions

Always emphasize proper movement first, without resistance. It is important for the student-athlete to demonstrate competence in each progression before moving to the next exercise. Sports and athletic movements require power that is initiated at floor level. The power snatch is a ground-based exercise that develops tremendous amounts of power, uses the whole kinetic chain, and improves athleticism. The power snatch and the squat snatch are important because they develop tremendous amounts of power that translates directly to sports activities and movements just as the clean does (6, 20). Before doing the snatch, the student-athlete must be competent in doing the overhead squat, because that is the catch position when doing the snatch.

Power snatch progressions are similar to the clean: muscle snatch, snatch from the power position, hang snatch, power snatch from the floor, advanced deep squat snatch from the floor. (4, 9). The progressions here are also top-down, as with the clean (4, 6, 7, 9, 18, 20).

Exercise Type

Multijoint

Primary Muscles Trained for the Power Snatch Progressions

Glutes, back, shoulders, thighs, hamstrings, calves (gluteus maximus, trapezius, deltoids, rectus femoris, vastus intermedius, vastus medialis, vastus lateralis, semitendinosus, semimembranosus, biceps femoris, soleus, gastrocnemius)

Muscle Snatch

Beginning Position

- Stand-upright holding a bar in the hands with a pronated hook grip and the hands outside of the legs with a snatch-width grip.
- Have the feet hip-width to a little wider apart, with the legs parallel and the toes turned out slightly and the weight distributed evenly over the whole foot.
- Keep the arms extended and the elbows rotated out, with the knuckles facing down.
- Keep the knees slightly flexed with a very slight hip hinge.
- Keep the torso upright, the back and the head neutral, and the gaze straight forward.

Movement Phases

1. It is important to keep the bar close to the body.

2. Extend the knees and hips and pull the bar up close to the body by shrugging the shoulders up while simultaneously pulling the elbows up to the height of the shoulders and above the hands (not seen in the photos).

3. Pull the bar up and over the head at this point and rotate the hands under the bar and hold it above the head.

4. Lower the bar back to the beginning position and repeat until the set is complete.

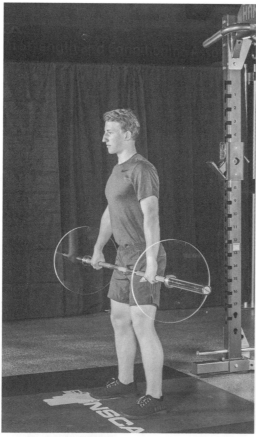

Beginning position

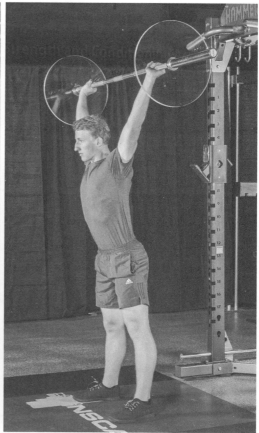

End position

Power Position Pull and Catch for the Snatch

Biomechanically, this is an incredibly powerful position for the body, and it needs to be practiced consistently.

Beginning Position

• The pronated hook grip for the bar is the same as for the muscle snatch, and the arms are extended with the elbows rotated outward.

• Have the feet flat and hip-width apart or slightly wider, with the toes turned out slightly or up to 5 to 10 degrees.

• Keep the knees slightly flexed, with the hips hinged slightly back just enough so that the shoulders are above but just a little in front of the bar.

• Rest the bar on the hip crease.

• Have the weight on the whole foot but concentrated more on the heels.

• Keep the chest spread, the torso upright, and the back and the head neutral, with the gaze straight ahead or a little bit up, looking at a spot on the horizon.

Movement Phases

1. Forcefully drive the legs and the hips straight up into extension while violently shrugging the shoulders up at the same time.

2. When the leg and hip drive are almost complete, immediately pull up on the bar with the shoulders and elbows so that the elbows rise slightly above the hands to shoulder height.

3. As the bar rises to shoulder height, pull under the bar to catch it.

4. While pulling under the bar, move the feet slightly wider to be able to catch the bar in an overhead squat position. Catching in a deep overhead squat position is preferable. Not everyone can achieve this depth right away, so catching in a power snatch position (legs slightly above parallel) is acceptable. The hips should be the

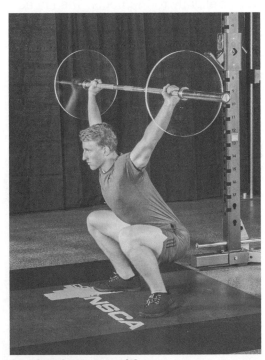

Overhead squat position

first part of the body to drop under the bar, dropping straight down between the legs and the heels.

5. Catch the bar above the head with a snatch grip.

6. Once the weight is caught, immediately push up on the weight with arms fully extended before attempting to stand up. Once control of the bar and the weight is achieved, forcefully extend the hips and the legs while keeping the upper torso upright and rigid and the arms extended and pushing up until standing. When the repetition is completed, safely drop the weight in front of the body to the floor and repeat until the set is complete.

7. Extend the arms to reset, and once again flex the knees and do a hip hinge to the beginning position. Repeat until the set is complete.

Hang Snatch

Movement Phases

1. Assume the high knee (hang) position by starting in the power position and lowering the bar against the thighs while the hips hinge further back and down until the bar is right above the knees.

2. Keep the chest spread, the torso rigid, and the back and the head neutral.

3. Push the knees back while lowering the bar to above the kneecaps so that the shins are vertical and the weight is on the middle of the foot.

4. Have the head and shoulders somewhat in front of the bar, with the arms extended and the scapula and shoulders retracted and depressed.

5. Have the shoulders higher than the hips and the hips a little above the knees.

6. Keep the bar close to the body with a pronated hook snatch grip and begin the ascent with an aggressive pull and a forceful leg and hip extension.

7. As the bar rises up the thighs to the hip crease (the power position), shift the weight slightly to the heels. The knees will go slightly forward as the torso rises, right before full extension.

8. The catch and finish are the same as for the power position catch and finish.

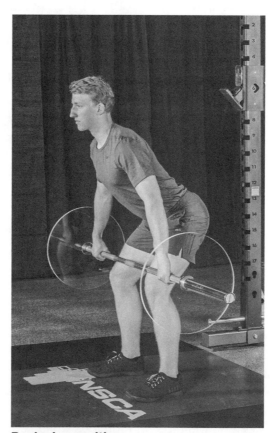

Beginning position

Power Snatch

A power movement is one in which the weight is pulled from the floor and caught overhead with both arms in full extension and the thighs just above parallel. An advanced catch is a deep squat snatch catch with the hips below parallel and the body upright and the torso rigid.

Beginning Position

It can be difficult for untrained and inexperienced student-athletes to lower themselves down to the bar with proper form to do the power snatch. This is a challenging position for those with flexibility issues. To address this, the lock and load procedure described for the power clean exercise (see page 148) can be used to help assure that the start of an exercise will be correct and consistent.

Lock Position to Set up the Load (or Beginning) Position Correctly

• Walk up to the bar so that the bar is above the ball of the foot.

• Stand with a hip-width or slightly wider stance, with the toes turned out slightly or up to 5 to 10 degrees.

• Hip hinge back and grab the knees with the hands. While holding on to the knees, get into the lock position by extending the arms to lock the back and torso into a strong, rigid position with the chest spread, the scapula retracted, and the back neutral. The head is neutral and slightly up in correct position for the load (or beginning) position.

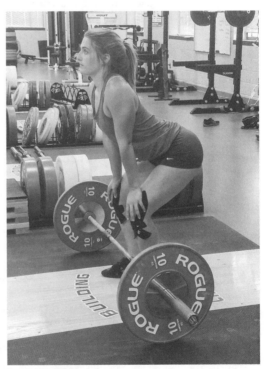

Lock position

Load (or Beginning) Position

• Lower to the bar by simultaneously flexing and lowering the hips and the knees (hip hinge deeper) to a position where the bar can be grasped with a pronated hook grip. As the body is lowered, the shins and the knees come forward and in front of the bar.

• Grip width is the designated hook snatch grip that has been chosen (wider than the clean grip).

• The feet are hip-width to shoulder-width apart, with the toes pointing out 10 degrees or more. The knees should push out against the elbows and be tracking somewhat over the toes or a little wider if the hips are a little lower on account of the wider grip.

• Have the bar above the balls of the feet.

• Have the joint of the shoulders directly above the bar so the top of the shoulders and head are in front of the bar, more with the snatch than with the clean.

• Keep the chest spread and the back neutral with the scapula retracted and depressed and the torso rigid.

• Keep the head and the top part of the shoulders in front of the bar, the head neutral and slightly up, and the gaze straight ahead or slightly up.

• Keep the shoulders and the head higher than the hips. For most student-athletes the hips will be slightly higher than the knees.

• Have the arms extended, with the elbows rotated out and the knuckles down.

• Concentrate the body weight on the whole foot.

• Just before the exercise, very lightly pull up on the bar to put a little tension on it.

Movement Phases

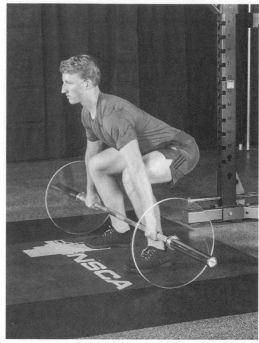

Beginning position

Phase 1: First Pull

1. Begin the ascent by forcefully driving the legs and knees into extension while keeping the feet flat on the floor.

2. As the bar begins to rise from the floor, drive the knees back until the shins are vertical (even more vertical than what is seen in the photo). Keep the bar tight to the body.

3. Retract and depress the scapula, keeping the spine neutral and the torso rigid.

4. The relationship and angle between the hips, the shoulders, and the floor must remain the same while the bar is pulled up to the top of the patellas. The shoulders and the hips rise together; do not raise the hips first.

5. Keep the arms extended with the elbows out.

6. Pull the bar to the top of the kneecaps.

Transition

1. Continue powerful knee and hip extension as the bar rises above the knees. It is very important to keep the shoulders in front of and over the bar until it is about mid-thigh.

2. Keep the back neutral and the torso rigid as the bar and the torso rise.

3. Keep the arms extended.

4. Although keeping the pressure on the whole foot, shift the weight to

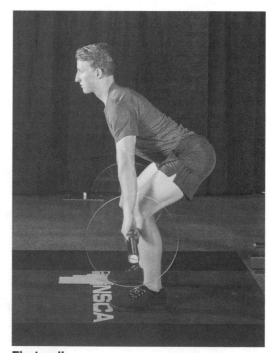

First pull

the middle of the foot while pulling the bar back into the thighs toward the power position.

Phase 2: Second Pull from the Power Position

1. When the bar contacts the body at the hip crease (the power position), weight distribution is on the middle of the foot and the knees flex slightly forward, putting the body in the power position.

2. At this point the torso and the head are above and slightly in front of the bar and the gaze is forward and slightly up. The bar remains close to the body.

3. The legs and the hips drive straight up into full powerful extension while the foot remains in contact with the floor, but the weight is shifted toward the heels. If the legs and hips keep driving with extension now through the heels, the student-athlete can maximize the power that can be produced. The force produced should lead the upper part of the body and head to lean back slightly at the top.

4. As the legs and hips are driving and completing full extension with the bar tight to the body, the body will reach maximum height and velocity. (It is common at this point for the student-athlete to go into triple-joint extension or to the ball of the foot as a result of really hard leg and hip drive.)

5. As maximum height and velocity are reached, and the legs and the hips are fully extended, the feet and the legs will spread slightly to descend under the weight.

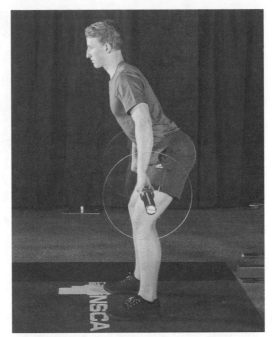

Transition

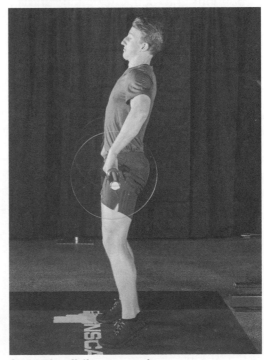

Second pull (in process)

Phase 3: Extension and Catch

1. To help the body descend under the bar for the catch, pull the body rapidly under the bar by powerfully shrugging the shoulders and trapezius and pulling the elbows up so they are near the height of the shoulders and above the hands (not shown in the photos).

2. As the body is being pulled under the bar, it is pulling the bar up over the head.

3. At the same time, the feet are moved out about a one-foot width wider, with the hips and the knees flexed so that the bar can be caught in a stance just

above parallel. (Catching the weight above the line of the thigh that is parallel with the floor is called a power snatch.)

4. This catch is complete when the bar is extended solidly above the head and the student-athlete is sitting tall with the arms extended, the feet solidly on the floor, and the torso upright.

5. Stand up with the weight and drop it to the floor by guiding it down in front of the body past the waist. Repeat again from the beginning position until the set is complete (3).

Breathing Guidelines

• Inhale just before lowering to grab the bar immediately prior to the pull. It is usual to hold the breath throughout the pull, the catch, and part of the ascent. Many will begin to exhale a little on the ascent, finishing the exhale at the completion of the exercise. Most athletes do this naturally.

• The Valsalva maneuver often takes place naturally. It is also often done on purpose. *Note*: The Valsalva maneuver should never be held for more than 2 seconds; doing so could be dangerous by raising blood pressure and creating dizziness.

Exercise Modification

The squat snatch is the most effective version of this exercise, the difference being that the catch is in a low or deep squat position. This develops more strength and flexibility and is more athletic.

Coaching Tips

• It is important toward the end of the pull to continue to drive the legs and the hips to achieve full extension and power.

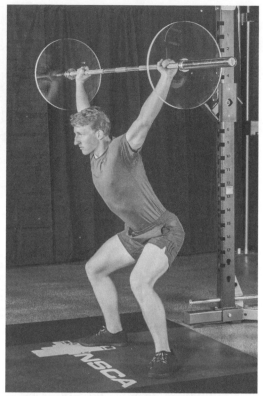

End (catch) position (above parallel)

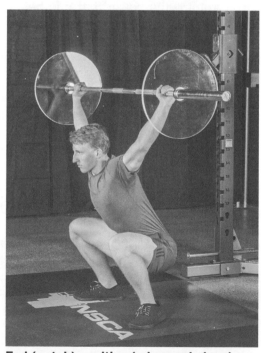

End (catch) position (advanced, deep)

• When the bar is caught, it is very important to squeeze the back, sit tall, and reach, driving the legs first or else the hips will come up first, causing the bar and the body to go forward.

5

Bodyweight Exercises

Jim Davis, EdM, MA, CSCS, RSCC*D

This chapter provides essential guidelines for bodyweight exercise theories and techniques. Safe and effective movement patterns are the cornerstone of any resistance training program. All athletes, from untrained and inexperienced to trained and experienced, benefit from increasing levels of competency in bodyweight training. Bodyweight exercises represent the essential components of movement, programmed to enhance performance. Though activities like gymnastics, plyometric training, yoga, and martial arts could all be considered bodyweight training, this chapter examines intentional movement patterns that are common to resistance training. When selected properly, they are patterns that stem from play and can be used to enhance it. Most of these movements can be performed without a spotter, though a spotter always helps if only to ensure proper technique. This is not an attempt to create an exhaustive list of bodyweight exercises, but the ones outlined here can serve as the bedrock of a strength program. A thoughtful strength and conditioning professional will expand this list to meet the needs and contexts of student-athletes (10, 11).

Fundamentals of Bodyweight Training

Bodyweight exercises often serve as an introduction to resistance training but are valuable for all student-athletes (9, 12). Bodyweight exercises should not be considered equipment-free variations of barbell-based movements, but human movement in its purest form: They are the pushes, hinges, and pulls that appear over and over in play (18). They are the essential building blocks of sport. When they are thoughtfully selected, they erupt from organic movement patterns to enhance the body's ability to meet future athletic demands. Bodyweight training is essential.

Student-athletes benefit from increased awareness of how their own body moves through space (22). When focus shifts away from external objects and heavy resistance, a student-athlete has the opportunity to pay specific attention to joint alignment, posture, breathing patterns, and other essential components of performance that might otherwise go overlooked. Building these capacities through bodyweight exercise can benefit performance and prevent injury (14, 28). Unstable and concerning movement patterns can be identified during bodyweight training, which can be used as a diagnostic movement screen. Concerns such as lack of balance on one leg, a weak core, and limited range of motion in a specific joint should be addressed before the student-athlete is subjected to the additional demands of resistance and speed.

All recommendations herein are intended to be helpful guidelines but should be adjusted based on the needs of the student-athlete. The specific expectations of each movement should be based on an athlete's individual anatomy. For example, if two student-athletes have significantly different femur lengths, their torsos will be at different angles during many of the lower body movements. In this example, a student-athlete with long femurs and a short torso will have to lean forward to keep their chest and shoulders over the base of their feet during a squat; a student-athlete with shorter femurs and a long torso would have a more vertical posture when performing the squat movement. An individual anthropometric evaluation will ultimately dictate the way a movement is performed (7, 19). The directions in this chapter attempt to take many of those considerations into account. Still, the strength and conditioning professional should always be diligent in observing the specific needs of individual student-athletes and adjusting as necessary.

The movement patterns described in this chapter can be accomplished by almost all healthy student-athletes. Even difficult ones, like pull-ups, can be performed by any student-athlete. Pull-ups refer to a bodyweight-resisted vertical pull. This movement can be made more or less difficult depending on equipment, spotters, and other forms of support, but the vertical pull is a movement that can be performed by all healthy student-athletes. For some student-athletes, their own body weight is too much resistance for the movement to be safely performed. In this case, the strength and conditioning professional should take note and adjust as needed. A spotter can help them through the movement until they can perform it on their own. If the student-athlete is still having trouble, variations (like an eccentric focus or isometric holds at different stages of the movement) can be performed until the full movement pattern can be achieved. Kipping variations have been met with varied response by members of the strength community and require wider incorporation of the body's structures, slightly changing muscle activation (8). Lat pulldown machines offer a great way to enhance the musculature of the vertical pull before student-athletes can manage their own bodyweight, but the variations outlined above serve the same function. A thoughtful coach or strength and conditioning professional should remove the stigma surrounding pull-ups and other exercises, offer creative solutions to student-athletes, and focus on healthy movement patterns. A few of these variations are listed for each movement in the second half of the chapter.

One of the key psychological benefits of bodyweight training is an appreciation of movement. It is not only fun to move and move well, but it is healthy, it is safe, and it will lead to improved performance. If strength and conditioning professionals can instill an appreciation for movement in their student-athletes, their long-term development will surely benefit.

Posture and Base

If bodyweight exercises are the building blocks of athletic performance, posture is the foundation. Poor posture can lead to injury. Poor posture can signal an existing injury or imbalance. Unfortunately, poor posture, especially in the cervical and thoracic spine, is a progressively likely occurrence; it seems that the increasing prevalence of advanced handheld technologies like smartphones has forced many people, especially young people, into slumped postures. The first step of bodyweight movement should be to move the body into a stable position. Step one: improve posture (15, 16).

Definitions of posture vary, but a working definition includes physical alignments that support one's naturally occurring, individualized skeletal structure. Most conversations surrounding posture focus on the spine. Common postural concerns are lumbar lordosis (excessive curvature of the lumbar vertebrae), kyphosis (over-arching of the thoracic vertebrae), and excessive abduction of the scapulae (shoulders rolled forward with shoulder blades flared) (5, 16). The good news is that focus on posture will not only improve performance, but performance of bodyweight exercise is often used to improve posture (15). One enhances the other for reciprocal benefit. Postural concerns are often attributed to weak muscles in the associated region and tight muscles in the antagonist muscle group. These concerns can be addressed through thoughtful exercise selection (5, 15).

The exercise descriptions in this chapter use terms like *neutral spine*, *stable torso*, and *stable posture*. *Neutral spine* refers to posture without excessive variation from the natural curvature of the spine; that is, uniform amounts of stress are placed on each of the vertebrae and intervertebral discs. To accomplish a neutral spine, one will need a stable torso or stable posture; *stable* is the operative word. The musculature of the torso (especially the abdomen and lower back) activates so the torso is firm and supported while maintaining the ability to move. It must be strong but not immobile; it must be stable (17, 20, 27).

Stability is a quality in constant conversation with gravity. Athletes should take care to establish a stable base before performing these movements (17, 19, 24). For most movements, the base is defined by the lateral width of a student-athlete's stance and the depth of their feet (distance from the front toe to the rear heel). In a standard squat movement, the base might be hip-width apart and as deep as a foot. In a lunge, the base is still hip-width apart but is now as long as the stride of the lunge. When the weight of the torso is above the base, the position is stable. Common terms in the description of these positions often refer to the joints as anatomical landmarks. When joints are stacked, they are aligned vertically, and when joints are planked, they are aligned horizontally. These provide visual cues for strength and conditioning professionals and proprioceptive awareness for the student-athlete to understand the relationship of one joint to another (22). Once an athlete has gained a minimum level of expertise while training on a stable floor, variations of the bodyweight movements can be made more challenging by increased unilateral focus, as well as using balance pads and other equipment (1, 3, 6).

Breathing

Inhalation and exhalation change the position of the torso and adjust posture. Generally speaking, posture should remain constant through the movements. A held inhalation not only allows the student-athlete to maintain posture, but it also pressurizes the abdomen. When pressure is created in the abdomen by filling the diaphragm with air, the spine is supported (4, 13, 16, 17). A student-athlete should inhale before exertion. This is especially important in the transition between the initial movement and secondary movement. In a movement like the squat, the most important moment is in the transition from the eccentric phase (down) to the concentric phase (up). A student-athlete's spine is most vulnerable at the bottom of the squat as they transition from one phase to the other. In that moment, the student-athlete should have a rigid torso. Inhaling is a contraction of the diaphragm that fills the lungs with air and increases pressure in the abdomen; this combined effect creates a rigid torso that supports the spine (4, 13). After exertion, or through it, many student-athletes begin to exhale (25). In bodyweight training, this exchange is less obvious than in heavy resistance training, but it is no less important. For example, a conditioned student-athlete could easily hold his or her breath through 5 to 10 push-ups. If that same student-athlete was breathing through a heavy bench press (the same movement pattern but with a significant increase in level of difficulty), breathing would play a much larger role. In a 1RM attempt a powerlifter might have a strict breathing routine, including but not limited to the Valsalva maneuver, but that same person might breathe fairly leisurely during bodyweight movements. One of the benefits of bodyweight training is that it can prepare good habits and sound techniques in a lower-intensity environment, which map on to future moments in training and play when intensity is increased.

Many advancing theories exist on breathing in both training and sport. As usual, one size does not fit all. Strength and conditioning professionals should work to enhance a student-athlete's awareness around breathing as it pertains to posture, kinesthetic awareness, and the rhythms of each movement pattern. The thoughtful strength and conditioning professional will keep an eye on advancing science and techniques to adapt as necessary to meet the needs and contexts of individual student-athletes.

Bedrock: Set the Foundation

Bodyweight training comes down to intentional coaching and execution. Exercise selection and position should not fall to any specific doctrine but intentionally align with the desired training effect. The primary outcome of any training program should be student-athlete safety. Safety should be prioritized both immediately (in training) and predictively (that is, in anticipation of the demands of the sport). A bodyweight training program should account for immediate safety concerns by creating a safe physical space, ensuring proper technique, and adapting exertion expectations (intensity and duration of the workout) based on the ability of the student-athlete. Predictive safety includes accounting for the potential demands of the sport or activity in which the student-athlete hopes to be involved. A lacrosse player, a cross-country runner, and a powerlifter can all benefit from bodyweight training, but the demands of their sport are vastly different.

It is the job of the strength and conditioning professional to predict those demands and appropriately adjust the training. The movement patterns will not change, but the way in which the movements are performed should be specific to the desired training outcomes. In addition to a deep understanding of the practical application of bodyweight exercises, posture, and breathing, the thoughtful professional will work to understand the specific adaptations that occur alongside specific muscle actions (eccentric, concentric, and isometric) as well as the repetitions, sets, and rest times associated with specific training outcomes (2, 10, 12).

Bodyweight training offers an opportunity for a strength and conditioning professional to set clear expectations, provide regular feedback, improve a student-athlete's technique, increase their self-awareness, and improve performance. These are the bedrock concepts of a training program. Bodyweight movements are not simply easy versions of heavy resistance exercises; they are the essential building blocks of sport. When they are thoughtfully selected, they erupt from organic movement patterns to enhance the body's ability to meet future athletic demands and set the foundation for future demonstrations of athleticism. Serious professionals understand that the weight room is a classroom. Bodyweight training is an essential lesson.

Exercise Finder

Push-Up

Primary Muscles Trained

Pectoralis major, anterior deltoids, triceps brachii

Setup

- The standard push-up requires little to no setup; all that is needed is space and a stable floor.

Beginning Position

- Set the open hands on the floor, slightly wider than shoulder-width apart.
- The arms should be fully extended and the scapulae reduced to maintain a neutral spine position and stable posture.
- The joints of the arm should be stacked from the wrist through the elbow to the shoulder.
- Set the toes hip-width apart and rise into plank alignment (straight line from the ankles through the knees, hips, shoulders, and jaw), with the arms fully extended.
- Return to this position before every repetition.

Initial Movement

1. All components of stable posture (back, torso, hips and glutes, and knees) should maintain their beginning position as the elbows flex.
2. The forearms should remain perpendicular to the floor and parallel to each other throughout the movement.
3. Descend until the elbow angle between the upper arm and forearm is less than 90 degrees.
4. If floor contact occurs, it should be at the mid- to lower sternum.

Secondary Movement

1. Apply force to the floor through the hands as the elbows extend.
2. As the body rises, all components of posture (back, torso, hips and glutes, and knees) should maintain their position.
3. Press until the joints of the arm are stacked from the wrist through the elbow to the shoulder, returning to the beginning position.

Exercise Modifications and Variations

- *Push-up on knees.* This variation begins on the hands and knees. This new beginning position requires the joints to be aligned from shoulder to knees, which decreases the amount of resistance and challenge during the push. This is an especially valuable variation, since so many components of the movement are essentially the same. It is valuable as a teaching tool for untrained and inexperienced athletes, but it can also be used with trained and experienced athletes to complete the total of volume of prescribed repetitions when form begins to waver.

• *Incline or decline push-up.* Tilting the body to different angles by putting the feet on a bench with hands on the floor, or hands on a bench with toes on the floor, will promote greater activation of the upper and lower chest, respectively. With hands on the floor and toes elevated, a student-athlete will work the upper chest and highlight the anterior deltoids. With toes on the floor and hands elevated, the student-athlete will work the lower chest and highlight the triceps. Aside from the body's alignment, there are no major adjustments in technique.

• *Scorpion push-up.* A student-athlete can work balance and proprioception by lifting one leg off the floor during the push-up. There is extra activation in the abdominals and glutes during this variation. Aside from the change in body position, there are no major adjustments in technique.

Coaching Tips

The push-up is one of the most common bodyweight exercises and also one of the most poorly performed exercises. Do not overprescribe push-ups. Untrained and inexperienced student-athletes should not be doing hundreds of push-ups; they should be doing push-ups in small sets (5-10 repetitions) until they can be done with great technique before advancing in volume or intensity. Create a space where a student-athlete feels comfortable doing push-ups one at a time if necessary, taking pride in form over total repetitions.

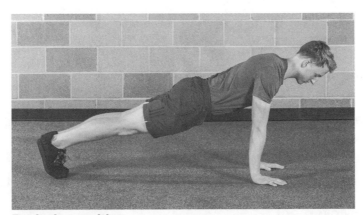

Beginning position

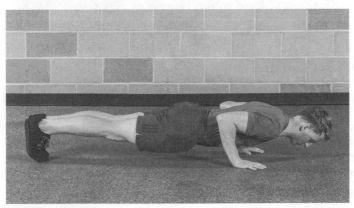

Bottom position

Bodyweight Row

Primary Muscles Trained

Latissimus dorsi, teres major, middle trapezius, rhomboids, posterior deltoids, rectus abdominis, transverse abdominis

Setup

• Set a barbell in a rack. The bar should be high enough that the student-athlete lying supine on the floor cannot reach it without lifting the scapulae off of the floor. This will allow for full extension of the arms when performing the movement.

• Set a bench parallel to the bar. The bench should be a distance from the bar that allows the student-athlete to set the heels on the bench while performing the movement.

Beginning Position

• Reach and grasp the bar with a pronated grip.

• The grip can vary but is most commonly at the edges of shoulder-width apart.

• Set the heels on the bench and lift the hips off the floor until there is plank alignment (straight line from the ankles through the knees, hips, shoulders, and jaw), with the arms fully extended.

• Maintain a neutral spine position.

• Return to this position before every repetition.

Initial Movement

1. Pull the chest toward the bar.

2. Maintain a plank position with a neutral spine throughout the movement.

3. The hips should neither lead the movement nor sag. The entire body should remain stable as the arms flex.

4. Touch the chest to the bar (unlike what is seen in the end position photo).

Secondary Movement

1. Lower the body back down to the beginning position.

2. Maintain a plank position with a neutral spine throughout the movement.

3. After the final repetition, maintain the grip and heel position, but set the glutes on the floor to rest.

Exercise Modifications and Variations

• *Feet on the floor.* If a student-athlete cannot perform the movement while maintaining posture, the challenge can be reduced by placing the feet on the floor instead of on a bench. In the beginning position for this variation, the feet should be flat on the floor and the joint alignment should include a straight line from the knee through the hips, shoulders, and jaw.

• *Start from the top.* If a student-athlete cannot perform the movement with the feet on a bench or on the floor, a spotter assists them into an arms-flexed position with the chest touching the bar. The focus should then be on the descent, using a controlled eccentric contraction as the elbows extend. Untrained and inexperienced student-athletes can also perform an isometric contraction at the top and hold for time instead of repetitions.

Coaching Tips

Watch for the same anatomical misalignments that one might find in an unstable push-up: elbows flared, excessive scapular abduction, and the hips above or below the plank position (arching or sagging). Like the push-up, remind the student-athlete that quality leads to performance faster than quantity. Instead of pumping out dozens of unstable repetitions, focus on doing one perfect repetition, then another. When a student-athlete gets used to the movement, experiment with eccentric and isometric variations to effectively improve torso stability.

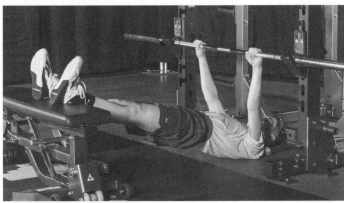

Beginning position

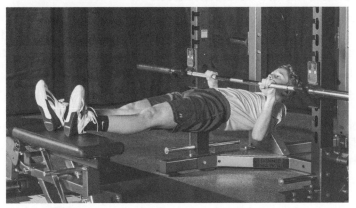

End position

Pull-Up

Primary Muscles Trained

Latissimus dorsi, teres major, middle trapezius, rhomboids, posterior deltoids, rectus abdominis

Setup

- Clear the area surrounding a pull-up bar for a safe descent after the movement has been completed.

Beginning Position

- Jump or climb to the bar, then grasp the bar with a pronated grip.
- The grip can vary but is most commonly at the edges of shoulder-width apart.

Initial Movement

1. Focus on contracting the latissimus dorsi as the elbows flex to initiate the movement.
2. Pull the upper chest toward the bar.
3. Retract the scapulae down and back at the peak of the movement.
4. Continue until the jawline is parallel with the bar or just above it.

Secondary Movement

1. Extend the arms with control and return to the beginning position.
2. After the final repetition, be aware of the surroundings and drop or climb down safely.

Exercise Modifications and Variations

- *Partner assisted.* If a student-athlete is having trouble performing the movement, a spotter can apply pressure to the thoracic region of the student-athlete's back, just below the scapulae. This will lessen the total resistance to the pull-up movement.

- *Band assisted.* If a student-athlete is having trouble performing the movement, a resistance band can be attached to the pull-up bar. A student-athlete can set a foot or a knee in the loop of the band to receive assistance at the bottom of the movement. The more tension on the band, the more assistance (less resistance) a student-athlete will experience.

• *Start from the top.* If a student-athlete cannot perform the movement, a spotter assists him or her into an arms-flexed position with their jaw aligned with the bar. The focus should then be on the descent, using a controlled eccentric contraction as the elbows extend. Untrained and inexperienced student-athletes can also perform an isometric contraction at the top and hold for time instead of repetitions.

Coaching Tips

Everyone can do pull-ups. If a student-athlete can reach up into the air as in an overhead press, direct them to retract their scapulae, flex their elbows, and bring their hands in line with their jaw. Then they can do a pull-up; it is a movement pattern. A pull-up is the name given to a bodyweight resisted vertical pull. Often, especially in untrained and inexperienced athletes, body weight proves to be more resistance than a student-athlete can manage. Lat pulldown machines offer a great way to enhance the musculature of the vertical pull before a student-athlete can manage their own body weight, but the variations outlined above serve the same function. Remove the stigma surrounding pull-ups for the student-athletes, and the results will follow.

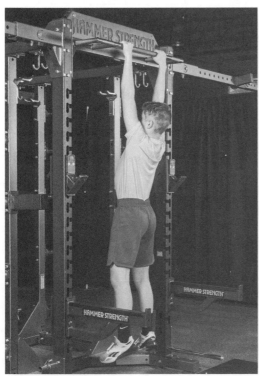 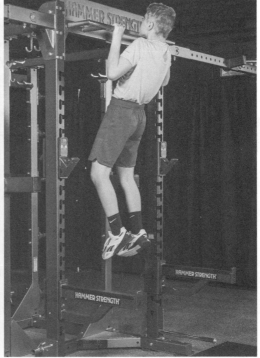

Beginning position   **End position**

Squat

Primary Muscles Trained

Gluteus maximus, biceps femoris, rectus femoris, vastus lateralis, vastus intermedius, vastus medialis

Setup

• The bodyweight squat requires little to no setup; all that is needed is space and a stable floor.

Beginning Position

• Begin from the floor up. Set the feet at the edge of hip-width apart. The toes should point forward or align with subtle external rotation.

• The joints of the body should be stacked in a straight line from the ankles through the knees, hips, shoulders, and jaw.

• Reduce the scapulae (pull the shoulder blades down and back) while keeping the bottom of the ribcage aimed down at the hips; do not tilt the ribcage.

• Look forward with a neutral spine and stable torso position.

• Keep either a 90-degree angle in the arms with the elbows close to the ribcage and hands in a ready position or extend the arms slightly forward to serve as a counterbalance for stability.

• Return to this position before every repetition.

Initial Movement

1. The hips and knees should flex while maintaining a stable torso position.

2. Look forward and keep a neutral spine. The thoracic and lumbar spine should not move throughout the squat, and the position of the cervical spine should have minimal variation, if any.

3. The chest and shoulders should maintain a consistent position above the base.

4. Though there will be subtle variation in weight distribution across the feet during the movement, they should remain flush to the floor.

5. Continue flexing the hips, knees, and ankles until the hips and knees are on the same flat plane parallel to the floor.

6. The knees should track over the feet between the middle toe and the instep.

Secondary Movement

1. The hips and knees should extend while maintaining a stable torso position.

2. The chest and shoulders should maintain a consistent position above the base as they rise.

3. Though there will be subtle variation in weight distribution across the feet during the movement, they should remain flush to the floor.

4. Continue through the movement until the joints are stacked in a straight line from the ankles through the knees, hips, shoulders, and jaw (beginning position).

Exercise Modifications and Variations

- *Jump prep/momentum squat.* Move the arms in coordination with the movement as though preparing to jump. On the initial descent, extend the arms backward. On the secondary movement, the arms should flex and pull forward. Aside from the arm movement, there are no major adjustments in technique.

- *Goblet squat.* A goblet squat position is one in which the arms are flexed, and the hands are together at chest level, as though holding a goblet in front of the body. This variation has additional stabilizing benefits through the core. Aside from the arm and hand position, there are no major adjustments in technique.

- *Overhead squat.* Retract the scapulae and extend the arms overhead into a position that resembles the letter Y. This variation has additional stabilizing benefits through the core and can be challenging for untrained and inexperienced student-athletes. Aside from the arm position, there are no major adjustments in technique.

Coaching Tips

Untrained and inexperienced student-athletes often think of the squat as a movement that goes down and up: When a student-athlete tries to go down, the knees often flex first and the heels lift off the floor. The simple cue of "hips back and hips through" reminds student-athletes to flex the hips first and sit back while keeping the weight of the torso over the base, which in turn allows equal pressure to distribute across the base.

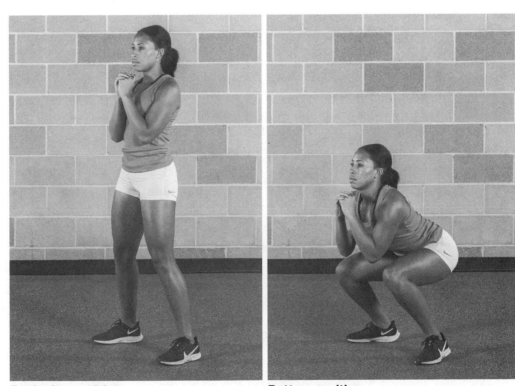

Beginning position   **Bottom position**

Rear Foot Elevated Squat

Primary Muscles Trained

Gluteus maximus, biceps femoris, rectus femoris, vastus lateralis, vastus intermedius, vastus medialis, semimembranosus, semitendinosus, iliopsoas

Setup

• Set up a bench or some other stable ledge that can support body weight.
• The front leg is the leg on the floor, and the back leg is the leg on the bench.

Beginning Position

• Stand less than one stride length in front of the bench and align the shoulders parallel to the bench.
• Set the back foot on the bench. Either dorsiflexion or plantarflexion is acceptable, as long as stability and safety are ensured.
• Set the front foot far enough away from the bench so that a unilateral squat can be performed.

Initial Movement

1. Flex the hip and knee of the front leg while maintaining a stable torso position.
2. Look forward and keep a neutral spine. The thoracic and lumbar spine should not move throughout the movement, and the position of the cervical spine should have minimal variation, if any.
3. The chest and shoulders should maintain a consistent position above the front foot.
4. The back leg functions primarily as a stabilizer, and its position should not significantly vary throughout the movement.
5. Though there will be subtle variation in weight distribution across the foot during the movement, it should remain flush to the floor.
6. Continue flexing the hip, knee, and ankle until the hip and knee are on the same flat plane, parallel to the floor.
7. The knee should track over the foot between the middle toe and the instep.

Secondary Movement

1. Extend the hip and knee while maintaining a stable torso position.
2. Apply force into the floor using the front foot, while the back foot functions primarily as a stabilizer.
3. The chest and shoulders should maintain a consistent position above the base as they rise.
4. Though there will be subtle variation in weight distribution across the foot during the movement, it should remain flush to the floor.
5. Continue through the movement until the joints are stacked in a straight line from the front ankle through the knees, hips, shoulders, and jaw (beginning position).

Exercise Modifications and Variations

• *Sprint mechanics:* Ideally, any split squat or unilateral lunge variation will also train upper body mechanics (arm actions), which align with running technique.

• *Overhead squat.* Retract the scapulae and extend the arms overhead into a position that resembles the letter Y. This variation has additional stabilizing benefits through the core and can be challenging for untrained and inexperienced athletes. Aside from the arm position, there are no major adjustments in technique.

Coaching Tips

This movement is an incredible diagnostic tool for weight distribution errors across the foot during a squat. Student-athletes will occasionally find that one knee tracks cleanly over their foot (between the middle toe of the foot and the instep) while the other might favor one direction or other. This occurs in untrained and inexperienced student-athletes, student-athletes who have experienced an injury, and student-athletes who have become overly accustomed to heavy, bilateral resistance training. When this happens, the student-athlete should slow down the repetitions and groove a movement pattern (repeat until it is smooth) on the leg in question.

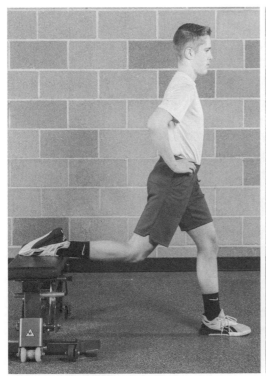
Beginning position

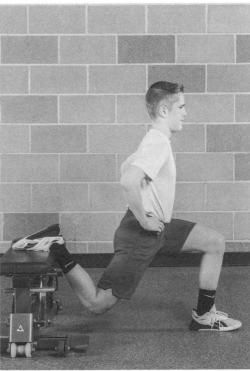
Bottom position

Forward Walking Lunge

Primary Muscles Trained

Gluteus maximus, semimembranosus, semitendinosus, biceps femoris, vastus lateralis, vastus intermedius, vastus medialis, rectus femoris, iliopsoas

Setup

• The walking lunge requires a cleared space through which a student-athlete may safely travel.

Beginning Position

• Begin from the floor up. Set the feet at hip-width and parallel to one another. The toes should point forward or align with subtle internal rotation.

• The joints of the body should be stacked in a straight line from the ankle through the knees, hips, shoulders, and jaw.

• Reduce the scapulae (pull the shoulder blades down and back) while keeping the bottom of the ribcage aimed down at the hips; do not "tilt" the ribcage.

• Look forward and keep a neutral spine and stable torso position.

Initial Movement

1. Drive the lead knee into the air and take a stride forward, landing with a flat foot and toes pointed forward. The length of the stride is determined by whether the shin can maintain its vertical position; do not significantly over-stride (which would create an obtuse angle with the femur) or under-stride (which would create an excessive acute angle to the femur).

2. Retain a stable torso position above the base of the feet.

3. The stride of the lunge should look similar to running technique, with the knee driving up in front of the hip and the toes of the lead foot pointed forward in dorsiflexion.

4. The knee of the back leg will flex slightly while striding forward.

5. The weight on the back leg should rise to the ball of the foot but not leave the floor.

6. In the landing (lunge) position, the knee and hip of the lead leg should be on the same flat plane, parallel to the floor.

7. In the lunge position, the alignment of the knee and hip of the back leg should be slightly behind the alignment of the knee and shoulder; this creates an angle only slightly larger than 180 degrees.

8. The bottom of the lunge is a coordinated isometric contraction; the knee of the back leg should not rest on the floor.

Secondary Movement

1. Repeat the initial movement from a lunge position instead of the beginning position.

2. Initiate the movement by pulling through the front leg and driving through the toe of the back leg.

3. The back leg should drive into the air and take a long stride forward, landing with a flat foot and the toes pointed forward.

4. Continue alternating legs and lunge forward for the prescribed distance or designated number of repetitions.

Exercise Modifications and Variations

• *Forward lunge.* The body positions and movement patterns will remain, but instead of walking forward, drive off of the front leg and pull through the back leg to return to the beginning position. This variation is preferred when space is limited.

• *Reverse lunge.* The forward lunge movement pattern will reverse in order. Step backward, leading with the toe and ball of the foot before settling into a lunge position. The isometric lunge position will look the same. The secondary movement requires pulling through the front leg and driving off the back toes to return to the beginning position.

• *Sprint mechanics.* Any lunge variation works the upper body mechanics (arm actions), which align with running technique.

Coaching Tips

Slow down, and change direction. Walking is easy. In walking lunges, student-athletes occasionally fall into the trap of traveling from point A to point B without paying close attention to technique. Coach a student-athlete to slow down and consider how their foot is striking the floor, how the weight shifts across the foot as they step, and whether one side feels more natural than the other. If this movement is too easy, do it in reverse. In reverse, many of the deeply engrained neurological patterns that create familiar locomotion unravel, and the student-athlete has to relearn the nuances of how to step, where to place the feet, and how long the strides should be.

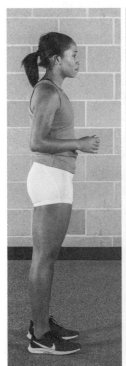 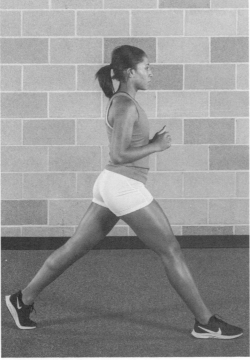 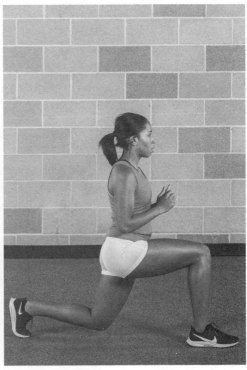

Beginning position   Middle of forward step   **Lunged position**

Step-Up

Primary Muscles Trained

Gluteus maximus, semimembranosus, semitendinosus, biceps femoris, vastus lateralis, vastus intermedius, vastus medialis, rectus femoris, iliopsoas

Setup

- Set a stable object like a bench or a plyo box in an open space.
- The height of the box may vary, but for most student-athletes it should start at approximately knee height.

Beginning Position

- Stand less than a full stride length away from the box (approximately 2 ft [61 cm]), facing it.
- Feet should be at hip-width apart and parallel to one another. The toes should point forward or align with subtle internal rotation.
- The joints of the body should be stacked in a straight line from the ankle through the knees, hips, shoulders, and jaw.
- Reduce the scapulae (pull the shoulder blades down and back) while keeping the bottom of the ribcage aimed down at the hips; do not "tilt" the ribcage.
- Look forward and keep a neutral spine and stable torso position.

Initial Movement

1. One leg at a time, drive the lead knee into the air and stride forward, landing on the box with a flat foot and the toes pointed straight ahead.
2. The torso should retain its position with no great variance and a stable posture.
3. The stride of the lunge should look similar to running technique, with the knee driving up in front of the hip and the toes of the lead foot pointed forward in dorsiflexion.

Secondary Movement

1. Initiate the movement by pulling through the front leg (on the box) with minimal drive through the toe of the back leg (on the floor).
2. Body weight should shift completely to the leg that is on the box and be evenly distributed across the foot.
3. As body weight shifts completely toward the front leg, the back leg should drive into the air with the knee aligned with the hip and the toes pointed forward in dorsiflexion above the box.

Tertiary Movement

1. Descend from the step-up position with caution.
2. Find the floor with the toe of the drive leg while the leg on the box controls the descent.
3. Return to the beginning position before each repetition.

Exercise Modifications and Variations

• *Sprint mechanics.* Any lunge or step-up variation works the upper body mechanics (arm actions), which align with running technique.

• *Overhead squat.* The scapulae should retract, and the arms should extend overhead into a position that resembles the letter Y. This variation will take all momentum out of the movement and has additional stabilizing benefits through the core. Aside from the arm position, there are no major adjustments in technique.

Coaching Tips

Assuming a coach has access to the necessary equipment and space, the step-up should be a core component of a student-athlete's training, especially if speed is an intended training outcome. The moment of exertion for the front leg relative to the rest of the body is difficult to accomplish with any other training method and uniquely replicates sprinting technique in the weight room. Student-athletes also seem to enjoy it, because it feels more like play than some of the more traditional bodyweight movements.

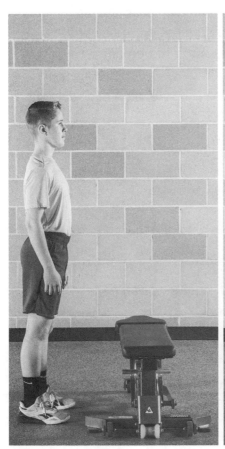

Beginning position

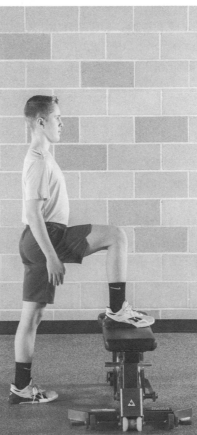

Foot placed on top of bench

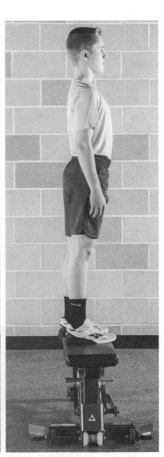

End position (one leg)

Single-Leg Romanian Deadlift (RDL)

Primary Muscles Trained
Gluteus maximus, semimembranosus, semitendinosus, biceps femoris, erector spinae

Setup
• The single-leg RDL requires little to no setup; all that is needed is space and a stable floor.
• The plant leg is the leg on the floor. The balance leg is the leg in the air.

Beginning Position
• Begin from the floor up. Set feet at hip-width apart and parallel to one another. The toes should point forward or align with subtle internal rotation.
• Reduce the scapulae (pull the shoulder blades down and back) while keeping the bottom of the ribcage aimed down at the hips; do not "tilt" the ribcage.
• Look forward and keep a neutral spine and stable torso position.
• Lift one foot off the floor and take a moment to stabilize on the plant foot.
• Maintain subtle flexion of the plant leg throughout the movement.
• Return to this position before every repetition.

Initial Movement
1. Flex, or hinge, at the hips.
2. The hips should shift backward slightly, and the lifted leg should serve as a counterbalance to the torso.
3. The heel of the balance foot should lead the path as it moves backward, activating the glutes on that leg.
4. Maintain a neutral spine as the chest closes the distance to the floor.
5. Although weight distribution will vary slightly through the movement, the plant foot should remain flush to the floor.
6. Continue until a stretch is felt in the glute and hamstrings of the plant leg.

Secondary Movement
1. When a stretch is felt in the glute and hamstrings of the plant leg, reverse the direction of the movement.
2. Focus on posterior chain activation and maintain a neutral spine as the chest returns to an upright position (*Note:* The end position photo shows the beginning of a common error where the student-athlete partially twists the torso to maintain balance.)
3. Although weight distribution will vary slightly through the movement, the plant foot should remain flush to the floor.
4. Return to the beginning position.
5. Complete an equal number of repetitions for each leg.

Exercise Modification and Variation

Corners of the square. Imagine a square drawn on the floor around the foot of the plant leg. Using the opposite hand, reach toward one corner of the square. On each subsequent repetition, touch a different corner of the square. This variation is often referred to as ankle prehab since it requires extra balance and stabilization of the ankle.

Coaching Tips

The bilateral RDL is an effective movement and can be used if the single-leg RDL is too difficult, though that is rare. The most common difficulties of the single-leg RDL have to do with coordination and attention to detail. This movement not only trains the posterior chain but enhances self-awareness and proprioception. Remind student-athletes to lead with the heel of the balance leg since the more they pay attention to the plant leg, the more they lose deliberate control of the other. The challenge of balance and attention can be as important to athletic performance as any physical training outcome.

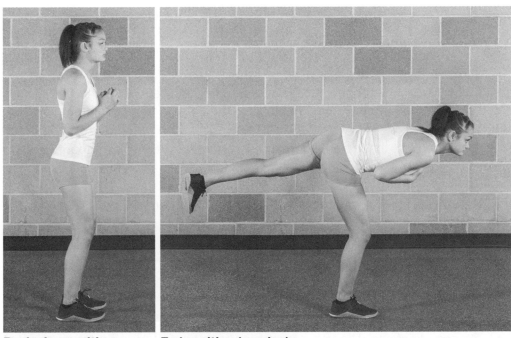

Beginning position   **End position (one leg)**

Glute Bridge

Primary Muscles Trained

Gluteus maximus, semimembranosus, semitendinosus, biceps femoris, erector spinae, transverse abdominis

Setup

• A mat can be set on the floor or padding can be added behind the head for comfort, but there is little to no setup required to perform the bodyweight glute bridge.

Beginning Position

• Lie in a supine position on the floor.

• Flex the knees until the feet are flat on the floor.

Initial Movement

1. Engage the glutes to extend the hips up into the air.

2. Apply pressure to the floor though the feet, focusing on the heel of each foot.

3. The ankle and knee should remain in alignment, traced vertically through the shin.

4. Maintain a consistent torso position, and do not lead with the belly. While the erector spinae should engage, the body should rise due to the floor pressure and activation of the glutes and hamstrings.

5. Continue until the knees, hips, and shoulders come into alignment.

Secondary Movement

1. Descend with control, engaging the glutes and hamstrings throughout the movement.

2. The lower back and top shelf of the glutes should touch the floor between repetitions without full disengagement.

3. Repeat for the prescribed number of repetitions.

Exercise Modifications and Variations

• *Stance variations.* The same movement can be performed from a variety of stances, such as slight internal rotation of the feet, a slightly wider stance, or a slightly tighter stance to enhance posterior chain activation.

• *Single-leg glute bridge.* An advanced version of the movement can include lifting one leg off the floor in the beginning position, perpendicular to the floor. The "up" leg should maintain its position throughout the movement, adding a balance component and additional strain on the leg planted on the floor, but there should be no other major variations.

• *Incline or decline glute bridge.* The same movement can be performed with either one or two feet elevated on a ledge (a short plyo box or an Olympic bumper plate) or with the upper body elevated on a bench.

Coaching Tip

Though it can be challenging to train the posterior chain without a barbell or other forms of external resistance, the glute bridge offers an easy way to enhance glute and hamstring activation (23). Since the movement itself is simple and straightforward, it provides an opportunity for the student-athlete to concentrate on muscle actions. One common prescription is a powerful concentric raise to bridge position, a brief isometric pause in the bridged position, followed by an eccentric descent to the floor.

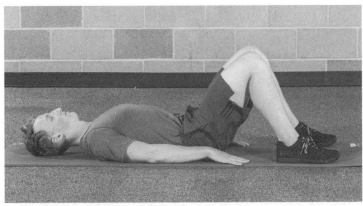

Beginning position

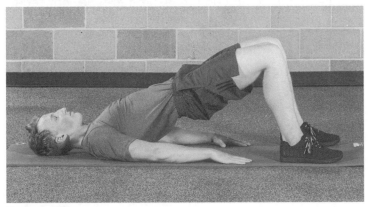

End position

Core Stability (Plank Variations)

Primary Muscles Trained

Rectus abdominus, erector spinae, transverse abdominis

Setup

- For the standard plank, no setup is required.

Beginning Position

- From a prone position, raise up on to the forearms and toes.
- The elbow should create a 90-degree angle from the forearm to the upper arm (humerus). The upper arms should be perpendicular to the floor.
- The joints from the jaw to the ankle (jaw, shoulder, hip, knee, ankle) should align in a plank position. (*Note*: The student-athlete in the photo is not as well aligned as is desired.)
- Slight abdominal contraction should ensure the bottom of the ribcage points directly down through the hips.
- Maintain a neutral spine and hold this position.

Initial Movement and Secondary Movement

The plank is an isometric contraction measured in time, not repetitions. There should be no movement during the standard plank.

Exercise Modifications and Variations

- *Side plank.* In the beginning position, rotate 90 degrees onto only one elbow until the chest is facing outward instead of pointed at the floor. The vertical line beginning at the elbow should now extend through the clavicle and into the other shoulder. The side plank is a common and well-researched method to support the musculature of the core and, oftentimes, relieve back pain (26).
- *Push-up plank.* Set the open hands on the floor, slightly wider than shoulder-width apart. Fully extend the arms and reduce the scapulae to maintain a neutral spine position and stable posture. The joints of the arm should be stacked from the wrists through the elbows to the shoulders.

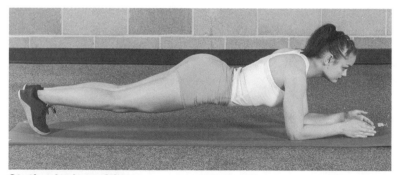

Static plank position

Coaching Tips

Plank variations provide a wealth of stabilizing benefits across all areas of the body, most notably in the trunk extensors (21). They provide many of the benefits of anti-rotational exercises, which are difficult to perform without equipment or a partner. Though the physical training benefits can be accomplished in a short amount of time, every now and then a coach can throw in a longer hold to safely test psychological resilience. While every compound movement provides room for error, there is little variance in this held position. In the case of absolute failure, the student-athlete would drop about 6 inches (15 cm) to the floor. Tests of longer holds offer a safe opportunity for a student-athlete to strain and build psychological capacity.

Core Exercises

Joe Lopez, CSCS, RSCC

To understand training the muscles of the anatomical core it is essential to define what is meant by the core area of the body. The **anatomical core** (simply called *core* in this chapter) is a group of muscles both superficial and deep that allow one to stabilize the spine, hips, and pelvis while also creating movement in the frontal, sagittal, and transverse planes of motion.

To categorize core exercises, we can sort them by their function as it relates to either stabilization or mobilization, or how it creates movement along the kinetic chain. The muscles such as the rectus abdominis, erector spinae, internal obliques, and external obliques are prime movers when flexing, extending, or rotating through the spine. The exercises that incorporate these muscles are referred to as *global mobilizers*.

The quadratus lumborum, piriformis, gluteus maximus, and multifidus are on the posterior side and allow extension, abduction, and rotation of the hips. On the anterior side hip flexor muscles such as the iliopsoas, tensor fasciae latae, pectineus, sartorius, adductors, gracilis, and rectus femoris all play a role in hip flexion, adduction, and rotation. The transverse abdominis, longissimus thoracis, pelvic floor, and even diaphragm play unique roles in the core because they act as stabilizers. Exercises that use these muscles are called *local stabilizers*. This entire group of muscles put together creates a solid core that allows one to transfer force throughout the upper and lower body efficiently (3).

Exercises or movements involving upper or lower extremities are known as *core-limb transfer exercises*. Without a solid core, one's movement patterns can be compromised, which can lead to more wear and tear on joints, ligaments, and tendons.

Categories of Core Exercises

When teaching core exercises to student-athletes, the strength and conditioning professional should break them up into three separate categories and teach them in this order of importance. Exercises should progress from simple to complex as the body adapts to the training stimulus.

The first category is bracing or creating tension within the core. This starts with teaching student-athletes to breathe properly by contracting the diaphragm and breathing from the belly rather than from the chest. Next, student-athletes need to learn to isometrically contract the correct muscles and stabilize the spine and pelvis.

The next category of core exercises to teach student-athletes are **anti-extension**, **anti-flexion**, and **anti-rotation**. These exercises are a form of bracing in which the student-athlete learns to resist movement against an external force, whether it is a weight, a band, or gravity. In athletics the ability to resist movement with a tightening of the core is extremely important. The core is the link between the lower and upper body. Without a tight core there is leakage in that kinetic chain, and everything the student-athlete does with the limbs will become weaker. So, without a tight core, student-athletes cannot throw a baseball 90 miles per hour or kick a penalty kick with velocity. The classic analogy is that you cannot fire a cannon out of a rowboat because it is unstable.

The last category of core exercise that student-athletes need to learn is **extension**, **flexion**, and **rotation**, or what many student-athletes probably consider standard core exercises. This is the classic abdominal routine to work on the rectus abdominis and obliques.

Instructing Core Exercises

Strength and conditioning professionals can do core work with large groups in two ways. They can do them either on command or on the clock. For on-command exercises, the strength and conditioning professional calls out "up" and "down," which signals when the student-athlete should contract and relax. The benefit of doing it this way is that the strength and conditioning professional can control the tempo of the exercise and can force the student-athletes into a longer isometric hold instead of allowing gravity to work. The second way, on the clock, means that instead of telling the student-athletes to do a certain number of repetitions, the strength and conditioning professional will put them on the clock and have them do as many repetitions as they can in a given period of time. This ensures that every student-athlete is challenged, and it makes it very obvious if a student-athlete is not doing the work.

Core training is multifaceted in that it uses so many muscles and planes of motion. The core is often overlooked, but that does not make it any less valuable. The ability of student-athletes to tighten their core directly affects the limbs' ability to deliver force. Because high school student-athletes are so young, it is advisable to start with the basics and slowly progress. Every exercise listed here has progressions and regressions (1). Core exercises have countless variations. Some will depend on equipment, space, or number of student-athletes.

Exercise Finder

Diaphragmatic Breathing

Exercise Category

Diaphragmatic breathing is a bracing exercise.

Primary Muscle Trained

Diaphragm

Body Position

- Lie on the back.
- Quiet the mind and focus on breathing.

Breathing Guidelines

- Place the hands on the stomach.
- Inhale and exhale deeply.
- Feel the stomach expand on the inhalation as if pressing the stomach into a belt.

Exercise Modifications and Variations

Practice this type of breathing from different positions in the weight room. Start with a bodyweight squat. Inhale and breathe through the belly at the top of the squat, and exhale while extending the hips to stand up.

Coaching Tips

This exercise can be used for a number of purposes. It can be used to teach the student-athlete to stiffen or to stabilize the core before an exercise, which will in turn protect the back from injury. It can also be used as a method of relaxation. This type of recovery breathing stimulates the parasympathetic nervous system, which slows down the heart rate and causes the body to relax. Student-athletes often find this useful and can practice this type of breathing as a means of meditation to help their bodies and minds recover from the stresses of performance. It has been correlated with lower levels of oxidative stress, lower levels of cortisol, and higher levels of melatonin (2).

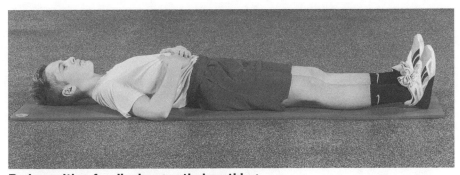

Body position for diaphragmatic breathing

Isometric V-Up

Exercise Category

The isometric V-up is a core flexion and extension exercise.

Primary Muscles Trained

Transverse abdominis, rectus abdominis, iliopsoas, tensor fascia latae, sartorius, pectineus, gracilis, rectus femoris

Static Position

1. Lie on the back with the arms by the sides.

2. Tuck the chin into the chest and raise the shoulder blades off the floor 6 to 8 inches (15-20 cm).

3. Tighten the quads by locking out the knees and raise the legs off the floor 6 to 8 inches (15-20 cm). The end position is similar to a *hollow body hold* in gymnastics.

4. This exercise can be done as a hold by stabilizing in that position.

Breathing Guidelines

Tighten the midsection without holding the breath.

Exercise Modifications and Variations

• To progress the exercise, raise the arms behind the head so that the biceps are framing the ears.

• Gently rock back and forth on the gluteus as if it were the fulcrum in a seesaw.

• To regress the exercise, slightly flex the knees. (Many student-athletes who lack core stability will instinctively do this anyway.)

Coaching Tips

This exercise can be rather dramatic at first. The student-athlete's body may shake as the neuromuscular demands are met. Start with one of the regressions and slowly progress. Typically, student-athletes will progress on this rather quickly. It is a spine-friendly exercise compared to the plank because it places the pelvis in a posterior tilt.

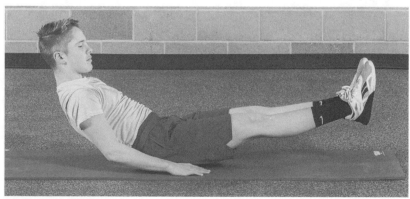

Static "V" position

Bird Dog

Exercise Category

The bird dog is a bracing exercise that uses both upper and lower extremity core–limb transfer muscles.

Primary Muscles Trained

Transverse abdominis, rectus abdominis, gluteus maximus, erector spinae, gluteus medius, external obliques, internal obliques, latissimus dorsi

Beginning Position

- Get on the hands and knees. The knees should be directly under the hips, and the wrists should be directly under the shoulders. (*Note:* The photos show a position with the hips and shoulders not quite *directly* over the knees and wrists.)
- Maintain a neutral spine.

Movement Phases

1. Extend one leg directly back as if trying to place the foot flat on the wall.
2. Extend the opposite arm as if trying to shake someone's hand.
3. Brace the core by pulling in the stomach and squeezing the glutes.
4. Maintain stiffness throughout the exercise.

Breathing Guidelines

Brace the core without holding the breath.

Exercise Modifications and Variations

- To regress the exercise, start with one arm rather than both the leg and arm.
- To progress the exercise, take the bottom knee slightly off the floor.
- Another progression is to extend the same-side arm and leg.

Coaching Tips

The bird dog looks rather easy, but it is in fact difficult for an untrained and inexperienced student-athlete to do correctly. One helpful cue for a strength and conditioning professional to give is to imagine someone is pulling the student-athlete's leg and someone else is pulling the arm as if trying to stretch the student-athlete out in both directions. Another cue is to squeeze the glute on the extended leg. Yet another is to pull in the stomach without holding the breath. The concept of bracing and squeezing certain muscles is difficult for many high school student-athletes. When they do it, they tend to hold their breath, so make sure they focus on bracing muscles and staying relaxed at the same time.

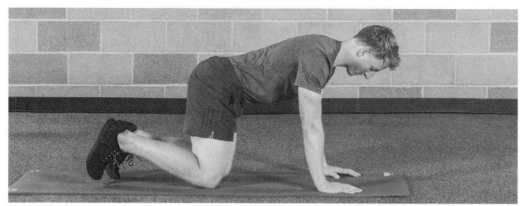

Beginning position

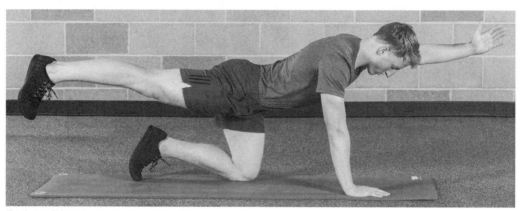

End position (one arm and leg)

Dead Bug

Exercise Category

Like the bird dog, the dead bug is a bracing exercise with the use of both upper and lower extremity core–limb transfer muscles.

Primary Muscles Trained

Transverse abdominis, rectus abdominis, external obliques, internal obliques, iliopsoas, pectineus, tensor fasciae latae, sartorius

Beginning Position

- Lie on the back.
- Flatten the lumbar spine and tighten the abdominals.

Movement Phases

1. Lying supine, raise the arms into the air with the wrists stacked over the elbows and shoulders.

2. Tuck the chin into the chest and raise the shoulder blades slightly off the floor (more than what is seen in the photos, for both positions).

3. Keeping the knees flexed at 90 degrees and the toes pointing up, raise the legs off the floor.

4. Slowly extend one arm and the opposite leg all the way out until the knee is locked out (the foot is 6 to 8 inches [15-20 cm] off of the floor) and the arm is extended behind the head.

5. Pause for a second, then return back to the beginning position.

6. Repeat with the opposite side.

Breathing Guidelines

Brace the core without holding the breath.

Exercise Modifications and Variations

- To regress the exercise, use only the arms or only the legs. Putting the feet flat against a wall can demonstrate that position while taking pressure off the lower half.

- To progress the exercise, add resistance. A mini-band around the feet works for the lower half, and a band wrapped around a sturdy object works for the upper half.

- To progress the exercise even further, extend both arms and both legs at the same time.

Coaching Tip

If at any point student-athletes feel anything in the lumbar spine, they should immediately stop and check their form. It could be that their abdominals are not strong enough yet and they need to choose a regression to build those muscles up.

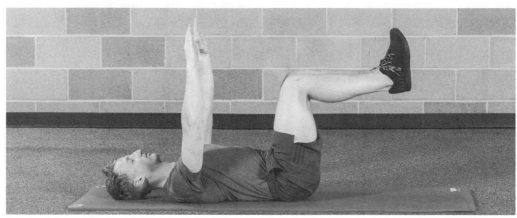

Beginning position with legs and arms raised

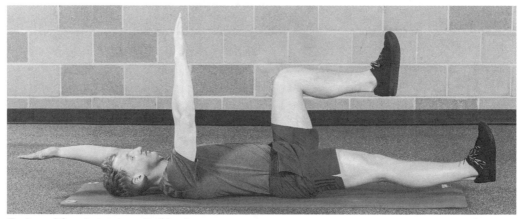

End position (one arm and leg)

Front Plank

Exercise Category

The front plank is a bracing exercise.

Primary Muscles Trained

Rectus abdominis, transverse abdominis, internal obliques, external obliques, rectus femoris, sartorius, vastus lateralis, vastus medialis, gluteus maximus, gluteus medius

Static Position

1. Lie prone with the hands next to the shoulders.

2. With the hands and elbows stacked directly under the shoulders, push the upper body up and lift the hips up toward the sky.

3. Remain as still as possible while bracing the entire body in a straight line.

Breathing Guidelines

Brace the core without holding the breath.

Exercise Modifications and Variations

• To regress the exercise, hold the position for a shorter period of time.

• Another regression is to move up to the hands as if at the top of a push-up.

• To progress the exercise, raise one limb off of the floor. This forces the center of mass to one side and therefore compensation by stabilizing the core.

• Another progression is to add weight. A strength and conditioning professional can add plates onto the student-athlete's back, forcing the student-athlete to tighten up against the added weight.

Coaching Tips

The goal should be intensity, not duration. If the student-athlete starts to compensate by arching the lower back and flexing at the knees, stop the exercise. The goal is to maintain strict rigidness for the duration of the exercise without any compensation.

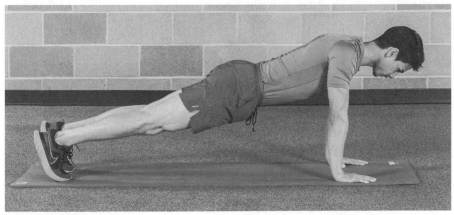

Static plank position

Side Plank

Exercise Category

The side plank is a bracing exercise.

Primary Muscles Trained

Internal obliques, external obliques, rectus abdominis, transverse abdominis, serratus anterior

Static Position

1. Lie on the side with the legs extended and one foot on top of the other.
2. With the forearm on the floor and the elbow stacked directly under the shoulder, lift the hips up toward the ceiling.
3. Remain as still as possible while bracing the entire body in a straight line.

Breathing Guidelines

Brace the core without holding the breath.

Exercise Modifications and Variations

- To regress the exercise, flex the knees. This shortens the lever point at the lower half.
- To progress the exercise, instead of holding the exercise, raise up and down as if doing a side sit-up.
- Another progression is to elevate the top leg onto a bench, which will start to fire the adductors.

Coaching Tip

The cue that is most effective for the side plank is the visual of having a rope around the waist that it is pulling the hips up toward the ceiling.

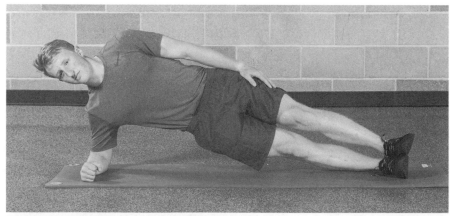

Static plank position (one side)

Pallof Press

Exercise Category

The Pallof press is an anti-flexion, anti-extension, and anti-rotation exercise.

Primary Muscles Trained

Internal obliques, external obliques, latissimus dorsi, pectoralis major

Beginning Position

• Stand perpendicular to a column with a cable or band attached to it.

• Flex the knees slightly in an athletic stance (not clearly seen in the photos) and grab the handle or end of the band, making sure the hand that is closer to the column is over the other hand.

Movement Phases

1. Extend the arms out in front in a smooth pattern.

2. Pause for a second with the arms extended.

3. Return to the beginning position.

Breathing Guidelines

The core should be braced, but breathing should be natural.

Exercise Modifications and Variations

• Kneeling
• Half kneeling
• Split stance
• Lunge
• Lateral
• Overhead

Coaching Tip

It is important that the strength and conditioning professional instructs

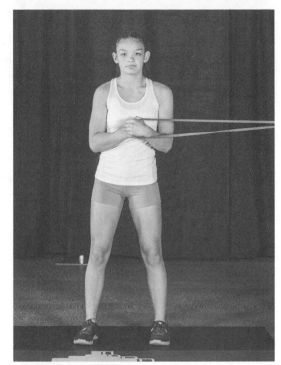

Beginning position

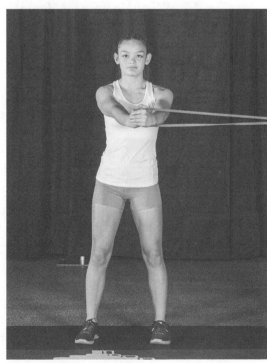

End position (one side)

the student-athlete to place the hand that is closest to the column on top of the other hand. This prevents the student-athlete from overusing the pectorals and forces the core to take over.

Loaded Carry

Exercise Category

Loaded carries are an anti-flexion, anti-extension, and anti-rotation exercise that uses lower extremity core–limb transfer muscles.

Primary Muscles Trained

Internal obliques, external obliques

Beginning Position

• The farmer's carry is the primary variation. Start with two heavy dumbbells, one in each hand.

Movement Phases

1. Grab two heavy dumbbells, one in each hand.
2. Maintain good posture by standing tall.
3. Extend the hips and brace the core.
4. Walk for either a specified period of time or a specified distance.

Breathing Guidelines

Brace the core without holding the breath.

Exercise Modifications and Variations

The loaded carry offers many variations.

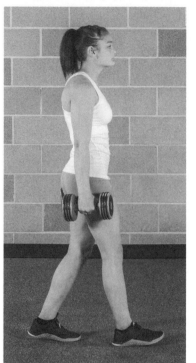

Loaded carry position

• *Trap bar carry.* Deadlift the weight up with good technique and walk with the weight.

• *Front-loaded carry.* Typically, this is done with a sandbag. Bear hug the bag and walk. Front-loading the weight will force the core to fire, similar to a heavy front squat.

• *Fireman's carry.* This can be done with a sandbag. Drape the sandbag over one shoulder with the arm on the top for stability. Alternate shoulders to eliminate imbalances and so as not to favor either side.

• *Yoke carry.* The yoke carry is a classic strongman exercise. Place the weight on the back similar to a back squat. If a yoke is not available, a barbell on the back works.

• *Barbell overhead carry.* This variation has great carryover to Olympic lifting. Carry the weight over the head in the lockout position.

• *Offset carry.* Loading only one side of the body forces bracing of the core. Different weighted options work well, including dumbbells and kettlebells. The weights can be carried in different positions, such as an offset suitcase carry or a kettlebell in the single-arm, front rack position or overhead.

Coaching Tips

This is one of the best core exercises an athlete can do because of its functional capabilities. The strength and conditioning professional can program this into regular training sessions as part of circuit training during periods of building work capacity. Adding in offset or front-loaded squats can add to the stimulus and teach the student-athlete how to brace the core in a variety of ways.

Superman

Exercise Category

The Superman is a bracing exercise that uses both upper and lower extremity core–limb transfer muscles.

Primary Muscles Trained

Erector spinae, gluteus maximus, gluteus medius

Static Position

1. Lie prone on the floor with the arms extended over the head.
2. Raise the arms and legs off the floor.
3. Remain as still as possible while bracing the entire body in a concave position.

Breathing Guidelines

Brace the core without holding the breath.

Exercise Modifications and Variations

• Raise and lower both arms and legs.

• Lift and hold while making sure to pause at the top for a second, then lower the arms and legs in a controlled manner.

• Execute swimmers by raising and lowering the opposite arm and leg at the same time (e.g., the right arm and left leg).

Coaching Tips

The strength and conditioning professional should make sure that student-athletes move slowly through this exercise and that they should feel it in their lower back and their gluteus. To make sure this happens, "up" and "down" can be called out to ensure that the movements are purposeful and that muscle relaxation and gravity are not the causes for lowering the body. A common fault for this exercise is to flex at the knees instead of extending the hips. If the student-athlete does not feel their gluteus contracting, that is probably the reason. The coaching cue is to move from the hips and not the knee.

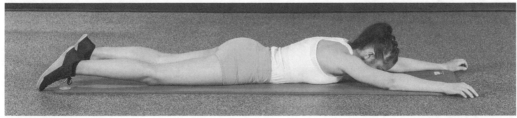

Beginning position

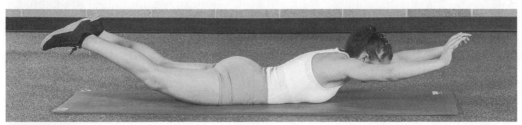

End position

Sit-Up

Exercise Category

The sit-up is a core flexion and extension exercise.

Primary Muscles Trained

Rectus abdominis, internal obliques, external obliques, iliopsoas

Beginning Position

• Lie supine with the knees flexed and back flat on the floor.

• Fold the arms across the chest and grab onto the opposite sides of the shirt or tank to avoid using the arms to build momentum.

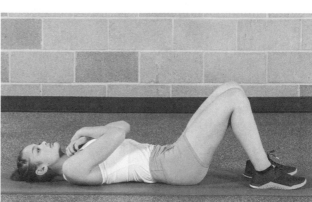

Beginning position

Movement Phases

Sit up so the shoulder blades come off the floor and the elbows touch the thighs above the midway point between the hip and the knee.

Breathing Guidelines

Exhale on the way up and inhale on the way down.

Exercise Modifications and Variations

• Butterfly the legs by externally rotating the hips

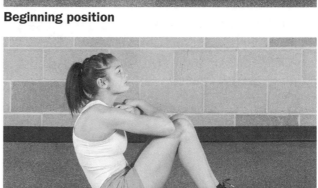

End position

and touching the soles of the feet. This eliminates the hip flexors from taking over some of the work of the abdominals.

• To regress the exercise, swing the arms to build momentum. This may allow for more sit-ups overall and for a weaker student-athlete to keep up with the group.

• To progress this exercise, grab a plate and hold it in the hands in front of the chest. While sitting up, reach the weight up toward the ceiling.

Coaching Tips

Part of coaching is teaching student-athletes where they should feel the exercise and where they should not. With any abdominal work the strength and conditioning professional should emphasize intensity rather than volume or duration. If at any point student-athletes feel the lower back starting to take over, they should stop and check their form.

Russian Twist

Exercise Category

The Russian twist is a global core mobilizer that uses trunk rotation.

Primary Muscles Trained

Internal obliques, external obliques

Beginning Position

• Sit on the floor with the legs crossed at the ankles and feet off the floor.

• Lean back slightly while keeping the spine neutral (more neutral than what is seen in the photos).

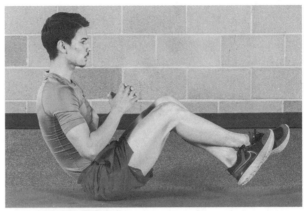
Beginning position

Movement Phases

Rotate the upper body through the shoulders to the right and to the left while keeping the hips through the lower body stationary.

Breathing Guidelines

Brace the core without holding the breath.

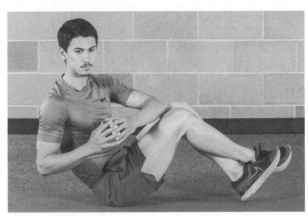
End position (one side)

Exercise Modifications and Variations

• To progress this exercise, rotate the upper body through the shoulders and the lower body through the hips in opposite movements.

• A weight plate, dumbbell, kettlebell, or weighted ball can be held in front of the chest and carried through the rotation.

Coaching Tip

If not using a weight, student-athletes should hold their hands together so that the upper body moves as a whole.

Leg Raise

Exercise Category

The leg raise is a core flexion and extension exercise.

Primary Muscles Trained

Rectus abdominis, external obliques

Beginning Position

1. Lie on the back.

2. Take the arch out of the lower back and remain as flat as possible in the lumbar spine.

3. Place the hands at the sides with palms down and tuck the chin into the chest while the shoulder blades are lifted slightly off the floor.

Movement Phases

1. While bracing the core and keeping the lumbar spine flat, raise the legs up to about 90 degrees, moving from the hips. The knees should be locked out and the ankles dorsiflexed throughout the entire movement.

2. When lowering the legs, remain under control to let the abdominals control the movement instead of letting gravity do the work.

Breathing Guidelines

Brace the core without holding the breath.

Exercise Modifications and Variations

• To regress the exercise, put the hands underneath the body, which gives a little more leverage.

• To progress the exercise, add an oblique twist. Change the angle to 45 degrees and complete the leg raise from the side.

• To progress the exercise further, hang from a pull-up bar and do the leg raises, starting with flexed knees and progressing to extended legs or even twisting to work the obliques.

Coaching Tips

The concept of bracing the core without holding the breath is a staple in a lot of core exercises. That is no different in the leg raise. The strength and conditioning professional can reinforce this by lightly touching the student-athlete's abdominals with a foam roller or something similar during the movement; the result is a reflexive bracing of the core.

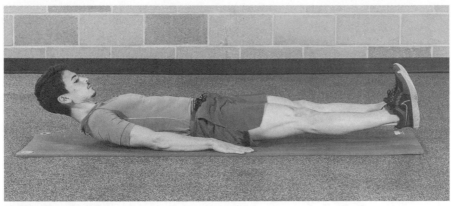

Beginning position

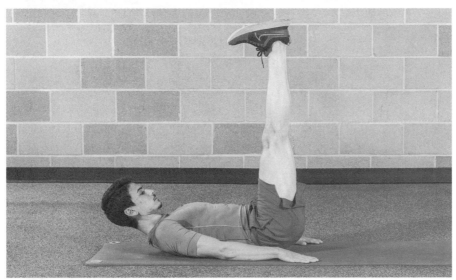

End position

7

Warm-Up

Darnell K. Clark, MPE, CSCS,*D, RSCC*D

Whether a physical education teacher, sport coach, strength and conditioning professional, or a parent who wants to train their child to become a better student-athlete, it is important to know that performance is multifaceted and requires a range of physical and skill capabilities. Subsequently, efficiency and effectiveness are critical in optimizing the training response (11). Developing an intentional and comprehensive warm-up is essential to cultivating the skills and capabilities required in movement and training.

Purpose and Benefit of a Warm-Up

Warm-up routines are performed to prepare the body to perform optimally during training or competition (1, 2, 5, 8, 16) and to prevent potential injuries during recreational or sport activities (5, 10, 16, 17). Additionally, because optimal performance does not solely depend on physiology, the student-athlete also must be psychologically prepared for activity. Psychological readiness depends on an individual's mental attention to the upcoming task or activity (11).

Traditional Warm-Up

A traditional warm-up has two phases: a **general warm-up** and a **specific warm-up**. The general warm-up commonly includes movements or exercises that involve the whole body, typically with an emphasis on the lower body such as walking, jogging, cycling, skipping, jumping jacks, shuffling, and backpedaling (9), followed by flexibility exercises that imitate the ranges of motion that are involved in the upcoming activity (14). The aim of this phase is to increase heart rate, breathing rate, sweat rate, blood flow, and deep muscle temperature (14, 15, 18).

Following the general warm-up, the specific warm-up includes movements similar to the upcoming workout. If the individual is warming up to do a specific sport, it is important that the specific warm-up also includes the movement patterns or skills of the sport (14). As a whole, the warm-up should include a combination of static and dynamic exercises (see later sections in this chapter), progress gradually, and provide sufficient intensity to increase muscle and core temperatures without causing fatigue or reducing energy stores (13).

Sport Performance Warm-Up

Although student-athletes may go through the two phases of a traditional warm-up, a more strategic warm-up is needed before doing a specific sport. To prepare student-athletes to be able to perform, a traditional warm-up is not sufficient by itself; instead, they need a period of intensification to build up to maximum performance. Therefore, there is a difference between a precompetition warm-up and a preworkout warm-up (14).

One such approach is the three-phase **Raise, Activate and Mobilize, and Potentiate (RAMP)** protocol (11). The first phase, raise, is similar to the traditional warm-up in that it begins with general activities that raise physiological and psychological alertness. It then progresses to specific activities that mimic the upcoming sport's movement or skill patterns or both. The result is that the student-athlete is specifically primed for the specific movement aspects and demands of the competition. The combination activation and mobilization phase typically involves **dynamic mobility** (actively moving through a range of motion [14]) exercises that reinforce both the warming effects of the first phase and the key movement patterns and motor control requirements of the upcoming sport. Then, to fully prepare the student-athlete for maximum performance, the potentiation phase uses movements that progress in their intensity until they match the intensity level that the student-athlete will experience in the competition. The potentiation phase is particularly important when the student-athlete's sport has critical power, speed, or strength demands.

Simply said, a traditional warm-up does not sufficiently prepare a student-athlete for the physiological and psychological requirements of competitive sport performance. It is only through the sequential RAMP phases that sufficient sport-specific intensification can occur.

Types of Stretches Included in a Warm-Up

A warm-up can include a combination of **static** (no movement) and **dynamic** (with movement) stretching exercises. Regarding the latter, sometimes the term *dynamic warm-up* is used (6), but the NSCA clarifies this to the more specific terms of *dynamic stretching* and *dynamic flexibility* (12).

Static Stretching

A static stretch includes the relaxation and concurrent elongation of the stretched muscle (7). Static stretching provides time for the sport coach, teacher, or strength and conditioning professional to instruct technique and form because the student-athlete is holding a fixed position. Further, static stretching enables student-athletes to work on their fundamental body positioning (e.g., an athletic stance that can be reinforced by adding an isometric squat hold). Research shows that static stretching effectively improves range of motion (2). Note, however, that static stretching can cause decreases in force production, power, speed, and reaction time in the subsequent activity or sport (14).

Stated another way, static stretching as part of a warm-up provides a strength and conditioning professional with an opportunity to teach a fundamental movement position of an associated exercise. When the movement is held (called the *hold*), the professional can teach, reinforce, and perfect the position with the student-athlete, and at the same time, the student-athlete's heart rate, blood flow, deep muscle temperature, and respiration rate increase in preparation for the upcoming workout or training session.

Exercise Finder: Static Stretching

Isometric Lunge

Primary Muscles Affected

Gluteus maximus, hamstrings, iliopsoas, quadriceps

Static Position

1. Start in a half-kneeling position with the forward foot firmly on the floor. The forward knee is at a 90-degree angle.

2. The resting knee should be on the floor directly aligned with the hip joint.

3. Put the hands on the hips and maintain a tall torso with the chest up.

4. Push through the heel of the forward foot until the resting (back) knee is 2 inches (5 cm) off the floor.

Breathing Guidelines

Inhale and hold the breath until reaching the desired position. Once in the desired position, exhale and begin to breathe normally.

Coaching Tip

Keep the head and torso upright and tall with the chest up, shoulders back, and hands on the hips.

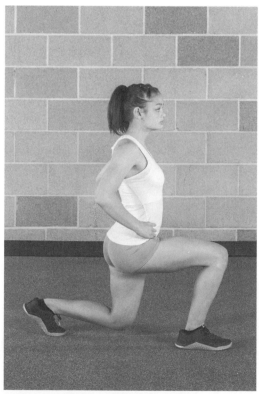

Static lunging position (one leg)

Isometric Push-Up Hold

Primary Muscles Affected

Pectorals, deltoids, triceps brachii

Static Position

1. Start in the prone position.

2. Extend the legs (as shown in the photo) or flex the knees, depending on the strength of the student-athlete, to balance the lower body on the toes or the knees, respectively.

3. Bring the chest off the floor until the elbow joints are at 90 degrees and hold that position.

Breathing Guidelines

Inhale and hold the breath until reaching the desired position. Once in the desired position, exhale and begin to breathe normally.

Coaching Tips

Use a wider hand placement to place a greater stress on the pectoral muscles and use a narrow hand placement to place a greater stress on the triceps.

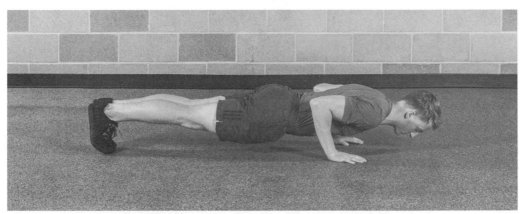

Static push-up position

Isometric Squat Hold

Primary Muscles Affected

Gluteus maximus, quadriceps, hamstrings

Static Position

1. Stand with feet slightly wider apart than shoulder width.
2. Turn the toes slightly out.
3. Flex the hips and knees until the quadriceps are parallel to the floor.

Breathing Guidelines

Inhale and hold the breath until reaching the desired position. Once in the desired position, exhale and begin to breathe normally.

Coaching Tips

Keep the head and torso upright and tall with the chest up, shoulders back, and arms and hands held in front of the torso. When in the bottom position, the knees should be vertically aligned over the midfoot and the toes.

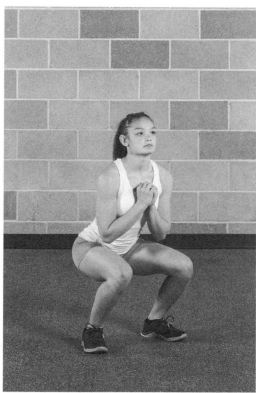

Static squatting position

Half-Kneeling Quadriceps Hold

Primary Muscles Affected

Quadriceps, iliopsoas

Static Position

1. Start in a half-kneeling position with the lead foot firmly on the floor one foot length in front of the lead knee.

2. The trailing knee should be on the floor directly aligned with the trailing hip joint.

3. Put the hands on the hips and maintain a tall torso with the chest up.

4. Push the hips forward until there is a sensation of stretching in the hip and the quadriceps of the trailing leg.

5. Hold the position when the lead knee joint is at a 90-degree angle.

Breathing Guidelines

Inhale and hold the breath until reaching the desired position. Once in the desired position, exhale and begin to breathe normally.

Coaching Tip

Keep the head and torso upright and tall, with the chest up, shoulders back, and hands on your hips.

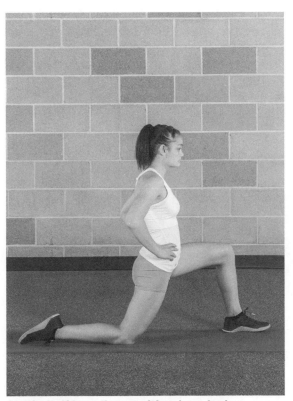

Static half-kneeling position (one leg)

Isometric Sumo Squat Hold

Primary Muscles Affected

Gluteus maximus, quadriceps, hamstrings, erector spinae, hip adductors

Static Position

1. Stand with the feet significantly wider apart than shoulder width.

2. Turn the toes slightly out.

3. Flex the hips and knees until the head, chest, and torso are upright.

4. Hold the position and place the palms flat on the floor (not shown in the photo).

Breathing Guidelines

Inhale and hold the breath until reaching the desired position. Once in the desired position, exhale and begin to breathe normally.

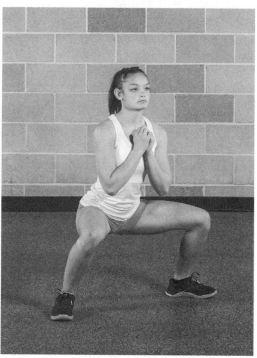

Static sumo squatting position

Coaching Tip

The foot placement will depend on individual hip flexibility. Widen the feet until the palms can be placed flat on the floor (not shown in the photo).

Dynamic Stretching

A dynamic stretch commonly involves (and progressively elongates) multiple muscle groups; actively places the body in a variety of positions; improves mobility, stability, and balance; and places an emphasis on the movement requirements of the sport or activity rather than isolated muscles (14). Dynamic stretching is also known to enhance performance in subsequent dynamic concentric muscle actions against an external resistance, thereby improving power, agility, sprint time, and vertical jump height (3). Further, it is a time-efficient way to warm up because a dynamic stretch includes multiple joints and muscle groups in one exercise (11).

Exercise Finder: Dynamic Stretching

Forward Lunge With Elbow to Instep and Rotation (World's Greatest Stretch)

Primary Muscles Affected

Gluteus maximus, hamstrings, iliopsoas, quadriceps, erector spinae, latissimus dorsi, internal obliques, external obliques, rectus femoris, soleus

Beginning Position

• Stand tall with the feet placed shoulder-width apart.

Movement Phases

1. Step forward with the right foot in a lunge position.

2. Place the left hand on the floor for balance and flex the right elbow and push the right forearm toward the floor inside the right foot. Hold for 3 seconds.

3. Move the right hand outside the right foot, and twist toward the right to reach the right arm toward the sky. Hold for 3 seconds.

4. Bring the left foot forward, stand tall, and start the process again, leading (lunging) with the left leg.

Breathing Guidelines

Breathe normally throughout the process.

Coaching Tips

• When in a lunge position and pushing the inside forearm to the floor, extend the back leg (more than what is shown in the photos) to intensify the stretch.

• When rotating and reaching to the sky, follow that hand with the eyes (not shown in the second photo). This will automatically rotate the torso properly.

• Think *right leg lunge, right forearm to the floor, right hand to the sky*. Then repeat: *left, left, left*.

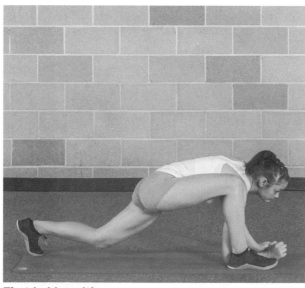

First held position

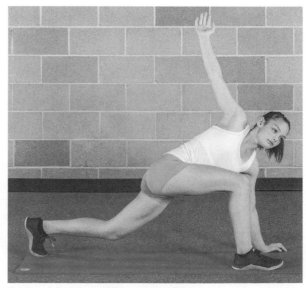

Second held position (one side)

Inverted Hamstring Walk

Primary Muscles Affected

Gluteus maximus, hamstrings

Beginning Position

- Stand tall with the feet shoulder-width apart.

Movement Phases

1. Standing tall, keep an extended, rigid posture, and flex forward at the waist, lifting the left foot off the floor while slightly flexing the knee of the planted leg. The result is a stretch in the hamstring of the planted leg.

2. Press both palms to the floor (not shown in the photos) while maintaining a neutral spine.

3. Bring the left foot down, stand tall (or step forward), and repeat the movement on the right side.

Breathing Guidelines

Breathe normally throughout the movement.

Coaching Tip

When flexing forward (and pushing the palms to the floor, if that is done), it is essential not to round the lower back to get the desired stretch of the hamstrings. Instead, maintain a neutral rigid spine throughout the movement.

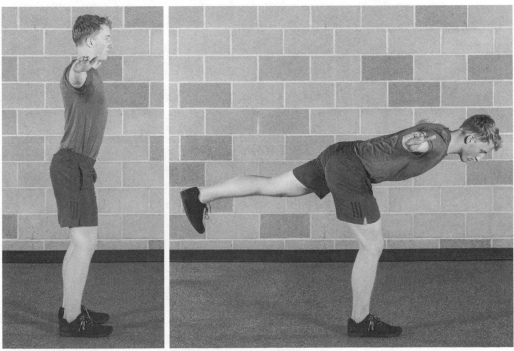

Beginning position   **End position (one leg)**

Forward Skip With Arm Circles

Primary Muscles Affected

Gluteus maximus, hamstrings, quadriceps, deltoids, latissimus dorsi, pectorals

Beginning Position

- Stand tall with the feet shoulder-width apart.

Movement Phases

1. Standing tall, keep an extended, rigid posture, and march in place with a focus on a high 90-degree knee angle.

2. After marching for 2 to 3 seconds, begin skipping in place for 2 to 3 seconds with a focus on a high 90-degree knee angle.

3. Start skipping forward while simultaneously rotating the arms forward in a large circular motion.

Breathing Guidelines

Breathe normally throughout the movement.

Coaching Tip

Starting with an in-place march to an in-place skip before moving forward helps develop the proper rhythm of skipping.

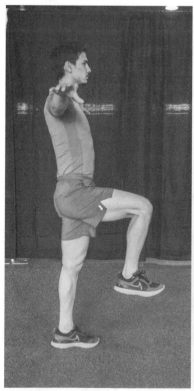
Marching

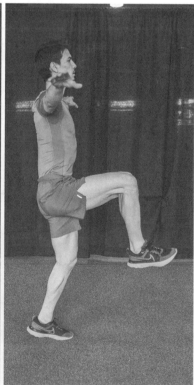
Skipping

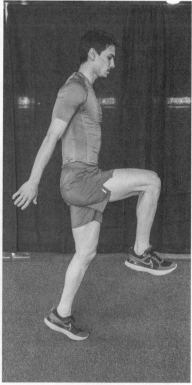
Forward skip with arm circles

Inchworm

Primary Muscles Affected

Gluteus maximus, hamstrings, soleus, anterior tibialis, erector spinae, deltoids, triceps brachii

Beginning Position

- Stand tall with the feet shoulder-width apart.

Movement Phases

1. Standing tall, keep the legs extended, and flex at the waist until both hands reach the floor.

2. Without flexing the knees, walk the hands forward until reaching a push-up position.

3. Keeping the legs locked at the knees, begin to take forward steps, with the ankles and feet providing the motion.

4. When walking the feet forward, stop the process when the knees can no longer be kept in the locked position (a photo of this position is not shown).

5. Repeat the process by walking the hands forward.

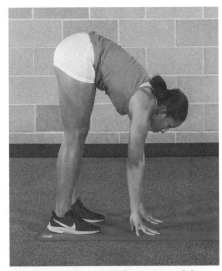

Breathing Guidelines

Breathe normally throughout the movement.

Coaching Tip

If it is not possible to reach the floor with extended legs, slightly flex the knees to approach the floor.

Beginning forward-flexed position

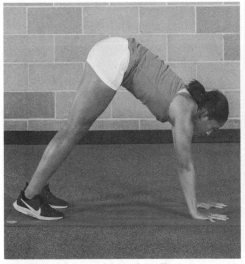 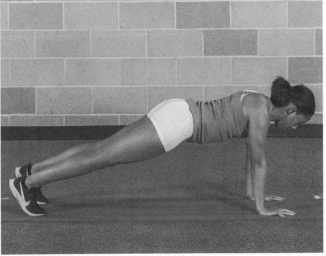

Middle of forward hand-walk movement   Push-up position

Lunge With Overhead Side Reach

Primary Muscles Affected

Gluteus maximus, hamstrings, iliopsoas, latissimus dorsi, internal obliques, external obliques, rectus femoris

Beginning Position

- Stand tall with the feet shoulder-width apart.

Movement Phases

1. Step forward with the left foot in a lunge position, keeping a 90-degree angle in the left knee.

2. The right knee should be flexed somewhat more than a 90-degree angle (this position varies based on the individual's flexibility) and positioned 2 to 3 inches (5-8 cm) from the floor.

3. Hold the lunge position and reach the right hand (i.e., opposite of the lunged leg) up to the ceiling.

4. While continuing to give effort to the "reaching" sensation, change the reach direction to reach over the head until the sensation of a stretch in the latissimus dorsi of the reaching side of the torso occurs.

5. After fully reaching, lower the right arm to the side, push through the lunge to stand tall, and repeat the motion with the right leg lunged forward and reaching up and over with the left hand.

Breathing Guidelines

Breathe normally throughout the movement.

Coaching Tip

Perform each movement deliberately, keeping each step separate. This will ensure the quality of the exercise movement.

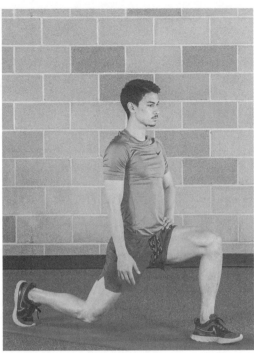

Beginning lunged position

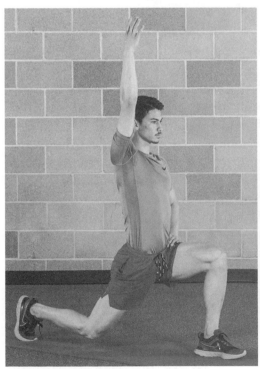

Lunged position with arm reach

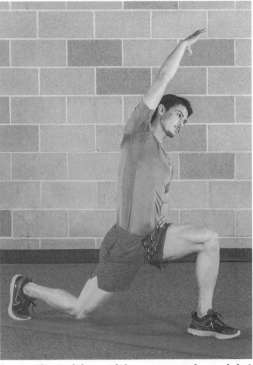

Lunged position with arm reach and lat stretch (one side)

Recommendations for Designing Warm-Up Routines

When warming up, it is important to consider the kinds of activities that will be performed during the training or activity session, previous injuries, and any tight or sore muscles or body areas. As with all forms of training, frequency, duration, and intensity are important issues in program design (4). A minimum of 10 to 20 minutes should be dedicated to a proper warm-up prior to any activity. This should include 5 to 10 minutes of general warm-up; four to six static stretches that focus on elongating the stretched muscles; and four to six dynamic stretches that focus on improving joint mobility, elasticity of the muscle, and the specific movements of the upcoming activity (9, 11, 14, 15, 18).

The strength and conditioning professional, whether in a classroom setting or an athletic setting, will have to contend with issues and factors that are unique to working with small and large classes, groups, or teams.

Considerations for Small Classes, Groups, and Teams

- *What type of session is it?* In a classroom setting, the teacher should choose warm-ups that reinforce movement qualities that are desired by the teacher or for the proceeding activity. For instance, if the lesson or drill involves jumping and landing mechanics, it would be beneficial to have the students perform an isometric squat hold. The squat hold will prime the necessary muscles in addition to reinforcing the basic positioning of jumping and landing mechanics. This is also the scenario when teaching takes precedence over performance. That is, a teacher may want to select fewer warm-up exercises and repeat them two or three times to reinforce the technique. In training and competition, a warm-up routine has been suggested to be critical in increasing the preparedness for subsequent effort and thus maximizing performance (14). In this setting, the strength and conditioning professional should choose exercises that focus on performance.

- *Is the warm-up inside or outside?* A teacher or strength and conditioning professional should consider the environment. Is there enough space to perform the warm-up? What is the desired temperature for the warm-up setting? Will the space be conducive for verbal instruction, or will there be distractions?

- *What type of equipment is available or needed?* Does the teacher or strength and conditioning professional use equipment like mini-bands, yoga blocks, or foam rollers? If so, activities should properly use these pieces of equipment to enhance the effect of the warm-up and the student-athlete's experience.

- *Is the student-athlete wearing restrictive equipment?* This is most relevant to student-athletes participating in an athletic practice or game. If the student-athlete has equipment, consider the range of motion restrictions. This may require creativity or performing the warm-up prior to putting the equipment on.

- *Does the team have a history of sport-specific injuries?* This is most relevant to student-athletes participating in an athletic practice or game. It is a good idea for the teacher or strength and conditioning professional to have a conversation with the sport coach or athletic trainer about the injury trends with a particular group or team. The answers will help guide the decisions about warm-up priorities. It is also helpful to record these decisions and revisit the list of warm-ups to see if the warm-up selection has an impact on the team's injury trends.

- *How much time is available for the warm-up?* Time will always be a factor. Choose warm-up exercises that focus on total body movement and find a way to get everyone engaged in the exercise at the same time instead of lines of two or three individuals.

Considerations for Large Classes, Groups, and Teams

For a large group or team, the considerations will be the same as those for small groups, but the decisions may differ based on the size of the group. For instance, if a group of 30 student-athletes is outside on a field performing dynamic stretching, the group may be set up in three horizontal lines of 10. The teacher or strength and conditioning professional may choose warm-ups that allow each group of 10 to move forward before the next group of 10 is released, and so on. Or if these 30 student-athletes are performing static stretching, each group of athletes may be in the same horizontal lines of 10 spread out 5 yards (5 m) apart. Thinking creatively about the setup of the warm-up will ensure that it is effective, efficient, and purposeful.

When instructing a large class or team, consider choosing a series of static stretches that elongate the muscles and focusing on holds that reinforce key positions, such as the athletic position. The held position of static stretches allows the teacher or strength and conditioning professional to move around and modify, correct, or praise the student-athlete's position. Additionally, it may be beneficial to follow with the dynamic version of the same exercise for positional reinforcement and demonstration of performing the exercise using a full range of motion.

- *Is the space restricted or unlimited?* If the area is restricted, choose activities or modifications of exercises that limit the need for space. If the space is unlimited, use the space to perform the warm-ups in various ways that keep the participants engaged in the activity. In both cases, position student-athletes in formations that allow good sight lines and walking lanes to maintain eye contact and move effectively while instructing.
- *Can student-athlete leaders (i.e., captains) run the warm-ups?* Warm-ups are an essential element of the training or performance preparation. If student-athletes run the warm-up, make sure there is a strength and conditioning professional present so error identification and correction of the participants' technique can be provided.

Examples of Simple Warm-Up Routines

The sample basic warm-up sequences—performed after a 5- to 10-minute general warm-up—reinforce the fundamental movement skills that are commonly used in many activities and begin to prepare the individual for the upcoming exercise or training session. (Note that the RAMP protocol is not applied or portrayed in the examples because the movements and exercises included would need to be tailored to that specific sport and therefore cannot be generalized here.)

Individuals

Here are examples of individual warm-up routines based on the relative size of available space (see pages 208-218 for descriptions of the proper technique for each exercise):

Restricted Space

Perform 1 or 2 sets of each exercise:

- Isometric squat hold: 20 seconds
- Bodyweight squat: 10 repetitions
- Isometric push-up hold: 10 seconds
- Push-up: 10 repetitions

- Isometric lunge: 10 seconds for each leg
- In-place forward or reverse lunge: 5 repetitions for each leg

Large Space

Perform 1 or 2 sets of each exercise:

- Forward skip with arm circles: 15 yards (or meters)
- Forward walking lunge with overhead reach: 10 yards (or meters)
- Inchworm: 10 yards (or meters)
- Forward lunge with elbow to instep and rotation: 10 yards (or meters)

Classes, Groups, and Teams

Of any aspect that affects the exercises selected for a warm-up routine for a class, group, or team, it is the relative size of the available space. (See pages 208-218 for descriptions of the proper technique for each exercise.)

Restricted Space

Perform 1 or 2 sets of each exercise:

- Isometric squat hold: 20 seconds
- Bodyweight squat: 10 repetitions
- Isometric push-up hold: 10 seconds
- Push-up: 10 repetitions
- Isometric lunge: 10 seconds for each leg
- In-place forward or reverse lunge: 5 repetitions for each leg
- Isometric sumo squat: 20 seconds
- Isometric quad stretch: 20 seconds
- Inchworm: Walk hands out and back for 5 repetitions

Large Space

Perform 1 or 2 sets of each exercise:

- Jog: 15 yards (or meters) out and back
- Forward skip with arm circles: 15 yards (or meters)
- High knees: 15 yards (or meters)
- Forward walking lunge with overhead reach: 10 yards (or meters)
- Inchworm: 10 yards (or meters)
- Walking quad stretch: 10 yards (or meters)
- Forward lunge with elbow to instep and rotation: 10 yards (or meters)
- Inverted hamstring walk: 10 yards (or meters)

Conclusion

For the teacher, sport coach, and strength and conditioning professional, the warm-up is an essential lead-in to a class, workout, practice, or competition. It physiologically prepares the body for the upcoming session and provides an opportunity to reinforce movement quality and skills. Further, the warm-up not only is essential for physical preparation but it also psychologically prepares the individual or group for more intense activity.

Resistance Training

Shana McKeever, MA, LAT, ATC, CSCS,*D
Rick Howard, DSc, CSCS,*D, FNSCA

The high school strength and conditioning professional has a vast yet interrelated number of variables to consider when designing a resistance training program for high school students and student-athletes. In addition to the nine variables of program design (47)—needs analysis, exercise selection, training frequency, exercise order, training load, repetitions, sets, rest periods, and progression—the high school strength and conditioning professional must be aware of how each variable is influenced by an individual's goals and abilities. Factors that contribute to participation in a resistance training program may include improving fitness, sport performance, or health and wellness; an interest in structured strength and conditioning; and previous experience with resistance training. Additionally, the strength and conditioning professional should consider the individual's grade in school and playing level (freshman, junior varsity, or varsity); developmental age, including the varying levels of physical and emotional maturity; and sport season variability or specialization.

The health and well-being of the student-athlete should be the central principle of the long-term strength and conditioning program (27). For students and student-athletes alike, program design should be individually tailored to improve performance and reduce the risk of injury, whether for physical education, organized sports, recreational pursuits, fitness, or general health. The National Standards for Physical Education (44) and the National Standards for Coaching (45) guide the educational outcomes and include the concept of physical literacy as the desired outcome in physical education long-term athletic development. Both physical literacy and long-term athletic development assume that everyone is an athlete within their given level of endowment and that plentiful, varied, and purposeful opportunities should be provided across the lifespan to encourage a physically literate society (table 8.1) (44, 45).

TABLE 8.1   National Standards for Coaching and Physical Education of the Physically Literate Individual

Standard	Coaching	Physical education
1	Develop and enact an athlete-centered coaching philosophy	Demonstrates competency in a variety of motor skills and movement patterns
2	Use long-term athlete development with the intent to develop athletic potential, enhance physical literacy, and encourage lifelong physical activity	Applies knowledge of concepts, principles, strategies, and tactics related to movement performance
3	Create a unified vision using strategic planning and goal-setting principles	Demonstrates the knowledge and skills to achieve and maintain a health-enhancing level of physical activity and fitness
4	Align program with all rules and regulations and needs of the community and the individual athletes	Exhibits responsible personal and social behavior that respects self and others
5	Manage program resources in a responsible manner	Recognizes the value of physical activity for health, enjoyment, challenge, self-expression, and social interaction

Adapted from SHAPE America (44) and SHAPE America (45).

High school strength and conditioning professionals should be aware of the following three popular long-term athletic development (LTAD) models.

1. Jean Côté's developmental model of sports participation (DMSP) (8) identifies three developmental phases of youth sports participation: non-age-determined sampling, specialization, and investing; this means that the level of coaching and program design should match the developmental phase of each participant.

2. Istvan Balyi's long-term athlete development model (3) identifies specific stages that athletes pass through, dividing them into either an elite performance track or a fitness-for-life pathway.

3. Rhodri Lloyd and Jon Oliver's youth physical development model (YPD) (29) highlights the importance of all youth training all 10 fitness attributes across all stages of development.

Pichardo and colleagues (38) overlaid the three most popular models of LTAD to guide the proper application of the variables of program design for all student-athletes under the watch of the strength and conditioning professional (figure 8.1). The LTAD models frame the developmental, physical, and psychosocial elements of positive youth development, from which high school strength and conditioning professionals can implement safe and effective student-centered strength and conditioning programs.

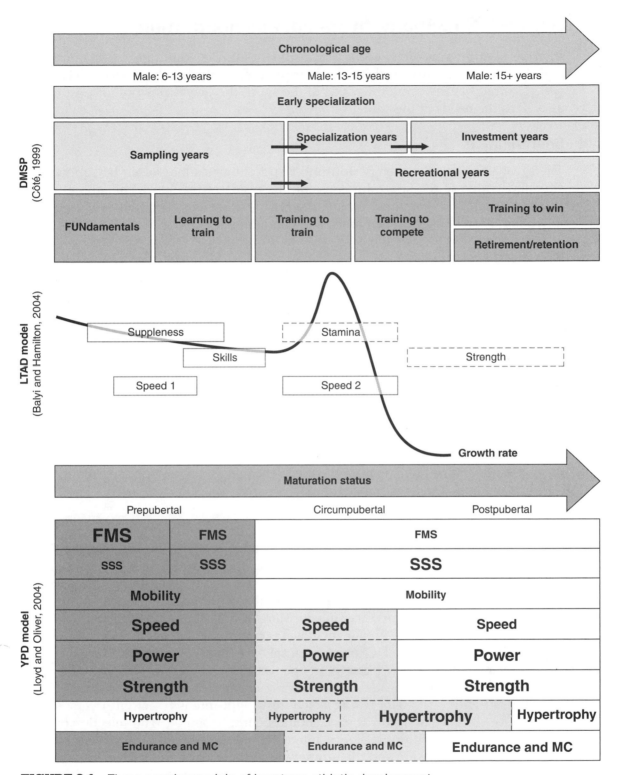

FIGURE 8.1   Three popular models of long-term athletic development.

DMSP = developmental model of sports participation; LTAD = long-term athlete development; YPD = youth physical development; FMS = fundamental movement skills; SSS = sport-specific skills; MC = metabolic conditioning

Reprinted by permission from Pichardo, Oliver, Harrison, et al. (2018).

Specificity, Overload, and Adaptation

In order to apply specificity to a sport or student-athlete's training, the strength and conditioning professional must perform a **needs analysis**, which is a two-step process aimed at assessing the needs of the sport, the player position or event, as well as the needs of the student-athlete.

Sport Analysis

The greatest reference when performing a sport analysis may often be simply watching video of the sport. In assessing the needs of the sport, the strength and conditioning professional should observe the sport with a mind to studying movements, physiological demands, and common injuries.

Mechanical Analysis

An assessment of sport mechanics should include observation of the joints and muscle groups involved, range of motion, movement velocity, rate of force development, and direction of movement (40, 46). These components should be noted both as general across many sports (e.g., running) and as specific to a single sport (e.g., swimming flip turn). For example, in a running-based sport such as cross country, the student-athletes may question why the strength and conditioning professional would prescribe upper body strengthening exercises. The simplest way to respond to this question may be in two parts: first, ask the student-athlete to run with their arms locked in place at their sides, then ask them to exaggerate their arm swing while running. It becomes clear that though the lower extremity is performing the propulsive work, the upper extremity has a strong influence on the movement of the lower extremity, thus identifying why the upper extremity should be included in a resistance training program.

Physiological Analysis

In working to understand a sport's physiological demand, it is important to consider not only the total duration but also the ebb and flow of intensities during competition. We must look at this from the perspective of what intensities are key to success and which energy system primarily contributes to those moments (40). For example, consider a soccer match: Many believe that soccer is an aerobic sport because at the high school level matches commonly last for 80 minutes in regulation time. However, if we observe closely, we find that soccer is a series of sprints, changes of direction, jogging, and periodic rest. Therefore, when training for soccer, a variety of repeated bouts of short-distance, high-intensity activity interspersed with periods of rest or active rest (light-intensity activity) versus running for distance at a slower pace should be implemented. The selection of running sets and repetitions, distance, intensity, and rest periods will vary based on the goals of the session and the timing within the sport season. This ensures that the body tissues and energy systems are trained to operate in a manner consistent with sport demands.

Injury Analysis

A priceless reference for learning about injury trends for both a sport and a specific team is the sports medicine staff, in most cases the certified athletic trainer

(AT). If an institution or team does not have access to an AT, the strength and conditioning professional should research common injuries of that sport and begin a discussion with the sport coaches to learn about injury trends specific to their team. Understanding injuries relevant to a sport or position is more important than simply noting that injuries have occurred.

Location of injury refers to the body area as well as to the specific tissues involved (muscle, tendon, bone, etc.). The strength and conditioning professional must consider whether the student-athlete had an existing weakness or other potentially predisposing factor within the tissues that led to specific tissues being damaged. It is important to recognize that gathering this information may be beyond the scope of the strength and conditioning professional and should be determined in collaboration with the AT.

The strength and conditioning professional, with input from the AT, should consider how the resistance training program can be programmed to reduce risk factors leading to injury.

Athlete Analysis

Beyond analysis of the sport, strength and conditioning professionals must consider the individual's current level of training and skill, both in their sport and with resistance training. They must also consider the primary goal of the resistance training program and how to implement resistance training activities to advance the student-athlete from their current state to the goal levels of training. It is important to note that it is not strictly resistance training that will bridge this gap. The application of an appropriate resistance training program in addition to various activities and movements (e.g., warm-up, mobility and assistance exercises, and sport training) will provide maximum benefit to the student-athlete.

Specificity

The human body is a remarkable entity that simultaneously filters and prioritizes countless signals. Imagine wearing a wristwatch for the first time: Initially, you will notice the presence of the watch, but with regular wearing the watch eventually becomes normal and you will no longer register its presence. However, one day you will inevitably forget the watch, and then you will notice its absence. In order to register the change, a stimulus must occur. To ensure that specific changes or adaptations are taking place, the strength and conditioning professional must appropriately time and implement changes in the resistance training and conditioning program. These changes in the resistance training program present in the form of the training frequency, exercise selection, exercise order, exercise intensity, sets and repetitions, and rest periods. **Specificity**, often used interchangeably with the principle of specific adaptations to imposed demands (**SAID principle**), highlights the fact that adaptations or training outcomes can be influenced by a training stimulus (9). Furthermore, specificity applies not to direct mimicking of sport skills but rather to applying movements and tasks that incorporate similar muscle groups, movement patterns, and the nature of the action, such as movement speed and force application (47).

Goodwin and Cleather (18) identified three ways that transfer of training may occur: primary, secondary, and tertiary transfer. Primary transfer involves high specificity and is expected to influence sport skills directly and so an improvement in training leads to a direct improvement in sport performance. Secondary transfer identifies the fact that improvements in training may not directly influence sport skills but may improve performance of specific sport activities, which may in turn improve sport performance. Tertiary transfer exists where there may not be any obvious transfer from training activities to sport performance, but the training activity may indirectly impact performance, for example, activities aimed at reducing the risk of injury.

Overload

To help student-athletes develop continuously, the strength and conditioning professional must consider the concept of **overload**: increasing the demand of the activity to apply stimuli that result in specific adaptations. Much like the wristwatch analogy, if there is not adequate change in the stimulus, the body recognizes the watch as a normal thing and prioritizes its attention elsewhere. However, by changing the stimulus—band material, watch size, watch weight, or not wearing the watch—the person will be more consciously aware of the presence or absence of the wristwatch. Much in the same way, if there is little change in the resistance training program, the body will begin to lack adequate stimuli to continue adapting. A common method of overload includes increasing the intensity or load of an exercise from week to week. Other methods of overload include altering the training frequency, sets, repetitions, and rest periods between exercises; emphasizing more technical or demanding exercises over simple ones; or any combination of these (47).

Adaptation

An important mantra for the high school strength and conditioning professional to understand is that *youth are not miniature adults* because it underscores the fact that strength and conditioning principles for adults should not be applied to youth and recognizes that youth resistance training should employ modified principles appropriate for the youth's age and skill level (1). In youth and adolescent student-athletes, the process of growth and maturation may mimic the effects of training, which complicates understanding the adaptations to training experienced by these individuals (36). A summary of the research on adaptations to resistance training programs for youth, presented in the NSCA position statement on youth resistance training (12), highlights that a properly designed and supervised resistance training program is not only relatively safe for youth but can enhance muscular strength and power, improve the cardiovascular risk profile, and improve motor skill performance. Additional benefits may include enhanced sport performance, increased resistance to sport-related injuries, improving psychosocial well-being, and promoting and developing exercise habits during childhood and adolescence.

Goals of a Resistance Training Program

In general, the goals of training are dependent on the goals of the student-athlete and the sport coach while the goals of the resistance training program vary depending primarily on the phase of training, analysis of the sport and the student-athlete, and what sport team activities are occurring. While sport team activities and their influence are discussed further in the Training Frequency section, the current focus will be the goals of the resistance training program and its phases.

Four general goals of resistance training have been identified: general fitness training, cosmetic training such as bodybuilding, training for competitive sport, and injury prevention and rehabilitation (50). Within the context of this chapter, these goals pertain most to improving fitness, enhancing sport training, and reducing the risk of injury. Muscular strength has been presented as a foundational component of training on which many other sporting characteristics are based, including but not limited to greater rates of force development, power, jumping, sprinting, and change of direction (56). For example, imagine two throwers with identical technique and biometrics: Thrower A has never resistance trained and has only trained her event while Thrower B has resistance trained two to three times per week in addition to her event training. With the consistent stimulus for strength, Thrower B is able to apply more force into the implement compared to Thrower A and therefore can throw the greater distance.

Improving a student-athlete's strength levels may improve their ability to both tolerate and produce greater forces involved with sport and has been shown to reduce the risk of injury (7, 25, 30) by way of improving bone mineral content (56) and the structural strength of ligaments, tendons, and their junctions, as well as joint cartilage (16). Compared to single-joint or machine-based exercises, the benefits of multijoint resistance training—particularly with free weights—include a greater targeting of stabilizing muscles, which can lead to increased coordination (57), faster maximal speeds, and improved repeated-sprint abilities (30). Because the nature of sport involves moments of high workloads and coordination, an appropriate resistance training program can be of great value in improving tolerance to increased workloads and body control (30). Improving a student-athlete's relative strength (strength in relationship to body mass) can manifest in the overall improvement of previously noted sporting characteristics through the individual's improved ability to move their own body mass or an external resistance (48). In a meta-analysis, researchers identified sufficient evidence to support resistance training as a superior intervention to reduce the risk of sport injuries compared to other injury reduction programs (25).

Program Design Guidelines

The 10 pillars of the NSCA position statement on long-term athletic development (27) can serve as guidelines for program design (table 8.2). Each of the guidelines for safe and effective strength and conditioning for the high school student and the student-athlete should be considered.

Developmental Age

Working with high school student-athletes requires high school strength and conditioning professionals to be aware of the existence of five developmental ages: chronological, biological, technical and tactical training, resistance exercise training, and psychological. It is reasonable to anticipate that each of these ages will play a role in the development of the resistance training program.

TABLE 8.2   The 10 Pillars of Long-Term Athletic Development for Coaches

Pillar	Recommendation for strength and conditioning professionals

Long-term athletic development pathways should accommodate for the highly individualized and non-linear nature of the growth and development of youth.	• Apply sound understanding of pediatric exercise science to
	    – prescribe training programs commensurate with the needs and abilities of the individual,
	    – distinguish between training-induced and growth-related adaptations (positive or negative) in performance, and
	    – understand how growth, maturation, and training interact.

Youth of all ages, abilities, and aspirations should engage in long-term athletic development programs that promote both physical fitness and psychosocial well-being.	• Appreciate the potential impact that other lifestyle factors (nutrition, rest and recovery, psychosocial health, and external pressures) have on physical fitness and physical activity. • Prescribe exercise intervention for muscle strength, motor skills, and athleticism. • Promote participation pathways for all youth to be able to transition between developmental pathways.
All youth should be encouraged to enhance physical fitness from early childhood, with a primary focus on motor skill and muscular strength development.	• Encourage an early start to free play and deliberate play (birth to 5-6 years) and developmentally appropriate strength and conditioning (starting at 6 or 7 years old). • View coordination and muscle strength as synergistic components of motor skill performance. • Prioritize neuromuscular training as part of the multidimensional strength and conditioning program.
Long-term athletic development pathways should encourage an early sampling approach for youth that promotes and enhances a broad range of motor skills.	• Promote sampling, an approach that encourages youth to be introduced to a variety of sports and activities and to participate in several positions within a given sport. • Focus on the *quality* of practice rather than on its *quantity*. • Refrain from early specialization, the year-round intensive training within a single sport or physical activity to the exclusion of other sports and activities.

The health and well-being of the child should always be the central tenet of long-term athletic development.	• Create a pleasurable and fulfilling culture of positive experiences in sport and physical activity that promote well-being by emphasizing
	    – a growth mindset,
	    – self-determined motivation,
	    – perceived competence,
	    – confidence, and
	    – resilience.
	• Focus on the long-term view of developing athleticism that includes chronic and sustainable adaptations.
	• Do not use physical activity as punishment or allow forced physical exertion.

Youth should participate in physical conditioning that helps reduce the risk of injury to ensure their on-going participation in long-term athletic development programs.	• Provide a well-rounded strength and conditioning program that includes resistance training, motor skill and balance training, speed and agility training, and appropriate rest. • Be sure that the strength and conditioning program is developmentally appropriate and suitably prepares youth for the demands of sport and physical activity. • Address underuse by providing a long-term program for athleticism for non-athletic youth.

Pillar	Recommendation for strength and conditioning professionals
Long-term athletic development programs should provide all youth with a range of training modes to enhance both health- and skill-related components of fitness.	• Recognize that both children and adolescents can make worthwhile improvements in all components of fitness irrespective of their stage of development.
Practitioners should use relevant monitoring and assessment tools as part of a long-term athletic development strategy.	• Collect quarterly measures of stature, limb length, and body mass to monitor growth and maturation. • Measure both the product (e.g., jump distance) and the process (e.g., how technically proficient the jumps are) when assessing physical capacities in youth. • Assess psychosocial well-being in youth with a validated instrument for children and youth.

Practitioners working with youth should systematically progress and individualize training programs for successful long-term athletic development.	• Adopt a progressive, individualized, and integrated approach to the programming of strength and conditioning activities.
	• Youth training programs should be dictated by the needs of the individual, the individual's technical competency, and the requirements of the relevant sports or activities.
	• Periodization represents the theoretical framework and involves sequential blocks of training to maximize the overall training response, and considers
	  – the accommodation of influential factors such as time and facilities available for training,
	  – the pressures of academic work,
	  – the need for socializing with family and friends,
	  – rest and recovery within and between sessions and as mandatory blocks within the periodization model,
	  – the scheduling of training and competitions, and
	  – the influence of growth and maturation for each youth.

Qualified professionals and sound pedagogical approaches are fundamental to the success of long-term athletic development programs.	• Strength and conditioning professionals need a solid understanding of
	  – pediatric exercise science,
	  – training principles,
	  – pedagogy,
	  – developmental appropriateness,
	  – coaching skills,
	  – cueing,
	  – providing motivation, and
	  – cultivating an environment that promotes intrinsic motivation and enjoyment.

Adapted by permission from Howard (2014).

Chronological Age

Chronological age is the age of the high school student-athlete by date of birth. Most youth sports are organized this way: Under-10, for example, is the group of children above the age of 8 years but not yet 10 years of age. The relative age effect, or birth date effect, informs coaches that children born closer to a critical cut-off period or date may have an advantage in athletics (51). For the strength and conditioning professional, this can lead to being responsible for student-athletes with large variances in physical and psychological maturity. A workout program that is not designed with multiple skill levels in mind could lead to increased risk of injury and decreased motivation to train if the program is developmentally inappropriate for some of the participants. High school strength and conditioning professionals who divide their programming by chronological age should also consider biological age.

Biological Age

Biological age, also called biological maturation, refers to progress toward a mature state (6) and varies in level (magnitude), timing (onset), and tempo (rate) of change (28). Age-related and maturity-related differences (e.g., skeletal, cardiovascular, respiratory, or endocrine systems) exist across childhood and adolescence. Strength and conditioning professionals must recognize that these systems develop at different rates and in a non-linear manner across childhood and adolescence (27). Youth can be classified as either biologically ahead of their chronological age (early maturing), at their chronological age (average maturing), or behind their chronological age (late maturing).

Physical maturity can be determined by means of a variety of measures such as X-ray or assessment of sexual maturity, both of which require a qualified medical practitioner to perform and analyze results. Somatic assessments that measure changes in overall growth or specific segments provide a practical method for strength and conditioning professionals to measure biological maturation. The somatic measure of years from **peak-height velocity** (PHV), defined as the accelerated rate of growth during the adolescent growth spurt, can be determined by calculating three body measurements (standing height, sitting height, and leg length), chronological age, and the interactions therein (34). There is substantial variability in the timing of when PHV occurs, suggesting that PHV is part of a dynamic process (20). When applied in the year prior to expected PHV, equation-based methods predicted the timing of PHV to be later than it actually occurred (33).

Most of the increase during PHV is due to acceleration in trunk growth; therefore, thoughtful planning of activities during this growth phase are crucial to successful participation in sport and other physical activities (59). Additionally, research on school-aged boys identified that consideration of a student-athlete's PHV may be beneficial in improving a training program's outcomes. The boys who were determined to be pre-PHV were found to have improvements in sprinting when the training program consisted of plyometric training or combined training (strength and plyometric training) (41). However, the post-PHV boys were found to have context-specific responses: for skills emphasizing concentric strength (acceleration and squat jump performance), both traditional resistance training and combined training programs demonstrated the greatest improvements; for skills emphasizing reactive strength (maximal running velocity and reactive strength index), both plyometric and combined training programs demonstrated the greatest improvements (41).

Therefore, in order to provide individualized resistance training and conditioning programs, biological age must be used in combination with other determinants of readiness, such as tactical and technical training age, resistance exercise training age, and psychological age.

Technical and Tactical Training Age

Technical and tactical training age (TTTA) refers to the amount of experience athletes have with their sport. **Technical age** relates to sport movement competence and the ability to solve movement problems in the sport; tactical competence applies to the decisions and actions during competition to gain an advantage, often thought of as game sense. **Tactical age** is developed during sport training and instruction from the sport coach, while technical age can be developed by the sport coach and the strength and conditioning professional. The high school strength and conditioning professional should work closely with the sport coach to determine the movements required of the sport (described in the Sport Analysis section) and include specific movements in the training program to improve the student-athlete's level of technical skill.

Resistance Exercise Training Age

Resistance exercise training age (RETA) is the amount of experience an athlete has specifically with resistance training exercises. RETA is differentiated from TTTA to help high school strength and conditioning professionals recognize that a high TTTA does not directly correspond to a high RETA. For example, a student-athlete who is a senior and has played a sport each year of high school may never have performed resistance training movements. That student-athlete's TTTA is at least four years, but their RETA is zero years. The resistance training program, therefore, must include basic weightlifting and resistance training exercises and appropriate progressions in line with the individual's resistance training experience. It is important to recognize that playing a sport for a given number of years does not automatically advance the student-athlete's ability to perform resistance training exercises.

High school strength and conditioning professionals should therefore take care to monitor a student-athlete's biological age whenever possible, rather than focusing solely on chronological age. Identifying an individual's RETA helps to create developmentally appropriate resistance training programs, regardless of TTTA. Careful consideration of these factors might show that it would not be appropriate for a freshman team to perform the same resistance training program at the same level of competence or intensity as the varsity team.

Psychological Age

Psychological age is the subjective age-equivalent of a person, or how old they feel (58). In teens, an advanced psychological age (feeling older and more mature than the chronological age) has been associated with achievement motivation and social maturity (58). Other psychological variables such as self-esteem, self-efficacy, and confidence should be factored into the structure of the strength and conditioning program. Other psychological and social factors, such as experimenting with roles and identities, mental performance, and grit—while leaving behind the archaic practice of "run them till they puke"—should also be considered when designing a developmentally appropriate resistance training program. When these complex psychological and social variables are considered, it should become clear that freshmen and seniors should not follow the same program, nor should different levels of teams within a single sport, with the exception of those who may be mentally and physically mature compared to their age-matched counterparts.

Exercise Selection

When designing a resistance training program, strength and conditioning professionals must observe a variety of considerations: facility size and open floor space, available equipment, ratio of coaches to student-athletes, session duration, and sport movements and demands, to name a few. Additionally, the strength and conditioning professional must also consider the range of both biological age and RETA of the individuals on a team. Each of these factors contributes to the strength and conditioning professional's mental workings to determine the feasibility of a workout. Before designing a resistance training program, to ensure student-athlete safety and the availability of desired or required equipment, it may first be necessary to take inventory of existing equipment (take special note of safety, warranty, and applicability to the vision and mission of the program), create a budget for equipment purchase and repair, and align equipment needs with the physical education curriculum and the athletic teams' goals and objectives.

It is not uncommon in the high school setting for a strength and conditioning professional to work with a team one to four times a week with durations ranging from 30 to 60 minutes, including the warm-up period. Therefore, although a strength and conditioning professional may have an idyllic facility with all imaginable equipment, it may not be advantageous to prescribe highly technical movements if a large team is training. Conversely, with a much smaller number of student-athletes it may be possible to successfully teach more complex movements and skills in line with the student-athletes' physical competence.

Commonly selected exercises include the weightlifting movements and their derivatives, core and assistance exercises, plyometrics, and trunk stability exercises.

Weightlifting Movements

The sport of weightlifting consists of two competition exercises: the snatch followed by the clean and jerk, where each exercise is performed to move the bar from resting on the floor to overhead, standing fully upright. The complexity of the full Olympic movements must not be undervalued and should be coached with a diligent eye to ensure safety and technical competence. A **weightlifting derivative** can be defined as a partial exercise that excludes some portion of the full snatch, clean, or jerk movements; these can be further broken down into catching and pulling derivatives, where pulling derivatives exclude the catch phase and finish with the completion of the second pull (53, 56). It is important to recognize that the emphasis on **triple extension** (simultaneous extension of the knee, hip, and ankle joints) that is associated with pulling derivatives may have the greatest transfer to sport performance when compared with catching derivatives (55). A common error with catching movements is known as "shorting the pull," which refers to incomplete triple extension of the lower extremity during the second pull phase in anticipation of dropping under the bar. This tendency may be combated by first using pulling derivatives to emphasize the rapid and powerful moment of triple extension before dropping under the bar.

Core and Assistance Exercises

Not to be confused with trunk stability exercises, which target the anterior, lateral, and posterior trunk muscles, **core exercises** refer to resistance training exercises that are primary features of a resistance training program. These exercises include multijoint movements of large muscle groups and more closely resemble sporting movements than assistance exercises (47). **Assistance exercises** are more isolated movements, focusing on a single joint or smaller muscle areas, and are considered less influential on sport performance (47); they may be considered most useful in targeting muscles of a sport-specific movement (e.g., shoulder exercises for overhead sports) or as exercises to reduce the risk of injury (47). When considering the level of transfer of training to sport performance, core exercises are commonly associated with primary and secondary transfer of training while assistance exercises are more commonly associated with tertiary transfer of training.

Plyometric and Ballistic Exercises

Prior to implementing plyometrics, the strength and conditioning professional must understand that, without adequate strength, plyometric exercises may negatively transfer to sport performance. This may manifest from the weaker student-athlete's inability to produce great enough force during the activity, resulting in greater time spent on the floor via an extended amortization phase (the time between eccentric and concentric contractions when performing a task), lower peak force, and higher and uncontrolled impact forces (19). However, when the student-athlete is strong enough to produce the forces that enable a rapid amortization phase, controlled impacts and landings, and greater peak forces, there can be great benefit from plyometrics as well as from other ballistic exercises. **Ballistic exercises** are those during which the student-athlete accelerates through the entire concentric phase of a movement; in resistance training this includes jump squats, medicine ball chest throws, and weightlifting derivatives such as the jump shrug and the hang high pull (57).

Trunk Stability

Whereas core exercises refer to the previously noted primary features of a resistance training program, trunk stability exercises refer to specific targeting of the trunk musculature. Common exercises fitting into this category include the following and their variations: planks, side planks, glute bridges, dead bugs, bird dogs, crunches, and so forth, and should aim to target the anterior, lateral, and posterior trunk. It is worth noting that when the core exercises are properly performed, the trunk musculature should be actively engaged. The student-athlete may therefore see training benefits from these movements despite the focus being on developing other muscle groups. However, it is still important to include trunk stability exercises to focalize training to specific trunk musculature that may not be adequately stimulated during the core exercises.

Training Frequency

The amount of time spent with a team varies greatly, depending on the priorities of the sport coach and the sport season. If the sport coach does not believe in the benefits of resistance training relating to reduced risk of injury, improved resilience against fatigue, and enhanced performance, they may not have their team scheduled to resistance train at all. However, if the sport coach does believe in the benefits of resistance training, the strength and conditioning professional may be allotted 30 to 60 minutes one to four times a week to work with that team. Challenges may be most present during the preseason and in-season with outdoor sports, particularly in regions where weather may greatly impact the training and competitive schedule on short notice. This may manifest to the strength and conditioning professional in the short term by a team trying to resistance train on short notice or the cancellation of a scheduled session to take advantage of being able to train outdoors.

It is important to note that training sessions of the same nature (e.g., resistance training) should not be performed on consecutive days but rather with 48 to 72 hours between sessions (12, 15, 25, 28). Separating the sessions by this amount of time allows both for an effective stimulus for strength and performance and for adequate recovery before the next session (15). If sessions are performed too closely to one another, the student-athlete may lose some of the benefits of the second workout due to soreness, fatigue, and impaired ability to work at the desired intensity. Although performing two different types of workouts (resistance training and sport training) in a single day or subsequent days is not ill-advised, it is recommended that consideration be given to the intensity of these closely scheduled workouts so as not to negatively affect performance of the following training session or increase the risk of injury due to fatigue.

An ideal scenario for the strength and conditioning professional would include working with a team or student-athlete throughout the full year and being able to implement an annual plan. The **annual plan** represents an outline of the sport year, where the various training phases can be sequentially programmed to ensure appropriate timing of training goals relative to the phases of the sport season: off-season, preseason, in-season, and postseason.

In the off-season, training priorities should focus on general fitness with a dash of sport skill practice; this may be referred to as the **general preparation phase**. It may include resistance training and conditioning sessions three to four times per week with one to two sessions per week of practicing sport skills on their own (figure 8.2). During this time, unorganized sport play or skill practice is still important, though largely de-emphasized; sport activity should not be eliminated during this time because it is important that the student-athlete be

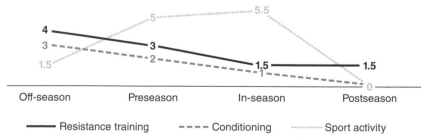

FIGURE 8.2 Estimated days per week by activity type by sport season.

able to translate the adaptations from resistance training and conditioning into the sport's skills.

As the end of the off-season nears, the fitness and resistance training characteristics should begin to reflect a slightly greater emphasis on sport demands and skills. As preseason dawns, sport activity should begin to increase in the number of skills sessions per week while the number of sessions for resistance training and conditioning decreases. The groundwork that has been laid in the off-season serves as the foundation for the preseason, where the emphasis should be on maximizing the transfer of the off-season work into improving power development, sport skills, and training and competition resilience.

Once in-season, the goals of the sport coach and student-athlete are primarily centered on improving technical skills and tactics while preparing for upcoming opposition; sport teams may meet for sport training or competition five or six days per week. During the in-season, the goals of the strength and conditioning professional should not be to develop strength and power but rather to prolong the strength and power characteristics that were developed during the off-season and the preseason. With that, teams may have resistance training sessions once or twice a week, where the exercises overall should be lighter in load and work through various ranges of motion. This is not to say that the strength and conditioning professional should not program strength-based exercises (i.e., including strength-based exercises in-season may assist in maintaining strength values) but rather to recognize that the emphasis should be on high-intensity yet lower fatigue-inducing programming.

Once the competitive season has ended, student-athletes should progress through the postseason for one to two weeks with little to no organized activity. Any organized activity of the student-athlete or team should promote recovery from the demands of the season and may occur one or two times per week. Examples of appropriate activities include foam rolling, stretching, walking, and so on, where the body is still active, though to a significantly reduced degree.

Exercise Order

According to the NSCA position statement on youth resistance training (12), exercise order should be based on the student-athlete's body size, fitness level, and exercise technique experience. For developing student-athletes, learning a variety of exercises using various implements helps to build an exercise library upon which future exercises can be built. Additionally, for those who are new to resistance training, it is appropriate to first introduce simple exercises and progress toward more complex, multijoint exercises as the RETA increases. High school student-athletes who meet minimum levels of accountability such as the **criterion repetition maximum** (13) can have exercise order adjusted accordingly. This decision should be made on an individual basis rather than based on the student-athlete's grade, team, or sex. Exercise circuits can be developed that alternate between upper body, lower body, and trunk musculature using a variety of exercise implements as well as body weight; these may be organized to emphasize upper body and lower body or push and pull. Bearing this in mind, the general principles of exercise order for resistance exercises (47) still apply.

After performing the dynamic warm-up, power exercises and other challenging movements (weightlifting movements, plyometrics, new exercises) should be performed early in a training session when the neuromuscular system is not yet fatigued. Performing these types of exercises at the end of the session when the individual is already fatigued may lead to injury, development or reinforcement of poor-quality technique, and likely the inability to perform at the desired intensity. Following power-based movements should be lower extremity multijoint movements, for example back squats and stiff-legged deadlifts (also known as the Romanian deadlift, or RDL). After the lower extremity multijoint movements have been performed, upper extremity multijoint movements such as the bench press and overhead press should occur. Following these, any additional assistance exercises should be implemented. Simply stated, exercise order should progress from the most taxing or neuromuscularly demanding to the least demanding.

Training Load

After determining which exercises will be prescribed in each block of training, the strength and conditioning professional must determine the most appropriate loads based on the goals both of the phase and of that exercise itself. Most simply, loading options should include consideration of the individual's strength and skill level, the force–velocity curve (52, 54), and the microcycle within a block. In the context of strength and conditioning, if an individual is weaker or less skilled, loading should be focused on improving strength and learning technique, whereas stronger or more skilled individuals may benefit from the inclusion of speed-based exercises to enhance power (15, 52).

It is important to recognize that intensity is not based strictly on load but also on velocity (15). For example, squatting 150 pounds (68 kg) at a moderate pace would have a lower intensity than squatting the same weight quickly. The number of prescribed repetitions also influence the load: If the level of exertion is equal, with increased repetitions the amount of weight lifted will inherently be less than when fewer repetitions are prescribed. Additionally, the goal of the individual exercise will influence the load; for example, speed- or power-based exercises may involve loads significantly less than the core exercises of the same workout. If a speed- or power-based exercise was prescribed at the same load as the core exercises, both speed of movement and technique may be compromised, depending on the movement itself (e.g., a jump shrug versus a power clean).

One-Repetition Maximum

Commonly, loads are prescribed using a percentage of the maximum amount of load that an individual can move for one repetition with good technique (i.e., the 1RM). However, in the high school setting it may be challenging or ill-advised to perform a 1RM assessment because of poor technique, time (number of individuals testing compared to coaches and spotters), and because a 1RM may change as skill and strength improve. Due to day-to-day fluctuations in fatigue and stresses, the 1RM is sometimes referred to as a fluid measurement and may not always be an accurate representation of a student-athlete's actual 1RM for that session (49). An alternative assessment to 1RM includes testing for a repetition maximum, or the amount that a student-athlete can lift with good technique for a single set of multiple repetitions, such as a 3RM (table 8.3). This may then be applied to estimate the student-athlete's 1RM while allowing a safer and more practical assessment to occur; for example, a 3RM is estimated to be 93% of a 1RM. It is important to consider the individual's RETA when applying loads based on 1RM because those with lower or intermediate RETAs will have more rapid increases in 1RM compared to those with higher RETAs.

TABLE 8.3 Percentage of the 1RM and Repetitions Allowed (% of the 1RM–Repetition Relationship)

% of the 1RM allowed	Number of repetitions
100	1
95	2
93	3
90	4
87	5
85	6
83	7
80	8
77	9
75	10
70	11
67	12
65	15

Reprinted by permission from Haff and Triplett (2016, p. 452).

Rating of Perceived Exertion and Repetitions in Reserve

Alternative methods of intensity prescription include the rating of perceived exertion, repetitions in reserve, and velocity-based training. Both **rating of perceived exertion** (RPE) and **repetitions in reserve** (RIR) represent subjective measures that reflect an individual's level of exertion; a benefit to this is the accommodation of fatigue: An individual who is less fatigued may be able to achieve greater loads than if they were highly fatigued with the same RPE or RIR prescription.

RPE is commonly used on the modified scale of 1 to 10, where 1 represents minimal and 10 reflects maximal exertion or effort. RIR represents the perceived number of repetitions an individual could theoretically continue to perform with good technique upon completion of a set (61). To describe this in further detail and with the RIR reflective of the final set's intensity: Although the load may be the same from set to set, the perceived intensity (meaning how difficult the repetitions are to complete) typically increases from set to set due to naturally occurring fatigue. RIR is based on, and has an inverse relationship with, RPE (table 8.4): If an individual completes a high-intensity squat for a set of 5 repetitions and upon completion of the set considers how many more repetitions they could complete beyond those 5, and identifies that they may complete one more repetition, this represents an RIR of 1 and an RPE of approximately 9. For example, in a 3 × 5 maximal strength block with a last-set goal RIR of 3, it is normal that without changing the load the first set's RIR may be 4, the second set's may be 3.5, and the third set's may be 3. A challenge that exists with the use of subjective-based intensity prescription is that accuracy increases with more experienced individuals; someone who is untrained and inexperienced may not know what it feels like to be at an RPE of 8 or 9 or an RIR of 1 or 2 (60) and accuracy with heavier loads (RIR 0-5) is greater than with lighter loads (RIR 7-10) (10, 21, 47).

TABLE 8.4 Methods of Subjective Loading and Correlated Relative Percentages

Load description[a]	Rating of perceived exertion[b]	Repetitions in reserve[b]	Relative percentage[a]
Maximal	10	0 repetitions remaining and no additional load; maximum effort	100
	9.5	0 repetitions remaining but could increase load	
Very heavy	9	1 repetition remaining	97.5
	8.5	1 or 2 repetitions remaining	95
Heavy	8	2 repetitions remaining	92.5
	7.5	2 or 3 repetitions remaining	90
Medium heavy	7	3 repetitions remaining	87.5
	5-6	3 or 4 repetitions remaining	85
Medium		4 repetitions remaining	82.5
		4 or 5 repetitions remaining	80
Light to medium		5 repetitions remaining	75
Light		5 or 6 repetitions remaining	70
Very light	3-4	Light effort	65
Very, very light	1-2	Little or no effort	60

[a] Adapted from DeWeese, Sams, and Serrano (2014). [b] Adapted by permission from Zourdos, Klemp, Dolan, et al. (2016).

An additional benefit to prescribing loads using RIR is that it may be possible to predict the **repetition maximum** (RM) and the 1RM from the load lifted (10, 11, 49). The RM reflects the greatest load that can be lifted for a specific number of repetitions. Strength and conditioning professionals can prescribe intensity using RIR, which correlates with an estimated percent of RM; this allows the individual to determine the appropriate load for a given exercise while accommodating for fatigue (10). For example, referring to table 8.3, a 5RM is determined to be approximately 87% of the 1RM (47); however, when considering acute fatigue accumulation as a workout progresses, one can expect that by the final set of 3×5 at an RIR of 0, the individual will not be able to maintain a load of 87% of the 1RM. Therefore, it is reasonable to estimate that when applied for multiple sets, an RIR of 0 (i.e., 100% of the RM) may be slightly below the estimated maximum percent of the 1RM from table 8.3. The strength and conditioning professional can calculate the estimated RM and 1RM using the following equation.

Estimated RM = (load lifted × 100) ÷ percent of RM

For example, if an individual performed a single set of back squats for 5 repetitions at 150 pounds (68 kg) with an RIR of 2, this would be equivalent to 92.5% of the 5RM. Therefore, this equation would be applied as (150 × 100) ÷ 92.5, which would equal approximately 162 pounds (73 kg) for the estimated 5RM.

Referring to table 8.3, a 5RM is equivalent to 87% of the 1RM. The same equation from above may yet again be applied with the new values to estimate the 1RM: (162 × 100) ÷ 87 equals approximately 186 pounds (84 kg).

Velocity

In **velocity-based training**, often abbreviated VBT, load and intensity are guided by measuring the speed of the movement as an objective gauge to match against velocity norms for various exercises and exertion. Because VBT requires the purchase of specific devices it may not be practical in the high school setting.

Ultimately, the method used to prescribe intensity should make sense both for the exercise program participants and for the strength and conditioning professional within the specific setting and budget.

Repetitions and Sets

When working with individuals new to resistance training, the focus should be on technique, with ample repetitions and light loads to teach the body to perform the movements correctly. Within this framework, it is recommended that low RETA individuals begin with 6 to 10 exercises, with 1 or 2 sets per exercise of 8 to 12 repetitions at 50% to 70% of the 1RM. Once technical competency progresses, the load should be increased while the number of sets and repetitions remains the same (28). Once the individual has progressed to the intermediate level, it would be appropriate to increase both the technical demand and the strength emphasis by decreasing repetitions and increasing load. Upon reaching the higher RETA the individual may be challenged through a greater spectrum of exercises, technical demands, sets, and repetitions, and these should be prescribed with consideration of the sport season (off-, pre-, in-, or postseason). Training age might not progress according to a specific timeline but should be based on the individual's abilities regarding sound technique, tolerance of increasing loads, and general skill throughout the resistance training program (table 8.5). It is possible that a student-athlete who is highly skilled in their sport may struggle to progress through their RETA while a student-athlete who is moderately skilled in their sport may advance more rapidly.

Off-Season

The off-season is the ideal period to focus on enhancing strength and **work capacity** (the ability to tolerate stress repeatedly). Here, the appropriate goals include strength-endurance with an additional goal of muscular hypertrophy. This phase of training—to use an analogy of washing a muddy vehicle—can be compared

TABLE 8.5 Examples of General Training Priorities by Training Age

	Untrained and inexperienced	Intermediate	Trained and experienced
Training age (years)	0-6 months	2-6 months, up to 1 year	≥6 months to 1 year
Focus or goal	Technique development; light load	Technique competence; increased load	Technique competence; increased load and intensity
Number of primary exercises	6-10	5-8	4-5
Sets	1-2	2-5	Depends on training phase
Repetitions	8-12	5-10	Depends on training phase

Adapted from Sheppard and Triplett (47) with data also from Lloyd et al. (28).

to the initial hosing down and soaping: It is not exactly one's favorite step, but without it, the following steps or phases would be much messier. It is important to recognize that developing strength-endurance serves as a foundation on which to build strength and the subsequent phases of strength-speed, speed-strength, and peaking. Training for both strength-endurance and hypertrophy involves 3-6 sets of 6-12 repetitions (table 8.6).

Strength-endurance should be the goal because training for strictly muscular endurance or hypertrophy may not adequately describe nor include the appropriate loading to enhance a student-athlete's work capacity in preparation for sport. Additionally, in training for transfer to sport it is important to intend to move quickly through the concentric phase of a movement. If the focus were strictly on muscular endurance, it would be prudent to prescribe repetitions in excess of 12 with light loads and brief rest periods. However, it is estimated that a 12RM is approximately 67% of the 1RM (47), while a stimulus for strength development has been identified to be greater than 60% of the 1RM (31). Therefore, unless near-fatigue loads are prescribed, the muscular endurance load may not be adequate to improve strength levels.

As the off-season begins to approach preseason, the strength and conditioning professional should shift the focus from strength-endurance toward maximal strength. In the car washing analogy, this involves hosing once more to remove the suds and subsequent drying. The vehicle has not yet met its best look, but it is significantly better looking than when it was caked in mud. To shift toward maximal strength, one must alter the sets and repetitions to reduce the volume and increase the load (intensity). This includes a range of 2-6 sets with repetitions of ≤6 and an increase in load to at least 85% of the 1RM (47) (table 8.6). While the

TABLE 8.6 Phases of Training With Appropriate Sets, Repetitions, and Percentages of the 1RM for Higher Training Ages

Sport season	Training goal	Sets	Repetitions	% of the 1RM	"MUDDY CAR WASH" Step	Goal
Off-season	Muscular endurance	2-3	≥12	≤67	Initial hosing and soaping	Rediscover the paint color
	Strength-endurance, hypertrophy	3-6	6-12	67-85		
	Strength	2-6	≤6	≥85	Hose off soap and dry	Prepare the vehicle for polish
Preseason	Power: single-effort event	3-5	1-2	80-90	Apply car polish	Transition from general to specific cleaning
	Power: multiple-effort event	3-5	3-5	75-85		
In-season	Maintain preseason strength and power	1-5	3-5	75-90	Buff the away the polish, wash windows	Make the vehicle as clean and shiny as possible
Postseason	Active rest; recover from season	0-3	1-5	Variable	Stand back and admire	Enjoy the completed work; relax

Adapted by permission from Haff and Triplett (2016, pp. 439-469).

primary goal is to increase strength, it is important to note that not all exercises during this phase must be oriented toward strength gains. One or more speed- or power-based movements should be included to further prepare the student-athlete for the coming preseason and competition.

Preseason

Just before or at the start of preseason, the resistance training focus should shift from maximizing strength to translating recent strength gains into moving heavy loads quickly. This phase may be referred to as strength-speed. As with applying car polish, there is still work to be done before the full beauty of the vehicle is reached. However, this is the phase where the work performed becomes more specific to the desired outcomes through the use of polish, tire shine, window cleaner, and more. Though the emphasis is still on strength, introducing velocity-based exercises may benefit the student-athlete by introducing stimuli that can translate into being able to perform more work faster.

In most sport competitions, the student-athlete or team that can produce the greatest forces in a shorter period will likely be the most successful. It is not enough simply to be strong; one must be both strong *and* able to produce maximal amounts of force quickly, maximizing one's rate of force development. For example, observe two sprinters capable of producing equal amounts of peak force. Sprinter A has a greater rate of force development and shortens the time on the ground with each foot contact while Sprinter B is unable to achieve the same force output in the same period and maintains a greater ground-contact time. Because Sprinter A can produce an equal force to Sprinter B with a shorter foot-contact time, Sprinter A moves down the track faster than Sprinter B.

In-Season

Following a period of strength-speed, a slight shift in focus toward speed-strength should occur. Just as the car polish needs to be buffed away to complete the car's washing, the in-season resistance training program should include exercises to promote maximal preparation for competition. This shift involves changing the emphasis from moving heavy loads quickly to moving light to moderate loads rapidly. The goal during this phase should be to prepare student-athletes to peak by enhancing the rate of force development. It is worth noting that while the emphasis should be on speed-strength, it is important to continue to include at least one or two strength-based exercises to maintain previous strength levels. If one were to program only speed-based exercises over the course of the season, a student-athlete's strength levels might decrease, thus reducing their ability to produce high forces quickly, and potentially increasing the risk of injury.

Postseason

When the competitive season is over, it is important for the health and well-being of the student-athlete to complete an active-rest period. This is akin to admiring the polished vehicle and enjoying a leisurely drive on a sunny day. Objectives during this phase include recovering from the previous competitive season and healing injuries incurred (42) while remaining active at a very light intensity.

A challenge for the high school strength and conditioning professional comes when a student-athlete transitions immediately from one sport season into the next, such as from the fall to the winter season. It may be challenging to "on-board" the sport coach to provide these transitioning student-athletes with reduced workloads at practice. Therefore, it may rest upon the strength and conditioning professional in conjunction with the AT to provide these student-athletes with an alternate workout of low- to moderate-intensity exercise exercise or recovery exercises during the first week or two after the season ends. The specific length of this period may vary by the individual's level of fatigue and injuries accumulated throughout the preceding sport season. An alternate workout program for this period might consist of dynamic stretching, foam rolling, and very light resistance training with an emphasis on range of motion.

Rest Periods

Rest periods may be one of the most undervalued components of the resistance training program, whether by student-athletes, sport coaches, or even strength and conditioning professionals. Adequate **interset rest periods** (the amount of time allotted for recovery between each set) may provide benefits by way of controlling acute fatigue while allowing the individual to maintain high-quality technique and greater loads (53) and permitting time for the strength and conditioning professional to provide feedback. To maximize the recovery benefits of interset rest periods, these should not be filled with additional exercises such as trunk stability or assistance exercises.

In the high school setting, maturation, training goals, and exercise intensity play a great role in determining appropriate rest periods. Adolescents may require an average of approximately 2 minutes of rest between sets, with lighter-intensity exercises requiring slightly less time while higher-intensity exercises require slightly more (15). Previous interset rest period recommendations have noted as little as 30 seconds (47) to 1 minute (24) of rest between sets during muscular endurance and hypertrophy phases of training, respectively (figure 8.3). However, it is important to consider that additional rest (between 2 and 3 minutes) has been shown to enable greater hypertrophy and strength benefits compared to shorter interset rest periods of 30 seconds to 1 minute (43). Therefore, it is recommended that longer rest periods between sets be implemented for improving the long-term benefits of hypertrophy, strength, and muscular power compared to short interset rest periods that may produce a muscular endurance effect (2, 22).

A method of incorporating rest periods during working sets includes **cluster sets**, where a high-repetition set may be broken into smaller portions of a single set. This method may be most beneficial for individuals who have a high training age and technical competence or for untrained or intermediate-trained individuals performing technically demanding or peak strength movements. For example, a set of 6 repetitions may be broken into 2 3-repetition sets: 1 set of 3 repetitions,

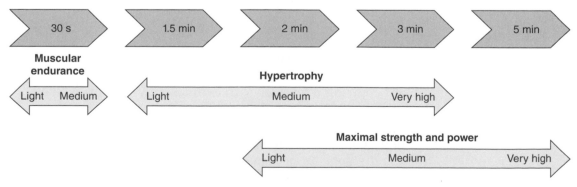

FIGURE 8.3 Appropriate rest periods by training goals and relative intensity.

Data from Schoenfeld et al. (43), Sheppard and Triplett (47), and Suchomel and Comfort (53).

brief rest period, followed by the remaining 3 repetitions before a longer interset rest period begins. This brief cluster rest period may range from 10 to 40 seconds (53), depending on the training phase goal. Another cluster method for a 6-repetition set may include 2 repetitions, brief rest period, 2 repetitions, brief rest period, and the final 2 repetitions. Depending on the cluster and interset rest periods and the number of student-athletes sharing the equipment, it may be more prudent to incorporate cluster sets during periods when there is a lower demand for equipment since a student-athlete may require more time with the equipment compared to a traditional set.

Progression

The principle of **progression** informs the strength and conditioning professional that the strength and conditioning program must be increased gradually to meet the specific demands placed upon developing students and student-athletes (14). The stress placed on the body should become progressively more challenging to continually stimulate adaptations consistent with the individual's needs and abilities to improve performance, reduce the risk of injury, and maintain interest in the program. Methods that can be used to provide more challenging stimuli include introducing appropriate exercises that the student-athlete has not yet performed, more complex movement patterns, adding sets per exercise, or additional resistance (figure 8.4) (14, 35).

The progression of strength and conditioning variables that follow a systematically varied program over time is known as **periodization** (12). The periodiza-

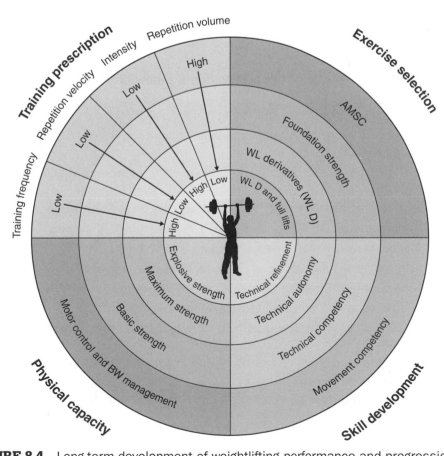

FIGURE 8.4 Long-term development of weightlifting performance and progression.

AMSC = athletic motor skill competencies; BW = bodyweight

tion model should prioritize training goals and systematically alter the training intensity, volume, rest periods, and exercise selection (12). In order to progress appropriately, general youth resistance training guidelines must be adhered to; these include beginning each session with a 5- to 10-minute dynamic warm-up, introducing new exercises with relatively light loads, focusing on correct exercise technique, and resistance training two to three times per week on nonconsecutive days (figure 8.5) (12, 15, 25, 28).

The NSCA has established program design variables for youth strength and power (tables 8.7 and 8.8) (12). While some variables for each training goal may be similar, it is important to recognize that as an individual progresses from one level to the next, overload occurs by altering intensity, number of sets and repetitions, training frequency, and the rest periods between sets and exercises. As the student-athlete progresses from untrained and inexperienced to trained and experienced, strength and conditioning professionals must observe safe transitions as the individual begins to adapt to the new stresses.

During the student-athlete's training to stimulate strength adaptations, the emphasis of moderate movement velocity coincides with the increased total volume of each selected exercise. Because it takes longer to complete each set, it is reasonable not to increase the body's stress further by cuing the individual to

---

General Youth Resistance Training Guidelines

- Provide qualified instruction and supervision
- Ensure the exercise environment is safe and free of hazards
- Start each training session with a 5- to 10-minute dynamic warm-up period
- Begin with relatively light loads and always focus on the correct exercise technique
- Perform 1-3 sets of 6-15 repetitions on a variety of upper and lower body strength exercises
- Include specific exercises that strengthen the abdominal and lower back region
- Focus on symmetrical muscular development and appropriate muscle balance around joints
- Perform 1-3 sets of 3-6 repetitions on a variety of upper and lower body power exercises
- Sensibly progress the training program depending on needs, goals, and abilities
- Increase the resistance gradually (5%-10%) as strength improves
- Cool down with less intense calisthenics and static stretching
- Listen to individual needs and concerns throughout each session
- Begin resistance training 2-3 times per week on nonconsecutive days
- Use individualized workout logs to monitor progress
- Keep the program fresh and challenging by systematically varying the training program
- Optimize performance and recovery with healthy nutrition, proper hydration, and adequate sleep
- Support and encouragement from instructors and parents will help maintain interest

FIGURE 8.5   General youth resistance training guidelines.

Reprinted by permission from Faigenbaum, Kraemer, Blimkie, et al. (2009).

move as quickly as possible. This cue may also detract from potential strength adaptations since the loads lifted may remain lighter in order to maintain faster movements; this is an unfavorable scenario as the goal of a strength phase is to increase the total amount of load lifted safely.

However, during a power phase, both velocity- and strength-based exercises should be incorporated. The NSCA recommends two separate loading strategies: light to moderate loads performed at rapid velocities and moderate to heavy loads for strength (12). As previously noted in the section on training load, velocity-based exercises allow the individual to take advantage of previously developed strength increases, applying a stimulus that may enhance the individual's ability to produce greater force more quickly, a trait that is beneficial in most sports. Strength exercises should also be included to maintain or continue to develop previous strength adaptations. The strength and conditioning professional should

TABLE 8.7   General Youth Resistance Training Guidelines for Strength

	Untrained and inexperienced	Intermediate	Trained and experienced
Intensity	50%-70% of the 1RM	60%-80% of the 1RM	70%-85% of the 1RM
Volume	1-2 sets × 10-15 reps	2-3 sets × 8-12 reps	≥3 sets × 6-10 reps
Exercise choice	Single- and multijoint	Single- and multijoint	Single- and multijoint
Muscle action	ECC and CON	ECC and CON	ECC and CON
Velocity	Moderate	Moderate	Moderate
Frequency (days/week)	2-3	2-3	3-4
Rest intervals (minutes)	1	1-2	2-3

Note: 1RM = 1-repetition maximum; ECC = eccentric; CON = concentric.

Reprinted by permission from Faigenbaum, Kraemer, Blimkie, et al. (2009).

TABLE 8.8   General Youth Resistance Training Guidelines for Power

	Untrained and inexperienced	Intermediate	Trained and experienced
Intensity	30%-60% of the 1RM (velocity)	30%-60% of the 1RM (velocity) 60%-70% of the 1RM (strength)	30%-60% of the 1RM (velocity) 70%-≥80% of the 1RM (strength)
Volume	1-2 sets × 3-6 reps	2-3 sets × 3-6 reps	≥3 sets × 1-6 reps
Exercise choice	Multijoint	Multijoint	Multijoint
Muscle action	ECC and CON	ECC and CON	ECC and CON
Velocity	Moderate to fast	Fast	Fast
Frequency (days/week)	2	2-3	2-3
Rest intervals (minutes)	1	1-2	2-3

Note: 1RM = 1-repetition maximum; ECC = eccentric; CON = concentric.

Reprinted by permission from Faigenbaum, Kraemer, Blimkie, et al. (2009).

keep in mind that the emphasis in a power phase should be to apply greater forces in a shorter period, not solely to continue developing strength or train for velocity. It is worth noting that, as previously discussed, the higher-training-age exercise prescription may be largely influenced by the sport season.

A simple tool to determine an individual's readiness to progress in a specific exercise is a **skill competency checklist**, which rates the student-athlete's proficiency while performing a specific exercise on a scale. A simple scale to assess skills is a 0 to 3 ranking, where 0 represents *developing*, 1 represents *capable*, 2 represents *basic*, and 3 represents *advanced*. The results can inform the strength and conditioning professional whether the individual is ready to progress to the next level of the exercise (an example using the back squat is shown in table 8.9) (14).

TABLE 8.9 Checklist for Back Squat Resistance Training Skill Competency

Phase	Desired action	Common error	Points possible	Score
Checkpoint	• Safe exercise area • Correct starting weight • Collars on the bar (if plates are used) and well-positioned safety rails	• Inadequate space • Incorrect weight selection • Lack of collars and poorly positioned safety rails	3	
Ready position	• Bar on shoulders and upper back • Head neutral and eyes forward • Feet wider than shoulder-width apart	• Bar positioned on neck • Head facing downward • Feet position too narrow	3	
Downward phase	• Flexed hips and knees • Thighs parallel to floor • Elbows under bar, knees over and in line with feet, torso erect, and feet flat	• Thighs not at proper depth • Trunk begins to flex forward • Knees inward or outward • Heels rise	3	
Upward phase	• Extend hips and knees • Torso upright, elbows under bar, knees over and in line with feet • Maintain bar control with firm grip until bar is racked	• Trunk begins to round forward • Elbows drift behind bar, knees move inward or outward • Firm grip is not maintained	3	
General demeanor	• Responsibility • Resourcefulness • Respect	• Does not follow safety rules • Unwilling to solve simple problems • Does not cooperate with others	3	
Total points			15	

Scoring scale: 3 points = *advanced*; 2 points = *basic*; 1 point = *capable*; and 0 points = *developing*.

Adapted by permission from Faigenbaum and McFarland (2016).

Sample Programs

The strength and conditioning professional has a variety of opportunities to improve the health and well-being of high school student-athletes. Whether before, during, or after school, the program should be consistent with the school's vision and mission. The strength and conditioning professional should create measurable goals and outcomes for the program that also align with those of the sport and the individual.

Multiple Fitness and Experience Levels

One of the complexities in high school strength and conditioning is that student-athletes have a wide range of fitness levels, varying RETAs (0-5+), and different levels of interest and motivation, from noncompliant and disinterested to extremely motivated and engaged (38). When working with individuals of varying skill and fitness levels in a group setting, it is helpful for the strength and conditioning professional to classify the range of skills and activities in order to identify common exercises where all skill levels are seamlessly accommodated (table 8.10).

TABLE 8.10   Sample Program for Varying Competency Levels

	Exercise type	Bronze	Silver	Gold	Volume
Field or court emphasis	Plyometric	Countermovement jump	Depth jump (low)	Depth jump (high)	3 × 3
		Single-leg drop (hold landing)	Single-leg jump	Single-leg depth jump	3 × 3 each leg
		Low-hurdle hop (rapid)	High-hurdle hop (hold landing)	High-hurdle hop (rapid)	3 × 5 each leg
	Speed	30-m sprint (submaximal intensity; maximum speed technique focus)	30-m sprint	30-m sled sprint	3 reps
		10-m sprint (submaximal intensity; maximum speed technique focus)	10-m sprint	10-m sled sprint	3 reps
		Float-fly-float (10-20-10)	Fly-float-fly (10-20-10)	Fly-float-fly (10-30-10)	3 reps
Weight room emphasis	Squat	Goblet squat	Box back squat	Back squat	5 × 3
	Horizontal push	Push-up	Dumbbell bench press	Bench press	5 × 3
	Pulling derivatives	Clean/snatch pull	Clean/snatch pull (<100% of the 1RM clean)	Clean/snatch pull (<100% of the 1RM clean)	5 × 3
	Clean variation	Hang clean	Clean from low blocks	Clean	5 × 3

Adapted by permission from Pichardo, Oliver, Harrison, et al. (2018b).

To address these challenges, it is important for high school strength and conditioning professionals to include all student-athletes in the process of creating programs that meet their interests and build on those interests toward improved health and well-being. Strength and conditioning professionals can have the student-athletes identify the types of activities, exercises, and sports they enjoy. The student-athletes can then create resistance programs based on their interests and experiences. This will offer broad appeal to student-athletes, class participants, and those who may be intimidated by the workout facility.

In-Class Programs

Physical education (PE) class at the high school level provides an excellent opportunity for students to learn about and create resistance training programs. The knowledge, skills, and abilities transfer to lifetime health and fitness and build on long-term athletic development pathways. The focus of high school PE class is the continued growth and development of every student. PE class provides an excellent opportunity to embrace cross-curricular activities with other subjects.

First, the strength and conditioning professional must identify which month and sport season the students and student-athletes are in at a given point of the school year (figure 8.6) and identify the appropriate timing and progression to teach each topic and activity throughout the semester (table 8.11).

Next, it is important to determine how much time the workout may take compared to the allotted class time (32) (table 8.12). The set duration indicates how much time it takes for two student-athletes to complete one set of an exercise. The time of year and how much class time is available will help determine the appropriate number of sets and repetitions from the provided ranges. Total time per exercise identifies the approximate time it would take to complete all the sets and repetitions of a single exercise. By adding the appropriate interset rest period, the total amount of class time needed can be determined. Due to class time constraints, it is important to select an appropriate number of sets to ensure that the appropriate number of repetitions can be performed. Once student-athletes have started the resistance training program, the strength and conditioning professional should closely monitor newly introduced exercises to ensure that proper technique is learned.

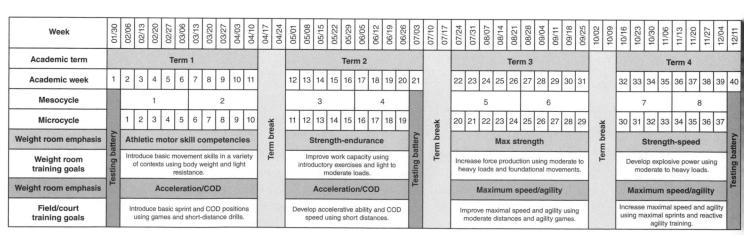

FIGURE 8.6 The academic year and weight training course progression.

COD = change of direction

Reprinted by permission from Pichardo, Oliver, Harrison, et al. (2018b).

TABLE 8.11 High School Introductory Weight Training Course Outline

Session number	Topic	Activity	Specifics
1-3	Intro to resistance training	Resistance exercise with body weight only to include chest, back, shoulders, arms, and legs; pretest for baseline if desired	Introduce bodyweight exercises; focus on form
4	Safe beginnings	Intro to machine exercises; safety and proper form; focus on muscular endurance	Four chest exercises, four back exercises
5	Intro to exercise technique	Student-athletes watch a demonstration and then practice exercises with a partner; no weight; 1 × 12 reps each	Four leg exercises; three shoulder exercises; one new chest exercise and one new back exercise
6	Intro to exercise technique	Student-athletes watch a demonstration and then practice exercises with a partner; no weight; 1 × 12 reps each	Two biceps exercises; two triceps exercises; repeat one new leg exercise and one new shoulder exercise
7	Intro to exercise technique	Student-athletes complete two exercises in each muscle group; large to small; 1 × 12-15 reps each	Student-athletes choose two back, two chest, one biceps, one triceps, and two leg exercises
8	Determining training loads	Student-athletes calculate beginning training loads	Determine training loads by percentage of body weight
9	Circuit training	Teacher-designed stations; 40 seconds with a partner, then switch	Focus on large muscle group exercises
10-11	Circuit training	Teacher-designed stations	Focus on small muscle group and trunk stability exercises
12-13	Circuit training	Teacher-designed stations	Focus on total body exercises
14	Training with accessory equipment	Stability ball workout	Teacher-led
15	Training with accessory equipment	Bands and balance exercises	Teacher-led; student-led
16	Flexibility	Discuss and participate in proper stretching; pros and cons of flexibility, proper application	Teacher-led
17	Muscular endurance program design	Student-athletes use personal goals to design their program, which must be 10 days long and must include all muscle groups	Focus on adding challenge of instability; must include warm-up and cooldown

> continued

TABLE 8.11   > *continued*

Session number	Topic	Activity	Specifics
18-28	Muscular endurance workout	Student-athletes participate in their own program	Student-led
29	Muscular strength program design	Introduction to resistance training programs to improve muscular strength; determine training loads and percentages	Determine training loads by estimating 1RM and 1RM percentages
30	Muscular strength	Discuss methods of designing strength programs; provide samples for student-athletes to study and find what best fits their goals	Teacher-led discussion
31-45	Muscular strength workout	Student-athletes participate in their own program	Student-athletes begin personal program
46-48	Cardiovascular conditioning	Discussion and program design; importance of using interval training with longer, less intense training	Teacher-led stations
49-54	Become an advocate	Partner with one other person in class; identify a family member or a friend for whom you will design a resistance training program	Teacher-led; follow guidelines provided or alter the activity to fit student-athletes' needs

Adapted by permission from Bertelsen and Thompson (2017).

TABLE 8.12   Examples of Estimated Time to Complete a Workout

Total session duration (min)	Total number of exercises	Number of sets	Number of repetitions	Set duration (min:sec)	Total time per exercise (min:sec)	Time between exercises (min:sec)
32	6	3	5-8	1:20	4:00	1:20
26	4	4		1:20	5:20	
30	5	3	5-10	1:30	4:30	1:30
30	4	4		1:30	6:00	
27	4	3	5-10	1:45	5:15	1:30
25	3	4		1:45	7:00	

The range of total session duration is based on the fewest and the greatest numbers of exercises, sets, and repetitions.

Source: P. McHenry (personal communication, February 20, 2020).

Before- and After-School Programs

It is the responsibility of the high school strength and conditioning professional to promote fitness and physical activity before, during, and after school. Before-school programs are sometimes referred to as "0 Period" because they are not part of the conventional school day but can be structured in such a way as to promote specific goals and objectives related to improved fitness or improved academic performance.

Dissociative exercises—exercises that lend themselves to thinking of things unrelated to the exercise itself (e.g., stationary bike riding, treadmill walking)—have a different effect on student-athletes' brains and have been linked with helping student-athletes learn vocabulary, math concepts, and other academic skills (4). **Associative exercises**—which involve focusing on the performance of the exercise, such as specific muscles used during an exercise or using coaching cues like "spread the floor when squatting"—should also be included. Depending on the period of the academic year (exams or other stressful periods) it is prudent to change the ratio of dissociative to associative exercises. The high school strength and conditioning professional can also program activities based on the three types of play (structured, semi-structured, and unstructured or free) so that student-athletes are engaged in and have an influence on the programming; this is critical to the buy-in to and success of the program. The three types of play can be categorized by the amount of adult influence.

- *Structured play* occurs under 100% supervision and control of adults making the rules, setting boundaries, and deciding who does what and when (37). Sports, resistance training, conditioning, and physical education are examples of structured play.

- *Semi-structured play* is controlled 50% by adults and 50% by youth. Adults set rules and boundaries and youth decide who does what and when within those rules and boundaries. Recess is an example of semi-structured play.

- *Unstructured play* can be defined as times when an adult is not structuring the interaction between children (26). Youth determine 100% of all aspects of play, which is why this is sometimes referred to as *free play*. Youth make decisions about the rules, settle disputes on their own, learn to solve problems, and form relationships (17).

Being mindful of the three types of play and the opportunity to reach the greater student population, resistance training programs can be developed and implemented for students and student-athletes of all high school grade levels and abilities. For sample resistance training, plyometric, and weightlifting models (38), see figure 8.7.

The high school strength and conditioning professional can be instrumental in reaching student-athletes before and after school. It is as important to apply the scientific principles of strength and conditioning during PE class sessions as it is during after-school training times (figure 8.8). For example, in track and field the high school strength and conditioning professional can tailor before- or after-school programs for student-athletes whose sports are in-season (table 8.13 and figure 8.9), preseason, off-season, or postseason.

In the likely event of non-athletes performing resistance training during the hours before or after school, it is important that the strength and conditioning professional provide them with guidance in order to ensure safety and proper exercise technique and to reinforce the individual's interest in participating in a resistance training program. These students should be approached tactfully and in a manner that does not discourage them from engaging in a safe resistance training program. Though the strength and conditioning professional supervising the workout facility may not necessarily have to plan a structured resistance training program for these individuals, they should offer guidance regarding the previously discussed scientific principles, assist with teaching new exercises, and provide appropriate cues to positively progress the student-athlete's technique and engagement.

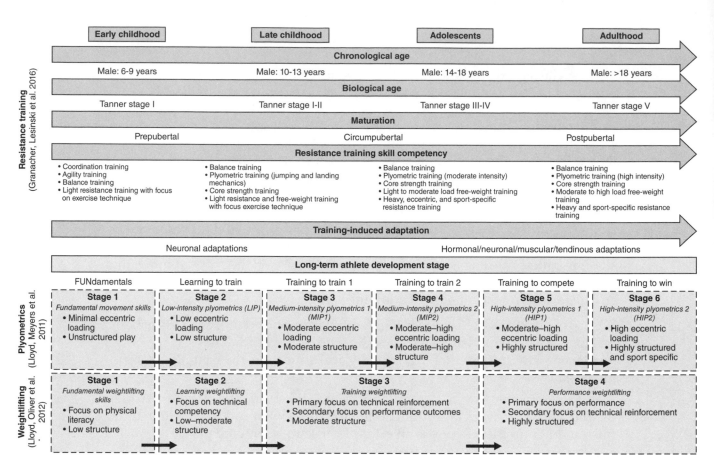

FIGURE 8.7 Sample models of resistance training, plyometric, and weightlifting.

Reprinted by permission from Pichardo, Oliver, Harrison, et al. (2018a).

Academic term	Term 4			Mesocycle	8		
Academic week	36			**Microcycle**	32		
Weight room emphasis	**Strength-speed**						
Field/court emphasis	**Maximum speed/agility**						
Day	Monday, 10/16	Tuesday, 10/17	Wednesday, 10/18	Thursday, 10/19	Friday, 10/20	Saturday, 10/21	Sunday, 10/22
AM	OFF	Clean derivative Squat UB H push UB H pull V plyometrics Acc/linear speed	OFF	OFF	OFF	Competition	OFF
PM	OFF	Sport training	OFF	Sport training	Snatch derivative Hinge UB V push UB V pull H plyometrics COD/agility	OFF	OFF

FIGURE 8.8 Sample microcycle program for PE class and after-school training.

UB = upper body; V = vertical; Acc = acceleration; H = horizontal; COD = change of direction

Reprinted by permission from Pichardo, Oliver, Harrison, et al. (2018b).

TABLE 8.13 Sample Plan for After-School Track and Field (Sprints and Jumps) During the Speed-Strength Phase (Outdoor In-Season)

Week of	April 20	April 27	May 4	May 11
Meets per week	1	1	1	1
Microcycle week number	7	8	9	10
Sessions per week[a]	2	2	2	2
Sets	3	3	3	3
Reps	3	3	3	3
Weightlifting/core exercises per session	4	4	4	4
Repetitions in reserve	4	3	2	5
Relative percentage[b] (% of the 1RM)	80-85	85-90	90-95	70-80

[a]Day 1 (push, in this order): push press, back squat, alternating dumbbell bench press, barbell lunge, hip strength exercises, and trunk stability exercises; day 2 (pull, in this order): jump shrug, stiff-legged deadlift, bent-over row, medball slam, hip mobility exercises, and trunk stability exercises.

[b]Based on RIR; using table 8.4, a range was created using one row above and one row below the RIR value given in this table.

Adapted from unpublished work created by Jacob Reed, PhD, CSCS. Used with permission.

TRACK and FIELD: Sprints & Jumps

NAME: _____

Outdoor Season Week 7

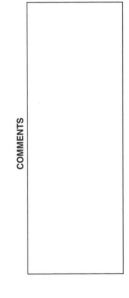

FIGURE 8.9 Part of a sample microcycle worksheet for the track and field student-athlete during the speed-strength phase.

e = each

Adapted from unpublished work created by Jacob Reed, PhD, CSCS. Used with permission.

Summer Programs

To ensure that all legal aspects of the program are complied with for the implementation of strength and conditioning programs, the strength and conditioning professional must first check with specific school district guidelines as well as state high school athletic association guidelines. Additionally, decisions need to be made as to whether the summer programs can be made available or promoted to incoming ninth graders, middle school students, or community youth. Using track and field as an example, table 8.14 shows how the phases of program design for summer programs can be clearly established and implemented.

TABLE 8.14 Sample Summer Plan for Off-Season Track and Field

Week of	July 8	July 15	July 22	July 29	August 5	August 12
TRAINING PHASE	RETURN TO FITNESS		STRENGTH-ENDURANCE			
Microcycle (week) number	1	2	3	4	5	6
Sessions per week	2[a]	2[a]	3[b]	3[b]	3[b]	3[b]
Sets	3	4	3	3	3	3
Reps	5	5	10	10	10	10
Core exercises per session (including weightlifting movements)	4	4	3	3	3	3
Repetitions in reserve	4	3	4	3	2	5
Relative percentage[c] (% of the 1RM)	80-85	85-90	80-85	85-90	90-95	70-80

[a]Day 1 (push, in this order): mid-thigh pull, deadlift (trap bar), dumbbell bench press, shoulder press, hip strength exercises, and trunk stability exercises; day 2 (pull, in this order): hang clean pull, stiff-legged deadlift, one-arm dumbbell row, hip mobility exercises, and trunk stability exercises

[b]Day 1 (push, in this order): push press, back squat, incline bench press, banded shoulder exercises, hip strength exercises, and trunk stability exercises; day 2 (pull, in this order): countermovement shrug, stiff-legged deadlift, inverted row, banded ankle exercises, hip mobility exercises, and core exercises; day 3 (mixed, in this order): clean pull from floor, one-arm dumbbell row, cable punch, hip strength exercises, and trunk stability exercises.

[c]Based on RIR; using table 8.4, a range was created using one row above and one row below the RIR value given in this table.

Adapted from unpublished work created by Jacob Reed, PhD, CSCS. Used with permission.

Conclusion

Program design for high school strength and conditioning professionals involves much more than sets and repetitions, increasing resistance from workout to workout, or following the program of a successful college team. Important considerations that must be addressed include determining the sport season, identifying the relevant training ages of the student-athletes, and individual and team goals and how to approach these. Taking into account the unique physical and psychosocial developmental needs of high school students, coupled with the appropriate level of resistance training and sports participation, the strength and conditioning professional can create individualized resistance training programs that meet each student-athlete at their development and focus on the health and well-being of each student and student-athlete, which will help develop lifetime habits of being physically active (figure 8.10).

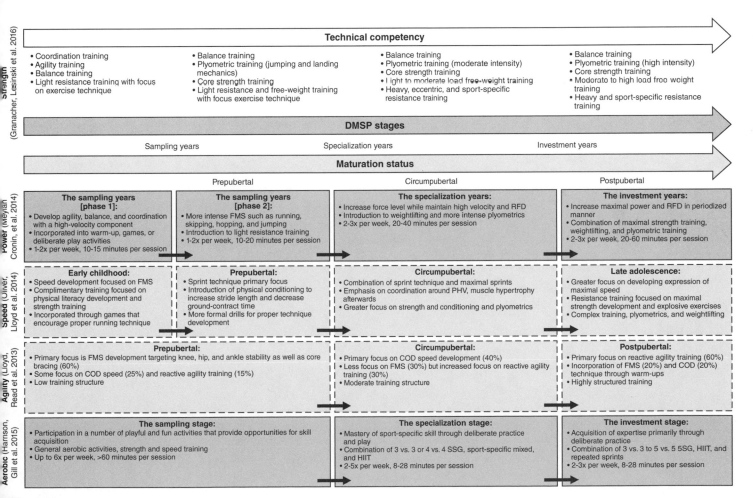

FIGURE 8.10 Summary of resistance training and power, speed, agility, and aerobic models.

The closed boxes are stages aligned to the DMSP while the dashed boxes are stages defined by maturation status. For reference see page 18 of www.research-gate.net/publication/326085544_Integrating_models_of_long-term_athletic_development_to_maximize_the_physical_development_of_youth

DMSP = developmental model of sports participation; FMS = fundamental movement skills; RFD= rate of force development; COD = change of direction; SSG: small sided games; HIIT = high intensity interval training

Reprinted by permission from Pichardo, Oliver, Harrison, et al. (2018a).

9

Plyometric Training

Samuel Melendrez, MS, CSCS,*D, RSCC

The use of plyometric training to improve qualities and characteristics that are essential to enhanced sport performance and reduced risk of sport-related injury is an accepted practice by strength and conditioning professionals (10). As with most training methods, the use of plyometrics has found its way into programs for the high school student-athlete as well. This chapter provides the tools the high school strength and conditioning professional, sport coach, and physical education teacher need to design and implement a safe and effective plyometric training program specifically for the high school student-athlete.

Program Design Guidelines

As with all types of training aimed at improving athletic performance, the high school strength and conditioning coach professional should be warned against implementing a plyometric program or plyometric exercises that are intended for more skilled or experienced athletes. The student-athletes' abilities and experience, as well as available equipment and space, must be carefully considered when designing a plyometric program. It may be tempting to try a drill or exercise seen on social media, for example, but the strength and conditioning professional's number one responsibility is the student-athlete's safety, and it is important to always evaluate one's practices against standards and guidelines outlined by professional organizations, such as the NSCA (10).

Age and Training Status Considerations

There is yet to be a universally accepted age deemed appropriate to begin a structured plyometric training program (10). Age-related concerns regarding plyometric training typically stem from a risk of damaging developing skeletal structures, such as the unclosed epiphyseal plates of prepubescent children. Very little evidence, however, supports the belief that plyometric training is dangerous to adolescents (8). Despite this, strength and conditioning professionals in the high school setting should be aware of these potential concerns from student-athletes' parents or guardians or other members of the school community, because an uneasiness about the methods of training used in any program can create problems with trust and compliance from the student-athletes being trained. Rather than being dismissive about these concerns from these important stakeholders in the high school setting, strength and conditioning professionals can help allay these concerns by providing educational resources (10) as well as being open about their diligence in designing age-appropriately designed plyometric programs.

General recommendations exist of requisite levels of strength determined by performance of a given intensity relative to body weight in a barbell-based exercise (the back squat for example), before beginning a plyometric program (6). These are less than reliable and even impractical for a few reasons. First, young children engage in activities during free play (e.g., skipping, hopping, bounding) that involve plyometric or plyometric-like characteristics on a regular basis (5), long before possessing an ability to demonstrate high levels of strength in a barbell exercise. Second, using a barbell back squat 1RM to assess readiness for plyometric training might be imprudent before the student-athletes have gone through the necessary progressions (see chapter 4 on resistance training and exercise technique). For many student-athletes, this may take a considerable amount of time to attain, if even attained at all while still in high school. Waiting for this to be the case before beginning a plyometric program may lead to a missed opportunity to use a type of training that has been proven to improve athletic performance markers such as agility and power (5) and reduce sport-related injuries (1, 3).

Perhaps a more reliable assessment of student-athletes' readiness to begin a structured plyometric program is their level of social and emotional maturity (10). The student-athlete must be able to focus on the coaching cues and other instructions given by the strength and conditioning professional and understand the value of this type of program as well as the potential risks (10). The high school strength and conditioning professional must keep in mind this level of readiness may vary from group to group, within each group, and even from day to day, especially in the high school setting. The strength and conditioning professional should also keep in mind that not all student-athletes will be ready for all the planned drills for that session, so appropriate plans should be in place that allow for safe exercise regressions or other modifications to the original plan.

Needs Analysis

A needs analysis requires the strength and conditioning professional to take into consideration the student-athlete's sport, position, and experience with the specific type of training before choosing appropriate drills (10). For many high school strength and conditioning professionals, evaluating specific demands of a sport or a position may be a challenge given that some of their student-athletes likely participate in multiple sports with varied demands. In this case it would be wise to choose drills that address general athletic characteristics and qualities (e.g., rate of force development) and common faulty movement patterns (e.g., knee valgus) that are in most need of improvement in this age group and with this untrained and inexperienced status (7). For the strength and conditioning professional working with student-athletes who participate in only one sport, considering these recommendations along with specific injury profiles and risks of that sport can help design a safe and effective plyometric program (10).

Exercise Type

The type of exercise refers to what part of the body is being trained. For simplicity purposes, plyometric exercises can be grouped into two main categories: upper body plyometrics and lower body plyometrics.

Upper body plyometrics are less researched and consequently less prevalent in most strength and conditioning programs; however, they can be an integral part of a program for student-athletes whose sports involve explosiveness through the torso, shoulders, and arms. Upper body drills often use medicine balls for throwing, catching, and passing exercises (10).

Lower body plyometrics have a more extensive list of exercises and terminology to describe the actions being performed. This is perhaps because so many sports require their athletes to produce a high amount of force quickly against the ground, floor, or another surface with their lower bodies, making these drills a great choice for not only improving these abilities, but for preparing the student-athletes' bodies for these demands (10). See table 9.1 for a breakdown of some of the basic categories and descriptions of lower body plyometrics.

Intensity

The intensity of a plyometric exercise or drill can be more challenging to quantify than that of a traditional resistance training exercise. Several generally agreed-upon factors should be considered when determining the intensity level of a plyometric exercise and whether it is the correct choice for a given group of student-athletes. For lower body drills these considerations include whether the drill is single leg or double leg, the velocity of the movements involved, the height or distance to be covered during the drill, and the body weight of the student-athlete performing the drill (10). Upper body plyometric intensity is delineated into low, medium, and high by the following factors: one arm versus two arm, the weight of the medicine ball, and the distance between partners or between the student-athlete and the ball's contact surface. An additional factor, especially relevant to working with younger, inexperienced, or less-trained athletes, is the technical demands and complexity of the exercise. Drills that require multiple steps or movements, higher balance demands, or control over the student-athlete's own body or an implement will increase the difficulty of the drill and should be programmed with careful consideration and appropriate progressions.

In this chapter plyometric exercises will be grouped into one of three categories based on intensity: *low-intensity drills* that have few steps and low velocities and amplitudes, are done in place or with limited distances and heights covered, and are aimed at teaching proper landing positions and ability to absorb and control force; *medium-intensity drills* with an increased demand for balance, control, and

TABLE 9.1   **Types of Basic Lower Body Plyometric Exercises**

Type of exercise	Description
Jump	Double-leg takeoff with a double-leg landing
Hop	Single-leg takeoff and landing on the same foot
Bound	Single-leg takeoff and landing on the opposite foot

speed, and that cover greater distances or heights; and *high-intensity drills* with progressively higher distances or heights that are covered with greater velocities than those in the low or medium categories.

Frequency

Frequency for plyometric training refers to the number of sessions per week. Several factors should be considered when determining how often to include this type of training in the weekly plan, including the level of intensity of the drills, the student-athlete's abilities, and whether the student-athlete is in-season or off-season (10). Along with this last consideration, the strength and conditioning professional should consider how much plyometric activity (jumping, hopping, bounding) is already included in the student-athlete's sport. For example, sports such as volleyball and basketball include a significant amount of these actions in their practices and games. For student-athletes in these types of sports, the strength and conditioning professional should consider including less frequent workouts and including low-intensity drills that emphasize controlling and absorbing forces in proper positions (11).

There is limited research on determining the optimal number of plyometric training sessions per week (10). Studies suggest adolescents can perform plyometric training two or three times per week on nonconsecutive days (2, 3). When considering frequency of plyometric training, recovery between sessions should be of utmost concern, and high school strength and conditioning professionals should err on the side of caution with less frequent (one or two sessions on nonconsecutive days), high-quality workouts that allow their student-athletes to properly recover from not only these sessions, but from any extra plyometric stimuli they are receiving outside of their time with the strength and conditioning professional.

Order

In general, plyometric exercises for high school student-athletes should be performed after a well-designed specific warm-up and movement preparation routine, but prior to other forms of resistance training to reduce risk of performing in a fatigued state. Doing so can increase the risk of injury due to poor position and can diminish the effectiveness of the drills due to the student-athletes' performance at less than maximal efforts. A select few of the most trained and experienced high school student-athletes may be able to gain benefits from combining a resistance training exercise with a plyometric exercise of similar movement pattern (e.g., a loaded squat followed by an unloaded jump squat). This organization of training is known as complex training and should be reserved only for student-athletes with a significant strength base and proficiency with plyometric techniques (10).

For the strength and conditioning professional who is limited with space or equipment and is training large groups of student-athletes, including plyometric training when it would be most effective in the session can be a challenging task. If a group of student-athletes must perform other forms of resistance training prior to plyometric drills due to the circumstances above, the strength and conditioning professional should choose resistance exercises that have as little impact on the plyometric exercise choices as possible. One option is for student-athletes to perform upper body resistance training exercises prior to lower body plyometric exercises or lower body resistance training exercises prior to upper body plyometric exercises.

Volume

The volume of a plyometric session is typically measured in the number of foot contacts for lower body drills (4) and number of catches or throws for upper body drills (10) per session. Recommendations for volumes in a plyometric program range from 60 to 100 foot contacts for untrained and inexperienced student-athletes during the off-season (10, 11). With such a large range, it can be challenging for the high school strength and conditioning professional to decide where to begin. Keep in mind that volume and intensity have an inverse relationship, meaning that the greater number and intensity of plyometric exercises included in a program, the more important it will be to stay on the low side of the volume recommendations, both per session and per week. Perhaps just as important is for strength and conditioning professionals to be aware of the total volume of all forms of training that is prescribed so they can make specific quantifiable adjustments and progressions to the program when needed.

The high school strength and conditioning professional must also consider the volume of plyometric exercises on an individual basis for their student-athletes. Student-athletes who are heavier, progressing at slower rates of technical proficiency at the drills, or have been recently exposed to excessive plyometric volumes outside of their session with the strength and conditioning professional may need even less volume than the above recommendations. The strength and conditioning professional must keep in mind that when it comes to plyometric training, the program design requires a quality-rather-than-quantity approach.

Rest Period

Rest in a plyometric program refers to the amount of time between sets of exercises or drills. Remember, the primary purpose of plyometric training is to improve muscular power, not endurance. Adequate rest must be given between sets to allow for proper recovery, maximize effectiveness, and ensure proper technique when performing this type of training. Recommended work-to-rest ratios range from 1:5 to 1:10 for plyometric exercises (10). For example, if a set of multiple broad jumps takes approximately 15 seconds, a proper rest period would be a minimum of 75 seconds and a maximum of 150 seconds before the subsequent set begins. Appropriate rest periods, even for low-intensity drills, are important to allow the high school student-athlete to be physically ready for the next set and for the student-athlete to be prepared mentally to display postural control and dynamic stability (11). For example, in a lower body plyometric drill, the student-athlete must be able to achieve a proper position (i.e., neutral spine, shoulders in line with the knees, and knees in line with toes) during the movement and while decelerating the movement or bringing the movement to a stop.

High school student-athletes may have a difficult time staying focused with exercises they do not deem to be sufficiently challenging, such as low-intensity plyometrics. It is a good practice to use the appropriate rest times to reinforce positional cues in order to remind the student-athletes of the specific objectives of the drills. For strength and conditioning professionals pressed for time or for those who typically do not like having idle time in between sets, one strategy is to insert a mobility or activation exercise (e.g., a quadruped leg raise to activate the muscles of the gluteal region) after each set of plyometric drills. This is not only an efficient use of time, but it will help keep the student-athlete from losing focus or engaging in behaviors that are not conducive to performing the next set to the expectations set forth by the strength and conditioning professional. If using this strategy, be sure to include mobility or activation exercises in low volumes and intensities that aid in the performance of the plyometric drill and do not take away from them. For example, after performing a set of multidirectional hops, the student-athlete can perform a set of 3 to 5 repetitions of a quadruped leg raise per leg or, for student-athletes with poor hamstring flexibility, a set of 3 to 5 repetitions of active extended leg raises per leg.

Progression

Like all forms of exercise, plyometric training must follow the general training principle of progressive overload (10). Progression of plyometric exercises involves making logical adjustments to the program variables (exercise selection, volume, and intensity) to make the program more challenging, with the goal of obtaining continued improvements in the desired adaptations from this type of training and reducing the likelihood of overtraining.

Progression may be the most misunderstood element of programming plyometric training for high school strength and conditioning professionals. General guidelines for appropriate progression for high school student-athletes include progressing from lower-intensity to higher-intensity drills and progressing volumes from low to moderate levels (8, 10, 11).

When planning progressions for student-athletes, high school strength and conditioning professionals should avoid following a predetermined timeline for when to progress exercises; instead, they should carefully evaluate their student-athletes' competencies before moving to the next level of progression (2). Additionally, the strength and conditioning professional should avoid feeling the need to move on too quickly from low-intensity lower body plyometric drills. The value of these drills (e.g., teaching body control, proper joint position, and the ability to absorb force) can help reduce the risk of lower extremity injury and lay a solid foundation of movement skills for subsequent higher-intensity drills and sport performance (11). With this in mind, it may be wise to include these drills, even with more trained and experienced high school student-athletes, throughout the training cycle as part of their movement preparation.

Safety Guidelines

The strength and conditioning professional's number one priority is student-athletes' safety. As with any type of exercise, plyometric training carries some inherent risk. It is strength and conditioning professionals' duty to mitigate these risks by following guidelines outlined in the earlier sections of this chapter as well as being diligent in seeking out other credible resources on the subject of plyometric training to ensure they are providing their student-athletes with the safest, most effective program possible. A few considerations for student-athlete safety specific

TABLE 9.2 Facility and Equipment Safety Considerations for Plyometric Training

Area of consideration	Safety guidelines to follow	Things to avoid
Surface	• Choose grass or turf fields, suspended floors, or rubber mats for plyometric drills.	• Do not perform drills on hard surfaces such as concrete due to poor shock absorption. • Avoid performing drills on mats that are too thick or soft for drills with repeated efforts, as they will increase floor contact time due to too much shock absorption.
Space	• Ensure more than enough space is provided for student-athletes to perform the drills without compromising position or actions. • Be sure the ceiling is high enough and the floor is unobstructed.	• Do not try to squeeze plyometric drills into congested areas with a lot of traffic or moving barbells, dumbbells, or other pieces of equipment.
Equipment	• Make sure that boxes are built from sturdy materials and have nonslip landing surfaces of at least 18 × 24 in. (46 × 61 cm). • For upper body plyometrics, use soft medicine balls to minimize the risk of an injury to a student-athlete attempting to catch the medicine ball or having too fast of a bounce off a wall for the student-athlete to safely catch. • Ensure that the wall that the student-athlete is throwing against is solid and free from hanging materials that may come loose during contact of the throw or pass.	• Do not use equipment not intended for the purposes of plyometric training (e.g., jumping, hopping, or bounding over or onto a weight room bench or other similar equipment). • Do not try to get as much use out of worn-out boxes, medicine balls, or other plyometric equipment before replacing them.

to plyometric training include teaching and demonstrating proper landing technique; providing proper supervision of the drills; and ensuring enough space, safe surfaces, and equipment for the drills. See table 9.2 for a summary of important safety facility- and equipment-specific considerations for plyometric training.

For high school student-athletes, mastering positions to absorb and control force is perhaps one of the greatest values of plyometric training. Before any jumps, hops, or bounds can be implemented into a program, the strength and conditioning professional must demonstrate the proper landing position. See figure 9.1 for a visual of the proper alignment of the shoulders in relation to the knees, the knees in relation to the toes, and alignment of the knees. This shows the student-athlete avoiding excessive inward (valgus) movement of the knees, which predisposes student-athletes to injury (10). While this landing position example is for a two-foot (leg) jump, single-leg drills like hops and bounds should

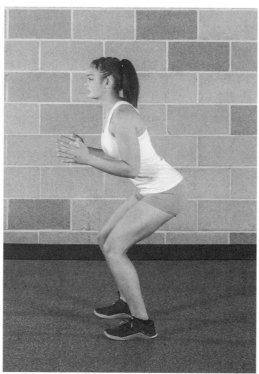

FIGURE 9.1   Proper landing position.

follow the same guidelines for position and can be more challenging to achieve due to the extra balance demand. The strength and conditioning professional must regularly provide cues to the untrained and inexperienced student-athlete to flex the ankles, knees, and hips and focus on staying engaged through the musculature of the torso.

Proper supervision during plyometric training is essential for a student-athlete's safety. The NSCA *Strength and Conditioning Professional Standards and Guidelines* document recommends a strength and conditioning professional-to-athlete ratio of 1:15 for the high school setting (9). This provides valuable insight on the level of importance of supervision during a training program. Perhaps as important as staying as close to this ratio as possible is that the strength and conditioning professional should actively coach these drills, not simply be physically present. Providing regular, timely feedback to student-athletes, especially about the landing positions, will not only improve the student-athlete's ability to perform the drills, but can decrease the risk of injury while performing them.

Another safety consideration for plyometric drills is the physical characteristics of the student-athletes. Student-athletes weighing more than 220 pounds (100 kg) should exercise caution when performing plyometric exercises because increased body mass results in higher compressive forces. As a result, avoiding high-volume and high-intensity plyometric exercises may be more appropriate for heavier athletes (10, 12).

Exercise Finder

Upper Body Exercises and Drills

The following upper body plyometric drills are a sample of options for the high school strength and conditioning professional; other variations exist (2, 10). As mentioned previously, upper body plyometric drills are less frequently used than lower body drills, but they are a valuable training method for student-athletes whose sport requires explosive upper body movements (10).

When deciding whether to use a partner or to throw against a wall with the following drills, the strength and conditioning professional must carefully consider the guidelines for space and equipment in table 9.2.

Medicine Ball Chest Pass

Type of Exercise or Drill

Passing or pushing action

Intensity Level

Low

Movement Direction

Forward

Equipment

Medicine ball (2-10 lbs [1-5 kg]) and a partner

Beginning Position

- A pair of student-athletes stands approximately 10 feet (3 m) apart. The space may be adjusted depending on each student-athlete's strength levels and abilities to throw the medicine ball.

- The student-athlete with the medicine ball begins in a square stance with feet shoulder-width apart, holding the medicine ball with outstretched arms for the preparatory countermovement (not shown in the first photo), which is bringing the medicine ball back toward the chest aggressively before the passing or pushing action.

- The partner begins in an alert position with eyes toward the passer.

Movement Phases

1. The student-athlete with the medicine ball brings it back toward the chest aggressively for the countermovement.

2. From the countermovement, the student-athlete quickly pushes the medicine ball forward toward the partner or the wall with as short of a transition time as possible.

3. The partner catches the medicine ball and repeats steps 1 and 2.

Coaching Tips

Emphasize to student-athletes that each movement needs to be a separate attempt to move the medicine ball as explosively as possible, and do not let them rush the repetitions. Inexperienced and untrained student-athletes tend to focus only on the pushing action of this drill and often eliminate the countermovement from the outstretched arm position; this should be corrected because it eliminates the student-athlete's ability to take advantage of the stretch reflex and the stored elastic energy in the muscle, making the subsequent passing action less powerful (1, 2). The strength and conditioning professional can increase the intensity of this drill by increasing the weight of the medicine ball, as long as the quality of the movement and speed of the throw does not decrease to the point where the drill becomes less valuable.

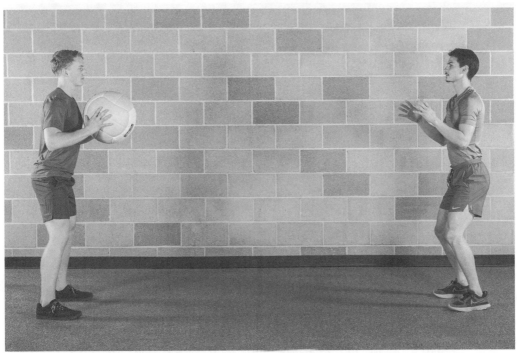

Beginning position (before preparing for the countermovement)

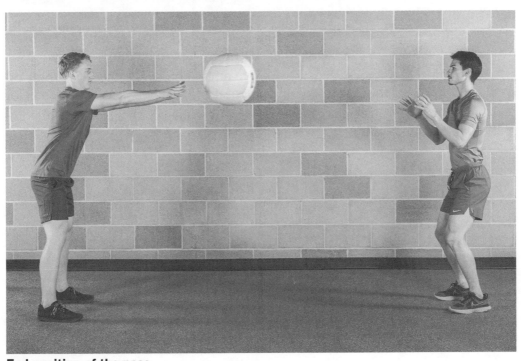

End position of the pass

Medicine Ball Two-Hand Overhead Throw

Type of Exercise or Drill
Throw

Intensity Level
Medium

Movement Direction
Forward and downward

Equipment
Medicine ball (2-10 lbs [1-5 kg]) and a partner

Beginning Position
- A pair of student-athletes stands 10 feet (3 m) apart or more as needed.
- The student-athlete with the medicine ball begins in a square stance with feet shoulder-width apart, holding the medicine ball overhead with both hands.
- The partner begins in an alert position with eyes toward the passer.

Movement Phases
1. The student-athlete with the medicine ball brings it back behind the head (while keeping the elbows extended) aggressively for the countermovement.

2. From the countermovement, the student-athlete throws the medicine ball forward and downward toward the floor in front of the partner as quickly as possible.

3. When the medicine ball comes to a slow roll, the partner picks up the ball and repeats steps 1 and 2.

Coaching Tips
Due to the backward momentum of the medicine ball during the countermovement, less experienced and weaker student-athletes may lose postural control in the lumbar spine and may even lose their grip on the medicine ball, letting it fly backward. Coach the student-athlete to maintain a neutral spine during the countermovement and to grip the ball tightly. Avoid letting student-athletes skip the countermovement and encourage them to make each throw a separate attempt to be as explosive as possible. This drill can be intensified by increasing the weight of the medicine ball.

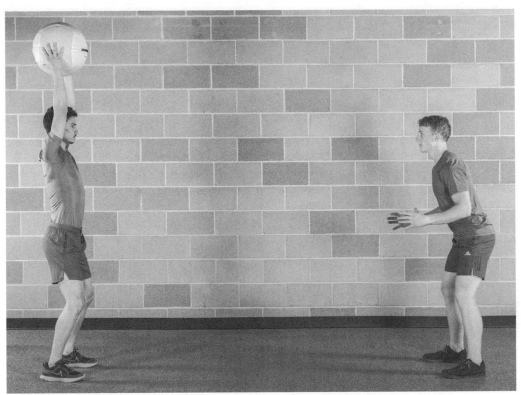

Beginning position (before preparing for the countermovement)

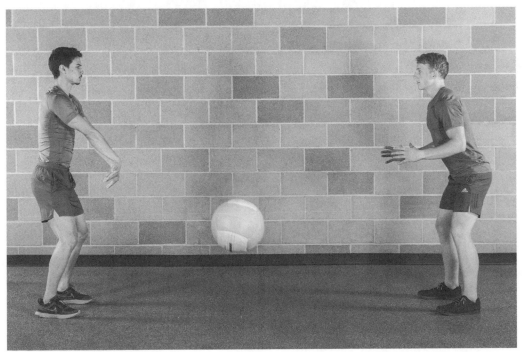

End position of the throw

Rotational Medicine Ball Throw

Type of Exercise or Drill
Throw

Intensity Level
High

Movement Direction
Sideways

Equipment
Medicine ball (2-10 lbs [1-5 kg]) and a solid wall against which to throw

Beginning Position
- Stand 2 to 3 feet (61-91 cm) away from a wall in an athletic stance with the shoulders perpendicular to the wall. Hold the medicine ball in front of the torso with arms fully extended in preparation for the countermovement.

Movement Phases
1. Begin with a countermovement of quickly bringing the medicine ball toward the hip that is away from the wall and slightly flexing the knees.

2. From the countermovement, push off of the foot farthest from the wall while rotating the hips and torso toward the wall. Release the medicine ball as quickly as possible with a powerful exhale.

3. Catch the rebound off the wall or allow the medicine ball to fall to the floor before repeating steps 1 and 2 for subsequent repetitions.

Coaching Tips
This is a more advanced drill than the previous upper body exercises. This exercise is for the core musculature with a high potential value for student-athletes in sports involving rotary power (i.e., sports with throwing, kicking, punching, etc.). Many student-athletes without experience in these sports or movements will struggle with this drill and will try to rely on their arms for the force of the throw, instead of applying force to the floor with the outside foot and driving through a powerful rotation of the hips and a stable torso. Coach the student-athletes to avoid excessive lumbar flexion and rotation during the countermovement and encourage them to flex their knees during this phase to have a more explosive throwing action. Whether the student-athlete is catching the ball on the rebound from the wall or letting it fall to the floor, they should start each repetition in the position outlined in step 1 to keep the subsequent repetitions from being rushed and performed with poor execution.

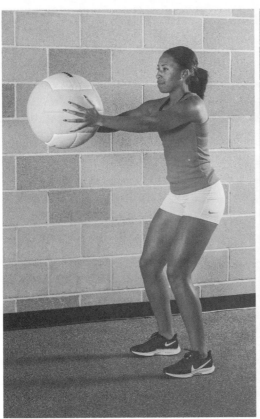

Beginning position

Countermovement

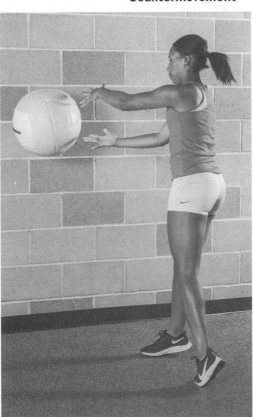

Throw (one side)

Lower Body Exercises and Drills

The following drills are by no means an exhaustive list of the available lower body plyometric drills; they are a sample of low-, medium-, and high-intensity drills that work well specifically with high school student-athletes in large group settings. The high school strength and conditioning professional should choose plyometric drills corresponding to student-athletes' skill levels, training statuses, and experience, especially early in their program progressions.

Snap Down to Two-Foot Landing

Type of Exercise or Drill

In place, two-foot landing

Intensity Level

Low

Movement Direction

In place, slight elevation of the body followed by a lowering into a two-foot landing position

Equipment

Appropriate landing surface

Beginning Position

• Begin with the feet slightly wider than shoulder-width apart, on the balls of the feet, with the heels off the floor. Arms are extended overhead, as if they are reaching for the ceiling.

Movement Phases

1. On a signal, open the stance to shoulder width, then bring the arms down to the sides while simultaneously dropping the body into a proper landing position with both feet in contact with the floor.

2. Hold the proper landing position until the strength and conditioning professional gives the signal to stand up (usually 1-3 seconds) and assume the beginning position.

3. Repeat the drill for the desired number of repetitions.

Coaching Tips

While this drill does not actually fit the definition of a plyometric exercise, it has potential value early in a teaching progression for two-foot landing mechanics and in being included in a movement preparatory phase of a workout for more trained and experienced student-athletes. While this drill is simple for even untrained and inexperienced student-athletes to execute, the strength and conditioning professional should be aware of several important technical errors.

First, many athletes will drop into a landing position that looks much different than that shown in figure 9.1. The strength and conditioning professional should look for stances that are too wide, excessive pronation of the ankles, and knee valgus. Second, many student-athletes will lose postural control and lean forward or lose a neutral spine in the landing position.

Having the student-athletes stay in the landing position for 1 to 3 seconds gives the strength and conditioning professional a chance to identify these issues, provide the student-athletes feedback, and strategize how to avoid these positions in this drill and future progressions.

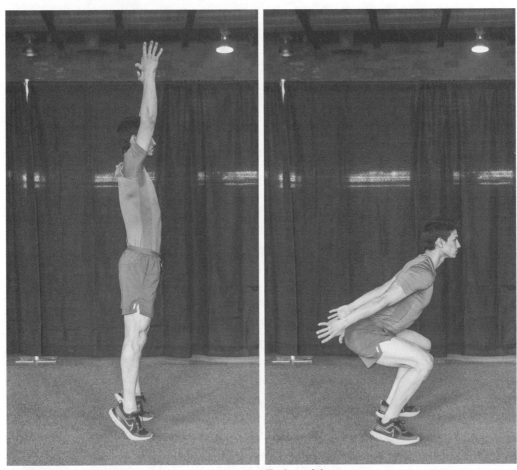

Beginning position   **End position**

Drop to Split Squat

Type of Exercise or Drill

In place, split-stance landing

Intensity Level

Low

Movement Direction

Forward with one leg backward and the other leg forward with a simultaneous lowering of the body into the bottom of a split squat

Equipment

An appropriate landing surface, 2 to 3 feet (61-91 cm) of unobstructed space in front and behind the student-athlete

Beginning Position

- Begin with the feet slightly closer than shoulder-width apart, with arms at the sides.

Movement Phases

1. On a signal, quickly move the right foot forward and the left foot backward, dropping the body into the near-bottom position of a split squat.

2. At the bottom position of the first repetition, the left knee should be close to the floor but not in contact with it (near a full range of motion split squat).

3. Hold the bottom position until the strength and conditioning professional tells the athlete to stand up (usually 1-3 seconds) and assume the beginning position.

4. Repeat the drill with the left foot moving forward and right foot moving backward, dropping into the near-bottom position of a split squat.

Coaching Tips

This drill can be viewed as the single-leg version of the snap down drill, with similar benefits and placement in a progression or phase of a workout. However, due to the balance component and coordination of the drop to split squat, this can be more challenging for some student-athletes than the snap down.

Student-athletes should strike the floor full-footed with their front leg, allow the knee to travel toward the toes (slight shin angle forward), and avoid knee valgus. Student-athletes inexperienced with this drill may collapse into this bottom position, with the back leg's knee hitting the floor to support their weight instead of controlling their body's momentum, ultimately eliminating the benefit of decelerating into a proper landing position. Strength and conditioning professionals should be diligent in keeping student-athletes from doing this and should consistently reinforce the importance of developing proper deceleration, timing, and body positions.

Instruct student-athletes to land with their hips over their back knee and to keep a neutral spine. Younger, inexperienced, or less-trained student-athletes often struggle not only with lower body landing mechanics but with postural control during phases of deceleration. This drill is simple with a low enough amplitude to help teach proper positions.

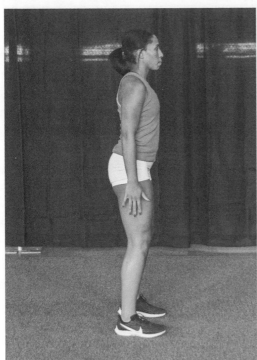

Beginning position

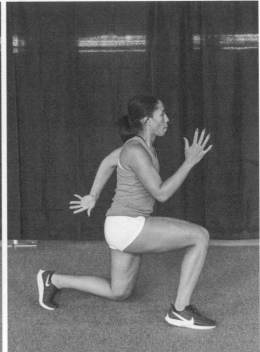

End position (right foot forward)

Multidirectional Jump

Type of Exercise or Drill

A series of noncountermovement jumps (two-leg takeoffs, two-leg landings) done within approximately a 6-foot (2 m) area.

Intensity Level

Low

Movement Directions

Vertical, sideways, rotational

Equipment

An appropriate landing surface, 2 to 3 feet (61-91 cm) of unobstructed space

Beginning Position

- Begin in the appropriate landing position seen in figure 9.1.

Movement Phases

1. On a signal, execute the first jump in the series by performing a submaximal noncountermovement vertical jump, driving upward with the arms, hips, knees, and ankles and landing in the beginning position.

2. On a signal, perform the jump in the same fashion and intensity as the first, this time in a sideways direction, approximately 2 to 3 feet (61-91 cm) to the right, landing again in the beginning position.

3. The next jump on a signal is sideways toward the left, landing in the area of the first jump and in the beginning position.

4. The next jump on a signal is done in place like the first one, this time rotating 90 degrees to the right while off the floor. Land in the beginning position.

5. The last jump is on a signal and again in place, this time rotating 90 degrees to the left to arrive back in the position that started the series and landing once again in the beginning position.

Coaching Tips

This is another drill intended to teach proper two-foot landing positions and is great for an early progression exercise or to be included in movement preparation. Multidirectional jumps are intended to introduce slightly higher forces in multiple planes of movement, helping student-athletes better learn to control forces in these planes. Many sports place forces on the body from multiple directions, and part of a robust program to help reduce the risk of injuries is to better prepare student-athletes to receive these forces in proper positions.

Many student-athletes (and sometimes strength and conditioning professionals) will get caught up in trying to jump too high, too far to the side, or over-rotate during this jump series. It is important for the strength and conditioning professional to keep in mind, and to communicate to student-athletes, that this drill is more about force control than force production. In fact, this is the reason for eliminating the countermovement to each of the jumps in the series. When inexperienced and untrained student-athletes concern themselves with the proper sequencing of the upper and lower body during the countermovement, they often disregard the proper landing position that is supposed to follow each jump or are unable to attain the proper landing position because too much force was produced due to the countermovement. (In fact, the student-athlete is displaying more knee valgus in the landing position photos than what is ideal.) For these reasons, it may be a good idea for the strength and conditioning professional to lead this drill with student-athletes as a group, giving them detailed directions of what percent of effort to give on each jump, how far to travel during the side jump, and what direction they should be facing at the end of each rotational jump. Before giving the signal to perform the next jump in the series, the strength and conditioning professional should hold the group in the proper landing position to reinforce the importance of this position and to identify student-athletes who are having difficulty with these positions. Along with deviations from the proper landing position shown in figure 9.1, strength and conditioning professionals should look for student-athletes who land with feet excessively pronated or supinated in the series because this can be the cause of other problematic positions (7).

When student-athletes begin to show proficiency in the landing positions, a microprogression of emphasizing upward arm drive and hip and knee extension can be added to this drill to begin teaching proper jump mechanics.

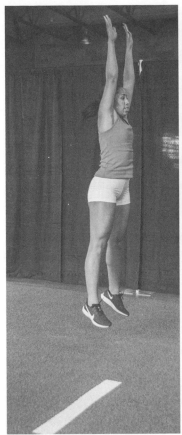 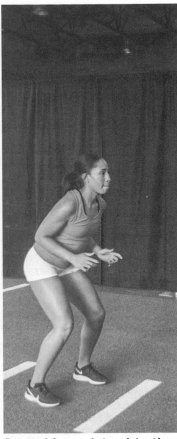

First jump: noncounter-movement vertical jump

Second jump: lateral to the right (end position)

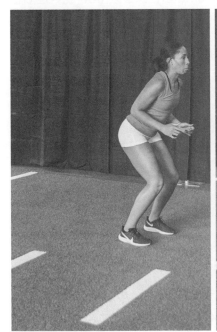 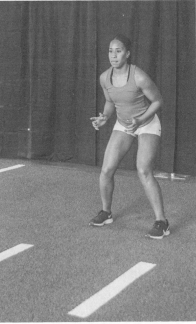 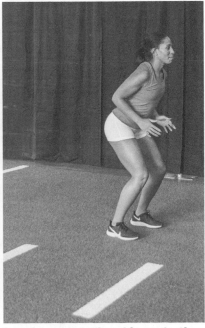

Third jump: lateral to the left (end position; see the note in the text)

Fourth jump: rotational jump to the right (end position)

Last jump: rotational jump to the left (end position)

Single-Leg Multidirectional Hop

Type of Exercise or Drill

A series of hops (single-leg takeoff, same-foot landing) done in place and within a 6-foot (2 m) area.

Intensity Level

Low

Movement Directions

Vertical, forward, sideways

Equipment

An appropriate landing surface and 6 feet (2 m) of unobstructed space

Beginning Position

• Stand on the right leg only, in essentially the single-leg version of the proper landing position in figure 9.1 (i.e., shoulder over the right knee, right knee over the right foot, knee slightly bent, right foot flat, and no inward movement of the right shin).

Movement Phases

1. On a signal, perform a submaximal noncountermovement vertical hop on the right leg, and land in the appropriate single-leg position on the right foot.

2. On a signal, perform a single-leg forward hop in the same fashion and intensity as the first one, this time approximately 1 to 2 feet (30-61 cm) in a slightly forward direction, landing in the appropriate single-leg landing position on the right foot.

3. The next single-leg hop on a signal is approximately 1 to 2 feet (30-61 cm) to the right side, landing in the appropriate single-leg landing position on the right foot.

4. The final single-leg hop in the series is approximately 1 to 2 feet (30-61 cm) to the left side, again landing on the right foot and in the appropriate single-leg landing position.

5. After completing all four hops on the right foot, repeat the series on the left foot.

Coaching Tips

Like multidirectional jumps, this drill helps student-athletes control forces in multiple planes of movement, now on one leg. This drill is slightly more demanding than its two-legged counterpart in that there are fewer points of contact on the floor and it has an added balance component. Therefore, student-athletes may struggle more with proficiency in this drill than the multidirectional jumps.

Also, like multidirectional jumps, student-athletes will often try to jump too high or too far in all directions of the drill and should be given explicit directions on effort, distance, and positions of landing. This is the reason for removing the countermovement action to this drill. Student-athletes who struggle with single-leg balance and control should be allowed to take a second small hop to help them regain posture and position, especially with the forward and side hops. With untrained and inexperienced student-athletes, it is better to have them add a second foot contact to help them learn to adjust body positions rather than to emphasize sticking the landing in a poor athletic position (7).

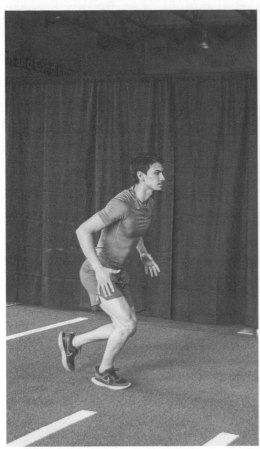

Beginning position

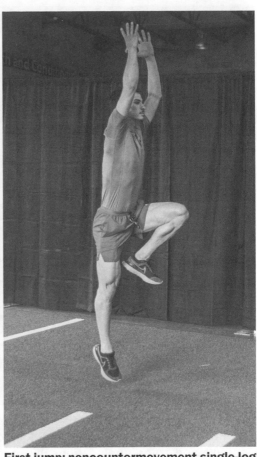

First jump: noncountermovement single-leg vertical hop

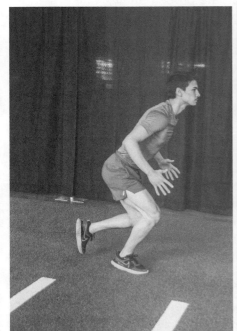

Second jump: single-leg forward hop (end position)

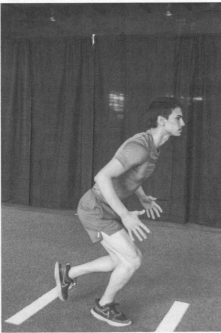

Third jump: single-leg hop to the right (end position)

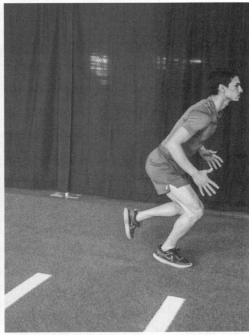

Fourth jump: single-leg hop to the left (end position)

Broad Jump and Stick Over Hurdle

Type of Exercise or Drill
Forward jump (two-legged takeoff, two-legged landing) over a hurdle, with a 1-second pause between each jump

Intensity Level
Medium

Movement Directions
Forward, vertical

Equipment
A hurdle between 6 and 18 inches (15-46 cm) tall, depending on the student-athlete's skill level and training status, and an appropriate landing surface

Beginning Position
• Begin approximately 2 feet (61 cm) in front of the hurdle in a tall position, with legs extended, feet shoulder-width apart, and arms (not shown in the first photo) extended above chest height in preparation for the countermovement of the forward jump.

Movement Phases
1. Perform the countermovement by quickly lowering into the proper landing position and transitioning from this position as explosively as possible into a forward jump over the hurdle.

2. Land with both feet on the opposite side of the hurdle in the proper landing position and hold the landing for 1 second before beginning the subsequent repetitions.

3. Depending on the space and setup, continue forward movement over the next hurdle, or turn around and jump back over.

4. Begin each repetition in the beginning position to use the countermovement for each jump.

Coaching Tips
This drill and similar variations are often added too early in a plyometric program progression and should be included only after student-athletes have shown proficiency in jumping and landing mechanics in the lower-intensity drills. This is a medium-intensity drill because student-athletes are tasked with generating more force in a shorter amount of time with the quick countermovement and subsequent concentric action into the jump, as well as covering a greater distance than the drills done in place without the countermovement.

In addition to decelerating into a proper landing position, one of the most important coaching points in this drill is helping student-athletes understand how to transition after the landing. When the landing and explosive point is emphasized, this drill can be effective in helping high school student-athletes improve their power.

Student-athletes may struggle with trying to clear the hurdle with hip and knee flexion instead of extension. This may be a result of the hurdle being too high or poor jumping mechanics. If this is the case, the strength and conditioning professional should start with shorter hurdles or regress the student-athlete to a lower-intensity drill that emphasizes proper jumping mechanics (i.e., full extension through the hips, knees, and ankles) before going any further with this drill.

Adding a vertical component to a broad jump (in this case, jumping over the hurdle) can decrease the amount of horizontal force placed on the student-athlete during the landing. If the student-athlete is simply asked to jump forward as far as possible without a vertical component, there may be too much force for the student-athlete to absorb safely and effectively (7). Outlining strict space parameters for this drill not only helps ensure quality of repetitions but can also help manage space in large group settings.

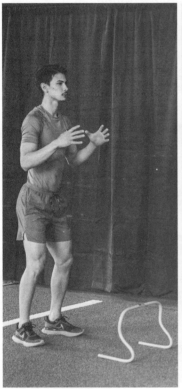
Beginning position

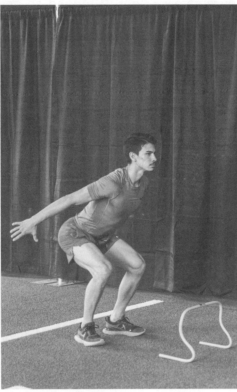
Countermovement

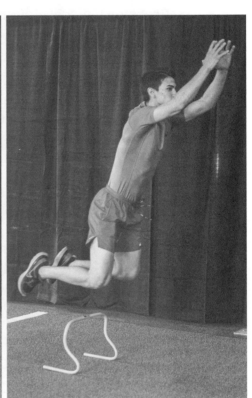
Jump

Lateral Bound and Stick

Type of Exercise or Drill

Bounding (take off on one leg and land on the other) from side to side, in place with a pause between each bound

Intensity Level

Medium

Movement Directions

Sideways, slightly vertical

Equipment

Unobstructed space of approximately 6 feet (2 m) and an appropriate landing surface

Beginning Position

• Stand tall on the left foot in the single-leg version of the proper landing position in figure 9.1 with the arms extended above chest height (not shown in the first photo) in preparation for the countermovement.

Movement Phases

1. Perform the countermovement by quickly lowering into the proper single-leg landing position, with the right knee slightly behind the hips, and transition from this position as explosively as possible into a slightly vertical and lateral movement to the right.

2. Land in the proper single-leg landing position on the right foot and hold the position (stick the landing) for 1 second.

3. After holding the landing position for 1 second, perform the next lateral bound (to the left) off the right foot the same fashion as the previous lateral bound, making sure to include the quick countermovement and subsequent explosive action in the slightly vertical and sideways movement.

4. After holding the single-leg landing position for 1 second on the left foot, repeat the drill for the prescribed number of repetitions.

Coaching Tips

This drill can build student-athletes' abilities to produce, control, and absorb force on one leg and in the sideways direction, because it introduces slightly more force than the multidirectional hops due to the countermovement.

Strength and conditioning professionals should carefully watch that student-athletes do not go into excessive knee valgus (i.e., knees collapsing inward) during this drill. If this continues to happen after feedback, the strength and conditioning professional should consider if the student-athlete may be deficient in strength levels and not ready for this progression in single-leg plyometrics.

Like the broad jump and stick over hurdle, strength and conditioning professionals with limited space or who need to ensure more quality control over this drill may want to provide student-athletes with specific distance guidelines (i.e., bound from this mark to this mark 2 to 2.5 feet [61-76 cm] away) or add a vertical component by placing a small (6 inch [15 cm]) hurdle to the student-athletes' sides to have them bound over it. In the latter example, be mindful of student-athletes using hip and knee flexion instead of extension to clear the hurdle. As student-athletes become proficient with this drill, the intensity can be increased by bounding slightly greater distances or over higher hurdles. However, the strength and conditioning professional should not lose sight of emphasizing a quick countermovement with an explosive transition into the bounding movement and, as always, a proper landing position that safely and effectively absorbs forces.

A common error is landing with little or no knee or hip flexion (or both) as seen in the landing position of the fourth photo (lateral bound to the left). One of the most important messages of this chapter is to convey that force absorption and proper landing positions should be paramount in programming lower body plyometrics for high school student-athletes.

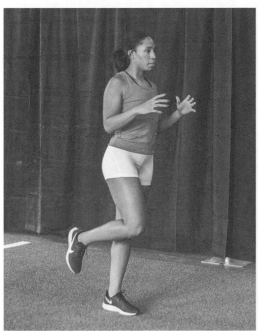

Beginning position

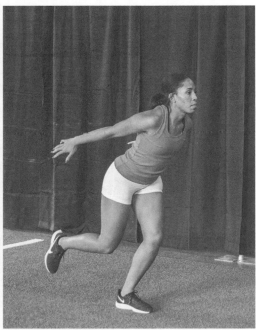

Countermovement

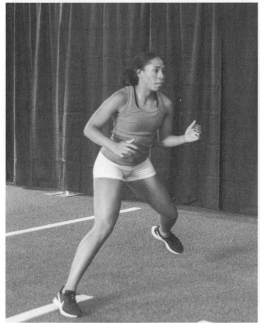

Landing the lateral bound to the right

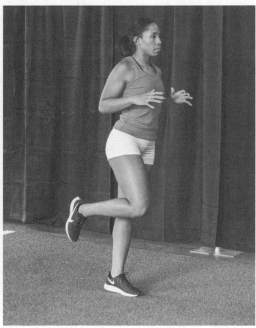

Lateral bound to the left (end position): Common error shown (see text)

Forward Bound and Stick

Type of Exercise or Drill
Bounding (i.e., take off from one leg and land on the other) forward with a pause between each bound

Intensity Level
Medium

Movement Directions
Forward, slightly vertical

Equipment
Depending on the number of repetitions and if this drill is performed stationary or with movement, several feet (a meter) to several yards (or several meters) of unobstructed space will be necessary

Beginning Position
• Stand tall on the left foot in the single-leg version of the proper landing position in figure 9.1 with the arms extended above chest height (not shown in the first photo) in preparation for the countermovement.

Movement Phases
1. Perform the countermovement (not shown in the photos) by quickly lowering into the proper single-leg landing position with the right knee slightly behind the hips, and transition from this position as explosively as possible into a slightly vertical and forward movement landing on the right foot.

2. Land in the proper single-leg position on the right foot and hold the position for 1 second.

3. After holding the landing position, perform the next forward bound off the right foot (to land on the left foot; not shown in the photos) in the same fashion as the previous forward bound, making sure to include the quick countermovement and subsequent explosive action in the slightly vertical and forward movement.

4. After holding the single-leg landing position on the left foot for 1 second, repeat the drill for the prescribed number of repetitions.

Coaching Tips
The forward bound and stick is the forward movement version of the lateral bound and stick and is also intended to help student-athletes learn to produce, control, and absorb force on one leg. Including a progression of plyometric drills in multiple directions is essential in preparing student-athletes for movements in various directions specific to their respective sports. Several of the same coaching tips from the lateral bound and stick apply to this drill too.

One challenge that student-athletes may face during this drill that is less common with the lateral version is postural control on the landing as they move forward explosively toward the opposite leg. The strength and conditioning professional should reinforce the cue to student-athletes to maintain a neutral spine and keep their shoulder over the knee of the leg that is on the floor when they stick the landing.

Another challenge is student-athletes' inability to land full-footed and instead placing too much initial impact toward their toes. Encourage these student-athletes to use a double hop to be able to gain control of the force and reestablish proper position.

For facilities with limited space, including the forward bound and stick drill can still be done simply by having the student-athlete jump, land, and turn around to perform the next repetition. This modification can reduce the space necessary for the drill from several yards (or several meters) down to several feet (a meter), or about the size of a standard lifting platform area, if the surface is appropriate and flush with the rest of the flooring.

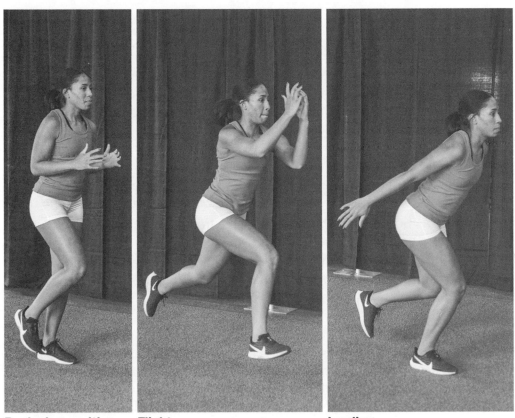

Beginning position   **Flight**   **Landing**

Multiple Broad Jumps and Stick

Type of Exercise or Drill
Multiple jumps (two-leg takeoff, two-leg landing with no pause between repetitions)

Intensity Level
High

Movement Directions
Forward, slightly vertical

Equipment
Several yards (or meters), depending on number of repetitions, of unobstructed space

Beginning Position
• Begin in a tall position with the arms extended above the chest (not shown in the first photo) in preparation for the countermovement.

Movement Phases
1. Quickly begin the countermovement, and as explosively as possible jump forward as far as possible, contacting the floor with both feet at the same time.

2. As soon as both feet hit the floor, begin the transition from landing to jumping forward for the next broad jump as quickly as possible.

3. Depending on the level of progression, either hold a proper landing position for 1 second after the second broad jump, ending the set, or begin the third repetition of broad jumps in the same fashion as step 2.

Coaching Tips
The multiple broad jumps and stick drill is a combination of related plyometric skills that should have been developed, if not mastered, by student-athletes early in the program with less intense drills. This drill is considered high intensity because it contains the added challenges of jumping for distance and repeating the effort for multiple jumps as quickly as possible. Therefore, the high school strength and conditioning professional should prescribe this drill carefully in a plyometric program and only to student-athletes who have demonstrated competency in the earlier phases of the program.

Many of the same coaching tips from the broad jump and stick over hurdle will be valuable in this drill; however, most of the coaching emphasis will be on having the student-athlete minimize the amount of time spent transitioning from the landing of the first jump to the takeoff of the second jump.

It may be necessary for the strength and conditioning professional to restrict the distance of the first broad jump in the series to a relatively short distance (3-5 yards [2.7-4.6 m]), especially with less experienced or capable groups. This allows student-athletes to learn to absorb the force in a position more conducive to short transition time, then allows student-athletes to jump as far as possible on the second jump in the series, holding the landing in a proper position to end the set.

If student-athletes become proficient with this drill, one way to increase intensity can be to add another broad jump to the series. For example, the student-athlete can perform three broad jumps, focusing on minimal transition time between jumps one through three, then finishing with a solid landing in the proper position after jump three. The strength and conditioning professional should be cautious about adding too many jumps to the series because the quality of repetitions can decrease as fatigue sets in.

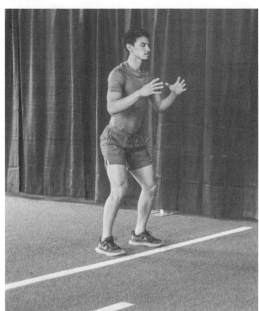

Beginning position

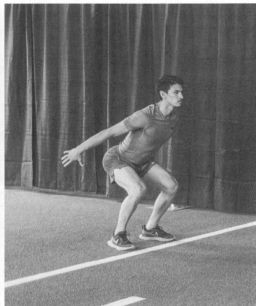

Countermovement

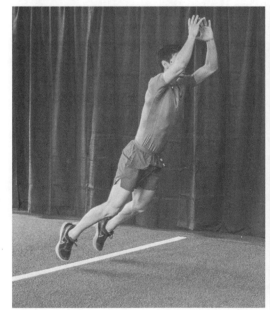

Flight

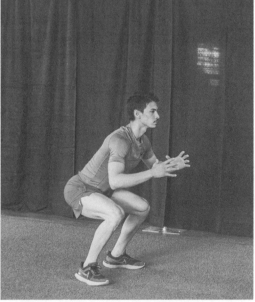

Landing (before countermovement of next jump)

Multiple Forward Bounds and Stick

Type of Exercise or Drill

Bounding (take off on one foot and land on the opposite with minimal pause during the first landing)

Intensity Level

High

Movement Directions

Forward, slightly vertical

Equipment

Several yards (or meters), depending on the number of repetitions, of unobstructed space

Beginning Position

• Stand tall on the left foot in the single-leg version of the proper landing position in figure 9.1 with the arms extended above chest height (not shown in the first photo) in preparation for the countermovement.

Movement Phases

1. Quickly begin the countermovement, and as explosively as possible, push off the left foot to land as far forward as possible, contacting the floor with only the right foot.

2. As soon as the right foot hits the floor, begin the transition from landing to pushing off the right foot forward to bound onto the left foot as quickly as possible.

3. When the left foot contacts the floor (not shown), hold the proper single-leg landing position for 1 second to demonstrate proficiency in decelerating the body.

4. Begin the second series of multiple bounds (not shown), this time in the beginning position on the right foot.

5. Repeat the drill, but start by pushing off with the right foot, bounding from the left foot to the right foot with minimal transition time, and hold the landing on the right foot for 1 second to demonstrate proficiency in decelerating on the right leg. This is considered 1 complete repetition.

6. Repeat steps 1 through 5 for the prescribed number of repetitions in the set.

Coaching Tips

The multiple forward bounds and stick is the highest-intensity drill outlined in this chapter and should be reserved for high school student-athletes with the highest degree of movement competency in the drills outlined in earlier progressions. Many high school strength and conditioning professionals add multiple bounds too early in student-athletes' plyometric programs. As the intensity of a drill or exercise increases, the volume or number of foot contacts for that drill should decrease. When programming multiple bounds for the high school student-athlete who has demonstrated proficiency in earlier progressions, err on the side of caution with regard to volume, and keep the number of total foot contacts low for this drill.

The strength and conditioning professional can use many of the same tips from the forward bound and stick for this drill, and like the multiple broad jumps and stick, be prepared to focus most of the coaching emphasis on minimizing the amount of time the student-athlete spends on the floor during the first landing. For student-athletes unable to make a quick, explosive transition, regress the drill and restrict the distance of the first bound to 1 to 3 yards (1-3 m). For student-athletes unable to hold the landing in a proper single-leg position after the second bound, allow them to take a second hop to adjust to the proper landing position until they become more proficient and can stick the landing.

Like the multiple broad jumps and stick, one way to intensify this drill is to add bounds to the series. In this progression the student-athlete starts on the left foot, bounds quickly off the right foot, then quickly bounds off the left foot, and finishes the drill in a proper landing position on the right foot. Again, multiple bounds are already a high-intensity drill, so be prudent when making the decision to include them in a plyometric program for high school student-athletes, and even more so when deciding to add an intensity progression.

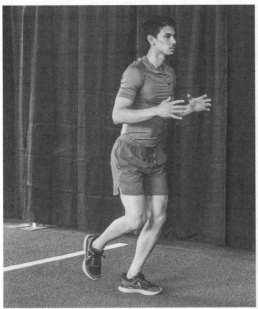

Beginning position

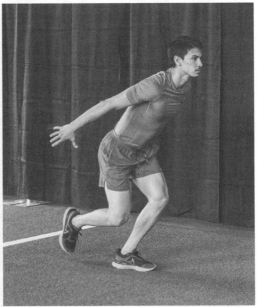

Countermovement

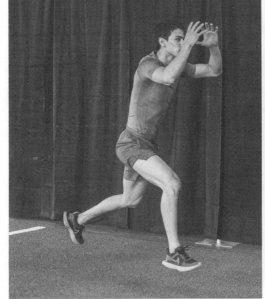

Flight

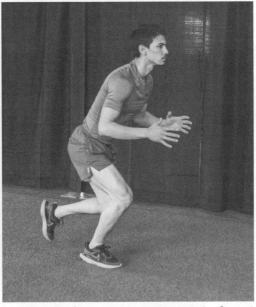

Landing (before countermovement of next bound)

Sample Plyometric Training Programs

Tables 9.3 through 9.6 provide four sample plyometric training programs of gradually progressing intensities and varying work-to-rest ratios.

TABLE 9.3   Sample Low-Intensity Plyometric Program

Work-to-rest ratio: 1:5		
DAY 1	**DAY 2**	**DAY 3**
LOWER BODY DRILLS	**UPPER BODY DRILLS**	**LOWER BODY DRILLS**
Snap down to two-foot landing 3 × 5	Half-kneeling medicine ball chest pass 3 × 5	Snap down to two-foot landing 3 × 5
Drop to split squat 3 × 3 on each leg	Half-kneeling medicine ball two-hand overhead throw 3 × 5	Drop to split squat 3 × 3 on each leg
Multidirectional jump 3 × 1 (each rep = all 5 jumps)	Half-kneeling rotational medicine ball throw 3 × 3 on each side	Multidirectional jump 3 × 1 (each rep = all 5 jumps)
Single-leg multidirectional hop 3 × 1 on each leg (each rep = all 4 hops)	Beginning in a half-kneeling position allows the student-athlete to gain competence in the countermovement of the shoulders and torso before progressing into a standing position and using the lower body.	Single-leg multidirectional hop 3 × 1 on each leg (each rep = all 4 hops)
Total foot contacts: 51	Total repetitions: 39	Total foot contacts: 51

TABLE 9.4   Sample Low- to Medium-Intensity Plyometric Program

Work-to-rest ratio: 1:7		
DAY 1	**DAY 2**	**DAY 3**
LOWER BODY DRILLS: SINGLE-LEG EMPHASIS	**UPPER BODY DRILLS**	**LOWER BODY DRILLS: TWO-LEG EMPHASIS**
Snap down to two-foot landing 1 × 5	Standing medicine ball chest pass 3 × 5	Snap down to two-foot landing 1 × 5
Drop to split squat 1 × 3 on each leg	Standing medicine ball two-hand overhead throw 3 × 5	Drop to split squat 1 × 3 on each leg
Multidirectional jump 1 × 1 (each rep = all 5 jumps)	Standing rotational medicine ball throw 4 × 3 on each side	Multidirectional jump 1 × 1 (each rep = all 5 jumps)
Single-leg multidirectional hop 1 × 1 on each leg (each rep = all 4 hops)	Progressing from a half-kneeling position to a standing position will increase intensity by allowing student-athletes to throw with more force from a position of higher stability.	Single-leg multidirectional hop 1 × 1 on each leg (each rep = all 4 hops)
Forward hurdle hop and stick 3 × 3 on each leg		Box jump 4 × 3
Side hurdle hop and stick 3 × 4 on each leg (2 reps right, 2 reps left = 1 set)		Loaded jump 4 × 3
		Loaded jumps can be done with a pair of dumbbells in the student-athlete's hands or with a hex bar. Loads should be light enough for the student-athlete to move explosively from the countermovement into the jump phase with a quick transition period.
Total foot contacts: 38	Total repetitions: 39	Total foot contacts: 41

TABLE 9.5   Sample Medium- to High-Intensity Plyometric Program

Work-to-rest ratio: 1:7		
DAY 1	**DAY 2**	**DAY 3**
LOWER BODY DRILLS: SINGLE-LEG EMPHASIS	**UPPER BODY DRILLS**	**LOWER BODY DRILLS: TWO-LEG EMPHASIS**
Snap down to two-foot landing 1 × 5	Standing medicine ball chest pass 3 × 5	Snap down to two-foot landing 1 × 5
Drop to split squat 1 × 3 on each leg	Standing medicine ball two-hand overhead throw 3 × 5	Drop to split squat 1 × 3 on each leg
Multidirectional jump 1 × 1 (each rep = all 5 jumps)	Standing rotational medicine ball throw 3 × 4 on each side	Multidirectional jump 1 × 1 (each rep = all 5 jumps)
Single-leg multidirectional hop 1 × 1 on each leg (each rep = all 4 hops)	Same upper body drills as table 9.4 but with an increase in total volume.	Single-leg multidirectional hop 1 × 1 on each leg (each rep = all 4 hops)
Forward bound and stick 4 × 3 on each leg (each set = 6 bounds)		Broad jump and stick over hurdle 4 × 3
Total foot contacts: 29	Total repetitions: 41	Total foot contacts: 29

TABLE 9.6   Sample High-Intensity Plyometric Program

Work-to-rest ratio: 1:10		
DAY 1	**DAY 2**	**DAY 3**
LOWER BODY DRILLS: SINGLE-LEG EMPHASIS	**UPPER BODY DRILLS**	**LOWER BODY DRILLS: TWO-LEG EMPHASIS**
Snap down to two-foot landing 1 × 5	Step-into medicine ball chest pass 3 × 5	Snap down to two-foot landing 1 × 5
Drop to split squat 1 × 3 on each leg	Step-into medicine ball two-hand overhead throw 3 × 5	Drop to split squat 1 × 3 on each leg
Multidirectional jump 1 × 1 (each rep = all 5 jumps)	Step-into rotational medicine ball throw 4 × 3 on each side	Multidirectional jump 1 × 1 (each rep = all 5 jumps)
Single-leg multidirectional hop 1 × 1 on each leg (each rep = all 4 hops)	The "step-into" modification allows the student-athlete to apply more force generated from the lower body into the pass, throw, and toss, adding intensity to the drill.	Single-leg multidirectional hop 1 × 1 on each leg (each rep = all 4 hops)
Multiple forward bounds and stick 4 × 2 on each leg (each rep = 2 bounds)		Multiple broad jumps and stick 4 × 2 (each rep = 2 broad jumps)
Total foot contacts: 23	Total repetitions: 41	Total foot contacts: 23

Conclusion

Plyometric training can be a safe and effective complement to the high school student-athlete's strength and conditioning program in developing several athletic qualities and characteristics as well as reducing the risk of sport-related injuries (10). The strength and conditioning professional must carefully consider programming variables such as intensity, frequency, volume, and progression as they relate specifically to the high school student-athlete's experience, training status, and skill level, and refrain from implementing a program or drills intended for more experienced and trained student-athletes. High school strength and conditioning professionals' number one priority should be the safety and well-being of student-athletes and they should have a foundational understanding of equipment and space guidelines to help ensure student-athletes' safety in plyometric training. They also should be focused on their student-athletes mastering proper technique with lower-intensity plyometric drills before progressing to more advanced, high-intensity drills.

10

Speed and Agility Training

Phil Tran, JD, MSEd, CSCS,*D
Ray Karvis, MSEd, CSCS

The saying "You can't coach speed" is a myth. For far too long, sport coaches have sought naturally fast athletes thinking they can coach everything but speed. Speed actually can and should be coached. A team can never have enough individual and collective speed. A proper training program will improve speed for all student-athletes at all levels of play (4).

For student-athletes to get faster on a linear plane or horizontal plane, they need to apply force and move correctly (12). The movements need to be fluid, and the strength and conditioning professional may challenge the genetic potential of student-athletes. This chapter will focus on developing speed, change of direction speed, acceleration, and other agility components on an introductory level. It will address maximum velocity drills that will assist in developing proper running form to enhance a student-athlete's top speed in a linear direction.

The ability to change direction as quickly as possible will have a dynamic correspondence with a student-athlete's sport. Agility is the ability to control one's body. In sport, the objective is to control the body while moving at maximum speed to achieve a competitive advantage over an opponent (12). This chapter includes simple drills that, when repeated and mastered, will challenge the student-athlete to become more agile during competition phases.

It is notable that the number of drills developed to improve speed and agility is large and ever expanding. High school sport coaches or strength and conditioning professionals can quickly and effectively implement the drills in this chapter. It is best to have a small playbook and master the fundamentals as opposed to having a large playbook containing drills that cannot be taught or that the student-athletes cannot perform effectively.

Program Design Guidelines

When designing a program for speed, it is very similar to designing any program; that is, begin with the end in mind. The demands of the sport will determine the outcomes. For example, a volleyball player does not have the same linear speed demands as a soccer player. So, knowing the end goal of training and working toward that goal is where a strength and conditioning professional should start when designing a program.

Periodization, the organization of training cycles, is a factor in designing a program. The changes that a student-athlete will undergo during the different phases and the amount of work done on a weekly plan should be the guide. Information should be collected prior to, during, and at the end of the program. This way the workouts can be changed based on how the student-athlete's performance varied. This can be done with a group or individually. When modifying a workout, consider which variables in the training are affecting the performance of the student-athlete.

All student-athletes should be trained to have proper running mechanics for all functional movements as well as any conditioning drills that focus on running or agility training. Setting up the program on progression blocks is an ideal guideline for speed and agility training. Here are some variables that should be considered:

- Distance covered in the drill: This will depend on the sport's primary energy system.
- Number of repetitions: This will depend on the focus of the drill.
- Sets: This will depend on the focus of the drill.
- Volume: This will depend on the focus of the drill and the time of year (season).
- Frequency: Consider sport demands in the off-season versus in-season.
- Intensity: This is based on the effort with good technique.
- Progression: Move from basic movements to more complex movements.
- Recovery: This depends on the time of year (season).
- Work-to-rest ratio. This depends on the system being trained.

Ultimately, the program design should provide a moderate progression from beginning to end. The examples in this chapter are starting points; additional resources (3, 7, 11, 13) can be consulted to make changes to the programs over time.

Age and Training Status Considerations

The ages of student-athletes, including those entering high school and those who are about to complete high school, typically range from 13 to 19 years. When designing a speed and agility program for high school student-athletes, an assessment of the student-athlete's developmental age is important to consider first (see page 229 in chapter 8).

Proper running form is essential, but first, a student-athlete will need to be classified as trained or untrained in both running and any type of resistance training. If the student-athlete is trained, some habits have already been created. Any bad habits must be corrected to maximize the potential of the speed development process.

No minimal age requirement exists for a young student-athlete to follow a training program except that the student-athlete needs to have the emotional maturity to follow directions (8). A pretraining medical exam is not mandatory, but student-athletes should be screened for injuries or illness that could hinder their safety (2).

The goals of youth resistance training programs should not only be about increasing strength but should also promote interest in physical activity that comes from speed and agility training. In addition to promoting a general interest in physical activity and fun experiences, reducing the risk of overuse injuries should also be considered (8, 14).

Different sports and positions within sports will have specific demands regarding speed and agility. Track student-athletes are different from field student-athletes. A field student-athlete will use the agility training and drills more than a track student-athlete will because the field student-athlete is constantly changing directions and accelerating out of those changes in direction. Goalies are different from position players in soccer and lacrosse. Goalies will require more focus on agility, while position players will do more linear speed work. It is important to individualize training as time and resources allow.

Intensity

The length and percentage of maximum effort will vary depending on the student-athlete's previous level of training. As a starting point, a percentage guideline can be used for the expectations for the student-athlete's intensity. For example, a strength and conditioning professional could use the gear method (see page 307). This can be as simple as levels 1 through 4. Gear 4 would be maximal effort, or 100 percent. Gear 3 could be 75 percent, or a stride. Gear 2 could be 50 percent, or half speed. Gear 1 would be 25 percent of maximum effort but still exhibiting the fundamentals of the running techniques described in this chapter.

Ultimately, training for speed or agility is not conditioning. To maximize the benefits of speed and agility training, the student-athlete must be fully recovered to perform without compromising technique and effort. Walking back after a repetition is completed for the recovery is acceptable.

Frequency

A helpful guideline is to have two speed training days and one agility training day. For example, Monday could focus on acceleration prior to a resistance training session, Tuesday could be an agility training day, and Wednesday could focus on maximum-velocity training or speed training. If a fourth day is done, it could be a speed endurance day or a conditioning day. (Conditioning is not discussed in this chapter.)

Agility drills can have components of speed and acceleration in them as well. A three-day plan is a great starting point for beginning high school student-athletes. Recovery is important, especially after the first week of the workout drills.

The sport-specific drills for each sport or position should be the basis for agility training. As a sport season approaches, running frequency only needs to be a few days per week but with a greater focus on maximal velocity. Further, testing is typically performed every four to eight weeks to monitor progress.

During the in-season, speed and agility training should be incorporated as well, such as at the beginning of a sport practice. After a dynamic warm-up, running form drills such as the ankling and high knee drill (see page 306) can be performed. At least once per week prior to competition, maximum velocity should be reached. Sprinting for even short distances during the competition phase of a sport is beneficial for the student-athlete in order to achieve that speed in contests or games.

Order

In a typical workout, speed and agility drills should be performed first after a proper dynamic warm-up routine. To achieve maximum rate of force production and have the body adapt to it, the body needs to be fresh, meaning that sufficient rest needs to be provided so a student-athlete can do the next repetition at maximum speed. After working on speed, the student-athlete will transition to working on the resistance training goal (for the training phase) in the weight room.

There will be times when, due to scheduling or facility space availability, speed and strength sessions need to be flipped. This is the reality in the high school setting and is not a big issue. Usually, a strength and conditioning professional should use conditioning workouts for these scenarios.

Because student-athletes will already be fatigued if a resistance training session was completed beforehand, any running done afterward should be performed at a moderate intensity between 50 and 75 percent, with time targets that are slower than the student-athletes' best times. The injury risk is heightened when student-athletes are fatigued and especially so for younger student-athletes who have limited training experience. Training at maximum intensity for speed development in a fatigued state will not develop the best results (11).

Volume

The volume of speed and agility work needed will be based off the unique needs of each sport. While speed and agility work and overall athleticism are of value for non-ground-based sports, such as ice hockey, swimming, and diving, these are not high priorities. Examples of ground-based sports that benefit from significant speed and agility training include football, baseball, softball, basketball, tennis, volleyball, field hockey, lacrosse, soccer, and track and field.

Work-to-Rest Ratio

The three main energy systems used for speed training are the phosphagen, glycolytic, and aerobic systems. The first two are for shorter distances that apply to almost every sport, and the third system needs to be trained more for aerobic endurance sports. Speed and acceleration primarily use ATP and creatine phosphate, so it is important not to mistake speed and agility training for conditioning.

The **work-to-rest ratio** is the comparison between how much time work is being done (e.g., sprinting, lifting weights, or doing high-intensity training) to the amount of time spent resting. For example, if a student-athlete completes a 10-second sprint and rests for 60 seconds, the work-to-rest ratio is 1:6. The ratio should vary based on the type of training and energy systems. It is typically lower (less proportional rest) for cardiovascular and muscular endurance training, and higher (more proportional rest) for strength and power training (6).

The work-to-rest ratio for speed and agility training should be 1:12 up to a 1:20 (6). For example, if a student-athlete exerts maximum effort or top speed for 5 to 10 seconds, the phosphagen system is used. The distances would be around 30 to 80 yards (27.4-73.2 m), the student-athlete would have 60 seconds with a 1:12 ratio in a 5 second sprint, up to 100 seconds of rest time (a 1:20 ratio) before the next sprint or exercise in the workout.

If the training segment uses the glycolytic cycle and the sprinting duration is 15 to 30 seconds (e.g., over 100 yards [91.4 m] but not to exceed 250 yards [228.6 m]), the work-to-rest ratios should be 1:3 or 1:5 (6). For example, if a student-athlete ran at top speed for 15 seconds using a 1:3 ratio, he or she would have 45 seconds to rest before running again.

If a student-athlete's form and mechanics break down or begin to look poor, allow more rest or end the session. If the strength and conditioning professional wants to incorporate these drills for a type of conditioning segment, the work-to-rest ratio would be shortened, which activates glycolysis. Again, the goal of speed development, even when incorporating conditioning, is for the student-athlete to repeat the sprinting form or ability with correct mechanics at maximum effort (12).

Progression

In progressing a student-athlete through a speed training session and program, it is important to emphasize recovery time between sets within a session and recovery time between sessions. If a student-athlete is unable to run at maximum speed in a speed training session, the student-athlete will not experience maximum gains. "Poor speed is poor quality" (13).

Every student-athlete is different based on a variety of factors such as training experience, injury history, stress, and genetics, and as such, total volume of work can be increased or decreased. As the student-athlete improves, volume can be increased; once a student-athlete is trained, volumes of up to 1,000 to 2,000 meters (1,094-2,187 yds) per week of acceleration and speed training are typical (13).

Exercises should be introduced to new student-athletes in order of difficulty level. The exercises presented in this chapter progress from easy to hard, and it is recommended that this order is followed before making adjustments to the program.

Safety Guidelines

Before beginning any training program, it is essential to have the student-athlete go through a screening and clearance process. In accordance with instructions specified by the American Academy of Family Physicians, American Academy of Pediatrics, American College of Sports Medicine, American Medical Society for Sports Medicine, American Orthopaedic Society for Sports Medicine, and American Osteopathic Academy of Sports Medicine Preparticipation Task Force (10) and other governing bodies related to high school athletic associations, a high school strength and conditioning professional can only work with student-athletes who have undergone health care provider screening (standard 1.1, page 74) (15).

Specifically related to speed and agility training, a primary consideration is the surface the student-athlete will use to perform the drills. Ideally, the surface should be the same or comparable to what the student-athlete experiences during the sport, if applicable. In addition to being free from obstacles and hazards, there needs to be sufficient space, especially for speed drills, so that a student-athlete can safely decelerate after the finish line (5).

Speed Mechanics

Speed is combination of **stride length** (distance traveled by each stride) and **stride frequency** (or *cadence*, the number of strides taken per second) (7). The more ground covered with each stride and the faster the legs can turnover, the faster an individual will be. Teaching correct mechanical techniques to increase stride length with the proper frequency will result in a student-athlete increasing speed.

Speed development comes down to mass and acceleration, which is also known as force. The rate of force development (also called the development of maximal force) in minimal time is an indicator of explosive strength (1). The force a student-athlete applies to the ground in a relatively short period of time relates to speed; a desired rapid production of high force rates can aid in the development of speed. Maximal velocity is desired for speed, whereas acceleration in some sports is more desirable. Acceleration is different from speed in that acceleration is a change in speed over a period of time. Speed requires the ability to accelerate and then reach maximal velocity. Agility requires a student-athlete's use of perceptual cognitive ability to decelerate and then accelerate again in a different direction (3).

A student-athlete needs to produce forces that overcome gravity and then be able to change speed in the desired direction. In mathematical terms, the force applied to the ground multiplied by how long the force is applied is **impulse**. A change in impulse results in a change in the momentum of a student-athlete and can demonstrate the student-athlete's ability either to speed up or slow down. With change of direction or agility drills, the impulse is similar, but the student-athlete often slows down to almost a complete stop before changing direction, in many instances, at a completely different angle. It is because of this degree of difficulty that the student-athlete's program also needs to include progressively developed plyometric and resistance training programs.

Training should be targeted at the stretch-shortening cycle (SSC) in which the muscle-tendon complexes are lengthened and shortened. The SSC is particularly important in sports that involve explosive movements at high speeds. Movements that are multijoint in nature and that produce the elastic and reflexive responses up the kinetic chain would be beneficial. To manage fatigue and get the most out of a training session, the explosive movements should be done in groups with ample work-to-rest ratios (3, 6).

Speed Drills

Many drills are designed to help improve linear speed and change-of-direction speed. The following drills can have other progressions added to enhance the development of the student-athlete's speed.

Exercise Finder

Arm Swing

Speaking at the NSCA Maryland State Clinic, Bryan Miller, associate football strength and conditioning coach for the United States Naval Academy, said, "We run with four legs" (9). But humans only have two legs. How can that be? The human body is interconnected. The faster the arms move in proper form, the faster the legs will move. By teaching proper arm movement, a young student-athlete will be on the right path.

Type of Drill

Running form

Beginning Position

- Stand and look straight ahead.
- The head is neutral and relaxed.
- The arms will be flexed at a 90-degree angle but relaxed.

Movement Phases

1. The arms will go up and down in alternating fashion with the palms open, relaxed, and facing inward in a neutral position.

2. The elbows stay tucked in and do not flare out in chicken wing fashion.

Coaching Tips

The coaching cue for the hands is, "Ear to hip." The hand will go to the hip on the downward movement, with the back elbow "smashing the wall" behind the student-athlete. The other hand on the upward motion does not actually touch the ear but is on an even plane with the ear. Some track coaches will teach "outside of the nose." In either case, track coaches generally agree that the hands never cross the midline of the body. As they say, "We are running, not skating."

As the student-athlete looks better at a slow pace, cue the student-athlete to go faster with the arm swings. The student-athlete must not compromise form while moving faster or at full speed. The arms should still show a full range of motion. There is a tendency for young student-athletes to cheat and fool themselves into moving faster by shortening their range of motion. The coaching cue is, "We are not chopping onions."

The elbows should stay flexed but relaxed. On the downswing at high speeds, the back arm angle may go from 90 degrees to an

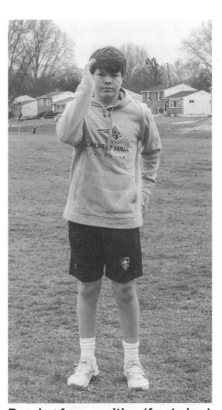

Running form position (front view)

obtuse angle. This is fine and natural. How-ever, a student-athlete who shows a fully extended back arm will need correction.

At maximum speed, the student-athlete should feel the arms propel the body upward. This is what is meant by "running with four legs."

Progressions

Progressions of the arm swing drill involve the student-athlete performing arm swings in lunge positions on both sides, performing one arm swing revolution on cue as fast as possible either in a standing or lunge stance, performing a walking lunge with proper arm swings, and combining one arm swing revo-lution with a jump lunge.

The lunge version is of great importance in speed development. Many issues in sprinting can be fixed by developing a proper lunge. It is taught with consideration of the population's needs and limitations but in such a way that it mimics the sprinting form:

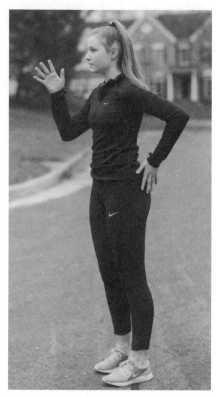

Running form position (side view)

• The lunge position should show approx-imately a 90-degree angle on the front leg and the back leg with the back knee hovering above the floor. The student-athlete should not overreach on the stride or take too short a stride so that the student-athlete is squatting instead.

• Instead, the student-athlete will move the trailing leg all the way through by first starting with a high knee then stepping through to a lunge (i.e., not pausing to bring both feet together before stepping forward).

• Lunge in a straight line and do not wobble and lose balance. It can be help-ful to have student-athletes straddle a line on the field to do walking lunges with arm swings.

The coaching phrases, cues, and directions include the following:

• Relax the head.

• Big chest.

• Upright torso.

• High knee.

• Dorsiflex the front ankle (i.e., point the toes upward, which is of great impor-tance).

• Opposite arm, opposite leg.

• Elbows tucked in; no chicken wings.

• Hands go ear to hip. The downward hand is at the hip, and the upward hand is not literally at the ear but on the same plane with the ear.

• Elbows are flexed but relaxed at a 90-degree angle. Some variation between a right angle and obtuse angle during the arm swing is allowable because the elbow has to be relaxed.

• Back elbow "smashes the wall behind." Pull the back elbow through.

• Shoulders and hips stay square. Do not reach with the upward arm swing.

• Plantarflex the back ankle (push off the back foot) to begin the lunge movement.

In the jump lunge with arm swing, the student-athlete will start in the lunge position, jump up as high as possible, rotate arms and legs in midair, and land in the opposite lunge position. Use a 1:12 work-to-rest ratio (6) so that the student-athlete exerts full effort and exhibit full range of motion.

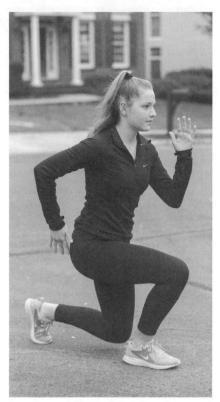

Lunge position (speed development version)

"A" March or Skip

This drill is a starting and acceleration drill to achieve proper sprinting form and technique.

Type of Drill

Running form

Beginning Position

Start with the hands at the side and the feet together.

Movement Phases

1. On a cue of "set," raise up on the toes or the balls of the feet.

2. On a cue of "go," flex the lead leg.

3. Move the opposite arm forward with elbow flexed at a 90-degree angle.

4. The front leg angle is approximately 90 degrees, and the rear leg angle is approximately 133 degrees or closer to an obtuse angle.

5. Alternate this motion for a set distance.

6. Stay on the toes or the balls of the feet and rotate at the shoulder with the arms.

7. The pace will be a march pace or slightly slower than walking.

Coaching Tips

The strength and conditioning professional should look for a good hip position (i.e., the hips are in the same direction) and an orientation of the trunk in the movement direction (i.e., the student-athlete steps forward, not laterally). The student-athlete should be relaxed and not too tense in the arms and shoulders, with good elbow flexion at 90 degrees, and the rotation of the arm should be at the shoulder, not the elbow. This drill can also be done against a wall or fence, which the student-athlete uses to stabilize with their arms to work on the mechanics of the drill. The drill can also be done in a backward motion.

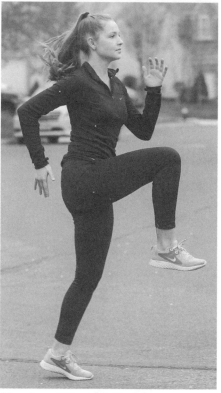

March or skip with first leg

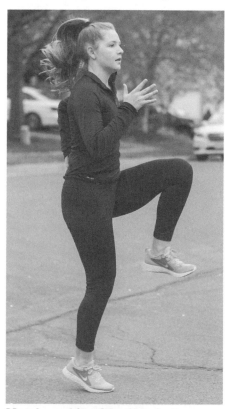

March or skip with other leg

Backward March or Skip

Just like how student-athletes need to learn how to stop moving a weight, they need to learn how to stop running forward. To accomplish this, student-athletes need to learn how to march and skip backward. Doing this well will not only make deceleration safer and more effective, but it will also translate to improved change-of-direction speed and agility.

Type of Drill

Deceleration

Beginning Position

Start with the hands at the side and the feet together.

Movement Phases

1. The backward march is simple; perform the "A" march while moving backward.
2. The same is true for the backward skip; perform the "A" skip while moving backward.

Coaching Tip

The form moving backward should be the same as if the student-athlete were moving forward.

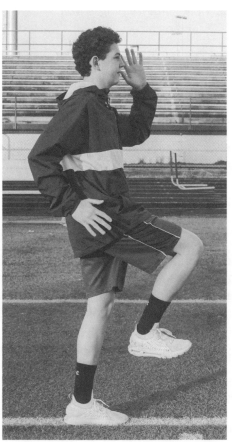

Backward march or skip body position

Ankling and High Knee

This is an acceleration drill to engage correct lines for linear speed and increased stride frequency. Ankling is referred to as *fast feet* or *quick feet* (12).

Type of Drill

Running form and acceleration

Beginning Position

Stand tall in a neutral position with feet together and hands at the side.

Movement Phases for Ankling

1. Lift one leg into knee flexion; the foot of that leg only reaches mid-shin height.

2. The opposite leg should be flexed slightly and toward the ball of the foot.

3. Alternate legs as quickly as possible while maintaining a tall posture.

4. The lifted leg should not go higher than mid-shin, and then it drives down violently.

5. The other leg in contact with the floor should be underneath the hips while maintaining a tall stance or posture.

Movement Phases for High Knee

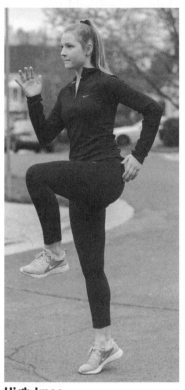

High knee

1. Lift one leg into knee flexion; the foot of that leg reaches a height above the opposite knee.

2. The opposite leg should be flexed slightly and toward the ball of the foot.

3. Alternate legs as quickly as possible while maintaining a tall posture.

4. The lifted leg rises above the opposite knee, and then it drives down forcefully.

5. The other leg in contact with the floor should be underneath the hips while maintaining a tall stance or posture.

Coaching Tips

The drills can be blended and a stride out or an "A" run can be performed for a total distance of 20 to 30 yards (18.3-27.4 m). For example, the student-athlete could do 5 yards (4.6 m) of ankling, then 5 yards (4.6 m) of jogging. That can be repeated for the desired technique and skill mastery. Then the student-athlete could do the high knee speed drill for 5 yards (4.6 m) and repeat for the desired technique and skill mastery. Then the student-athlete could perform ankling for 5 yards (4.6 m), then blend into a high knee for 5 yards (4.6 m), which can be repeated as well. Finally, the student-athlete could perform ankling for 5 yards (4.6 m), blending to high knee for 5 yards (4.6 m), and then run for 10 or 15 yards (9.1-13.7 m) and repeat for the desired technique and mastery of skill and training progression of the drill. This can be done every day. The "A" run is a burst of approximately 75 percent of maximum speed. It would be similar to a flying run or flying start. In the program template it may be noted as "flying 40s'" or "flying 10s." This means that any full exertion or maximum velocity occurs after a buildup. The student-athlete will increase speed, and when they reach the mark (or 20-yard [18 m] distance), he or she is at maximum velocity.

Gears

Gears drills can be used as a specific drill, or a collection of variations of the gears drill could be a full training segment that lasts up to 20 minutes, depending on the student-athlete's training status. The word *gears* is a term to compare the speed progression of a student-athlete to that of a car. Today some cars have up to eight gears. For the purposes of the gears speed drill, the focus will be on only four gears, with gear 4 being maximum velocity or top speed. Think of each gear as a percentage, so the first gear is 25 percent of maximum velocity, the second gear is 50 percent, the third gear is 75 percent, and the fourth gear is top speed or maximum velocity.

The running form should look the same in each gear. The student-athlete is just in contact with the ground longer and the strides are shorter. The real difference is the amount of time the feet are in contact with the ground and the length of the stride. In fourth gear, the student-athlete should exhibit proper running technique with minimal ground-contact time and as full or complete stride length as possible.

Some of the fastest runners in the world have a stride length of about 5 yards (4.6 m). In first gear, a student-athlete might only have a stride length of 1 yard (~1 m). In second gear, a student-athlete might have a stride length of up to 2 yards (1.8 m), but they would not be jogging. In third gear, also known as a *strider*, the stride length would be almost as full as it can be, but the contact time with the ground would be a bit longer than that of a student-athlete at top speed. The change in speed is easily recognizable from one gear to another. If it is not recognizable, the drill is not being done properly, and the student-athlete should repeat it after adequate rest.

Gears Drill

Type of Drill
Maximum velocity, acceleration, and deceleration on a linear plane

Beginning Position
- Begin in a crouched or three-point stance and look at the ground.
- On the strength and conditioning professional's cue, rise up slightly while still in the crouched sprinter position.
- The lead knee should be slightly over the toe.
- Elbows should be flexed to about 90 degrees, with the opposite arm back of the lead leg and foot.

Movement Phases
1. Push down with the lead or forward leg and lift the back leg to move forward.
2. Aggressively move the lead arm back.
3. Reach a good stride pace for 20 yards (18.3 m) or the desired distance.
4. Accelerate to reach maximum velocity at the cone or mark. The cone or mark should be visible to the student-athlete at intervals of 20 yards (18.3 m).
5. Stay at maximum velocity for the desired distance.
6. Stay in good form (upright sprint position) past the cone or mark.
7. Decelerate for the desired distance.

> *continued*

> *continued*

8. Accelerate again depending on the cued gear.

9. Finish all the way through the last cone.

Coaching Tips

This drill can be done after dynamic warm-ups and speed progressions such as marches, skips, ankling, and high knees. The distances or acceleration can be changed to simulate the demands of various sports.

For example, football players have different needs for different positions. An offensive lineman would only need 5 or 10 yards (4.6 or 9.1 m) between each cone to change speed or gears. A wide receiver or defensive back would run the entire 20 yards (18.3 m) between each cone and run a full 80 to 100 yards (73.2-91.4 m), whereas the lineman would only run a total of 40 or 50 yards (36.6 or 45.7 m) with speed changes. The strength and conditioning professional can alternate between different speed gears as well as the distances that the various speeds are run.

For example, if a strength and conditioning professional plans to have the student-athletes run six gears, eight student-athletes could run on a track, one in each lane. Groupings can be based on student-athletes' speed, positions, or grade level.

The strength and conditioning professional can tell the student-athletes what gears will be run between each cone. For example, if the professional calls out gears 1, 2, 3, and 4, the student-athletes know that this repetition is a buildup or progression to maximum velocity. After each group has completed that repetition, the coach could change the next repetition to be, for example, gears 2, 4, 1, and 3. In this case student-athletes start at half speed, work to full speed, decelerate to 25 percent without losing form, and then finish with a 75 percent stride. For the next four repetitions of the drill, the strength and conditioning professional can vary the numbers in different patterns depending on what the focus is for that day.

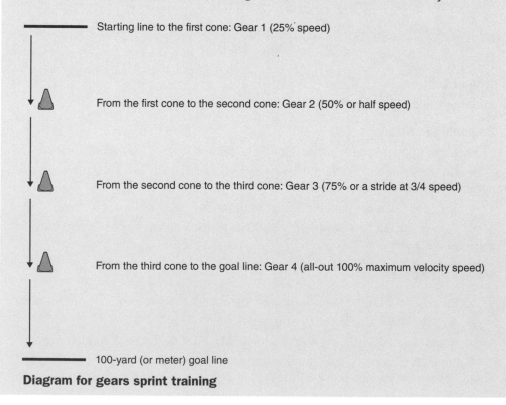

Starting line to the first cone: Gear 1 (25% speed)

From the first cone to the second cone: Gear 2 (50% or half speed)

From the second cone to the third cone: Gear 3 (75% or a stride at 3/4 speed)

From the third cone to the goal line: Gear 4 (all-out 100% maximum velocity speed)

100-yard (or meter) goal line

Diagram for gears sprint training

Agility Mechanics

Linear speed training helps a student-athlete run faster straight ahead; however, many sports require changing directions during the course of a play. In agility training the student-athlete is taught how to come to a near-sudden stop, change direction laterally, and rapidly reaccelerate to full speed in a different direction.

True agility is reactive. If two linebackers of the same size and talent are dropping back in pass coverage and the opposing quarterback tucks and runs, the linebacker fastest to react and change direction is the more agile linebacker. Reactive agility drills are called open agility drills. Too often, equipment or apparatus, most notably a floor ladder, are incorporated into a running-based drill and the drill is labeled as "agility drill" when, in actuality, it is not. That type of drill develops coordination and foot speed, both important traits, and has some value in developing agility, but a game on an open field has no preset landmarks or patterns, so that drill offers little game-based value. Those nonreactive agility drills are called closed agility drills because the student-athletes must perform a predetermined pattern with fixed landmarks.

To improve true reactive agility, student-athletes must be put in a simulated game environment where they need to read and react to a situation, lower the center of gravity, and quickly change direction.

Agility Drills

A wide variety of agility drills exist to improve acceleration with a change of direction. The following five drills can be modified for sport specificity.

Exercise Finder

Breakdown

Changing direction requires rapid deceleration and rapid acceleration. The backward skip progression is taught to improve deceleration (see the backward march or skip drill on page 305). Part of developing change of direction speed and agility is breaking down a forward sprint properly. Therefore, this drill does not have a beginning position like other drills; rather, the breakdown drill occurs at the end of a forward sprint.

Type of Drill

Change of direction

Movement Phases

1. Sprint forward and then rapidly pump the arms, chop the feet, and break down in an athletic position with the

- hips low and the hips, knees, and ankles flexed;
- knees over the feet;
- torso leaning forward;
- chest visible; and
- hands in a ready position.

2. The buffer from sprint to breakdown should be between 3 and 5 yards (2.7-4.6 m).

3. By the end of the breakdown, the body should be in an athletic stance.

Coaching Tips

In an actual game, the student-athlete obviously will not stop and freeze in an athletic position, but it is taught as a foundation of changing direction on the field of play. In a proper breakdown the student-athlete will rapidly decelerate moving in one direction and rapidly accelerate in a lateral direction.

Progressions

The first step in the progression is to have the student-athlete break down in an athletic position, chop the feet in place, and be ready for the next command to read and react. After that, the student-athlete will not show the athletic position at all because the student-athlete will put it all together and smoothly and rapidly move in a lateral direction after sprinting forward.

When changing direction in any angle, the student-athlete must show a low hip position with rapidly moving arms and feet in short strides. Breaking down in an athletic position will effectively teach the student-athlete how to come to a full stop after a forward sprint and immediately move left, right, or back.

After teaching the student-athlete how to decelerate and finish in an athletic position, the student-athlete needs to learn how to break down in a lateral lunge position. This will help the student-athlete reverse direction by 180 degrees while performing a forward sprint. The student-athlete should shorten the stride, pump the arms, chop the feet, and finish in a lateral lunge position with the back leg extended and touching the line. Toes should point forward in relationship to the body so that the hips can open in the opposite direction. Have the student-athletes perform this drill and stop in the lateral lunge position to determine proper foot placement. The back foot should be perpendicular to the direction the student-athlete wants to go, and the hip should be opened toward that direction.

Progress toward an actual sprint in the opposite direction upon command. In this case, the student-athlete will immediately sprint in the opposite direction on the line. If the student-athlete is not rounding out the turn and is changing directions in 180 degrees, the drill is being performed correctly.

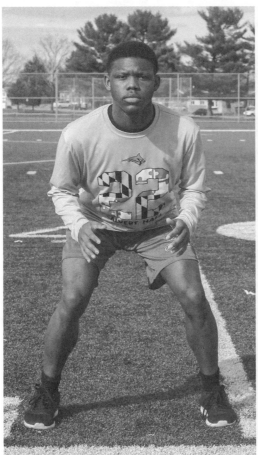

Athletic (body) position

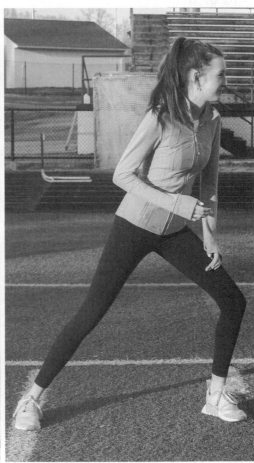

Change of direction body position

Lateral Walk, Lunge, and Skip

As presented by Marisa Viola at the NSCA Maryland State Clinic, a student-athlete needs to learn how to move laterally on the frontal plane to effectively change direction (16). This is accomplished with the progress of a lateral walk, lunge, and skip (16).

Type of Drill

Lateral agility

Movement Phases: Lateral Walk

1. Walk laterally; the front foot will reach out and step, and the back foot will come back to balance. The feet never cross over. The toes should always point forward and never to the side.

2. Do the lateral walk drill for 10 yards (9.1 m) in one direction, and then switch directions.

Movement Phases: Lateral Lunge

1. Following the same guidelines as the lateral walk, lunge while performing opposite arm and opposite leg movements. Finish with the hips low, the back leg extended, the front knee flexed and on top of the foot, and both sets of toes pointing forward.

2. Do the lateral lunge drill for 10 yards (9.1 m) in one direction, and then switch directions.

Movement Phases: Lateral Skip

1. Skip in place using proper arm movement.

2. Once comfortable with the rhythm, bounce off the back foot, land with front foot, bring the back foot back to balance, and immediately bounce again off the back foot.

3. Do the lateral skip drill for 10 yards (9.1 m) in one direction, and then switch directions.

Coaching Tips

An important coaching cue is to lead with the heel. The body will go where the hips tell the body to go. If the student-athlete points the toes toward the direction of the movement to pull the body through, the hip is in an open position and the foot is misaligned for a change of direction in 360 degrees. Lead with the heel by exaggerating the movement. Have the student-athlete pop the heel out before stepping. In an actual game, the student-athlete will not do this, but if properly trained, the student-athlete will exhibit proper technique on the field naturally.

Specific to the lateral skip drill, the knees need to be high on the skips, and the toes must point forward so the hips will not open in one direction. The arms and legs must move opposite from one another. The back foot never crosses over the front foot but returns to the same position under the same shoulder and bounces off the ground upon landing to continue the lateral skip.

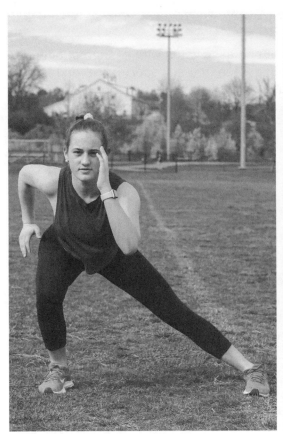

Start of lateral lunge or step

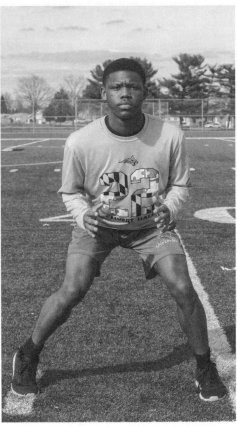

Popping out the heel before stepping

Pro Agility Drill

The pro agility drill is the most common drill associated with change of direction and is frequently used to test student-athletes in many sports. The drill is also referred to as the pro agility, short shuttle, pro shuttle, or a variation of the 5-10-5 drill. If the drill is tested, student-athletes should complete it in under 5 seconds.

The strength and conditioning professional will need cones or marked lines on a field, track, or flat surface that are 5 yards (4.6 m) apart and cover a total of 10 yards (9.1 m).

Type of Drill

Change of direction

Beginning Position

• Stand in front of cone 1 at the midpoint of the diagram with the feet straddling the midpoint line or the middle of the cone. (A student-athlete can start at the edge of cone 1 for practice or variations of the drill, but for the actual test and timing of the drill the student-athlete will start in the middle.)

• Get into a three-point stance or, if the drill is not timed, get into an athletic position.

Movement Phases

1. Start the drill with the left foot taking a step in the intended direction. This should be an open step, not a crossover step.

2. Sprint toward cone 2.

3. Touch the base of cone 2 with the left hand or foot.

4. Change direction, and sprint past cone 1 toward cone 3.

5. Touch the base of cone 3 with the right hand or foot.

6. Change direction, and sprint back to (and past) cone 1.

Coaching Tips

The student-athlete's movement to start the drill will be either to the left or to the right. The description describes movement to the left first, but the direction depends on the strength and conditioning professional's focus. The student-athlete should attempt to keep the shoulders facing square toward the direction of movement, plant the outside foot, and reach toward cones 2 and 3 with the outside hand. The student-athlete should not turn the entire body around to attempt to make a turn and change direction.

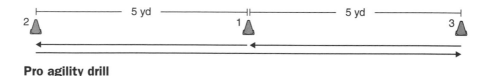

Pro agility drill

"L" Drill

Another common drill associated with change of direction is the "L" drill. It is beneficial for almost all sport athletes. The "L" drill is also referred to as the three-cone drill or a variation of the 5-10-5 drill since it deals with changing direction in those distances. The "L" drill is often used to train or test explosiveness out of a break or change of direction for football and soccer players but can easily be incorporated into testing or training sessions for many sports. The "L" drill is different from the pro agility drill because the "L" drill also measures angular acceleration. It therefore tests two components.

The strength and conditioning professional will need cones or marked lines on a field, track, or flat surface that are 5 yards (4.6 m) apart and cover a total of 10 yards (9.1 m).

"L" drill

Type of Drill

Rounding the corner

Beginning Position

• Stand in front of cone 1 facing cone 2 and get into a crouched sprinter stance or a sprinter stance. (A student-athlete can start at the edge or the outside of cone 1 if desired.)

• Get into an athletic position with the weight over the balls of the feet.

Movement Phases

1. Sprint toward cone 2, back to cone 1, back to cone 2, make a 90-degree cut to the right, and sprint to cone 3 (see letters *a* through *d* in the diagram).

2. Make a 180-degree turn around the inside and underneath of cone 3, and sprint back to cone 2 (see letters *d* through *f* in the diagram).

3. Make a 90-degree cut to the left around cone 2, and sprint back to (and past) cone 1 (see the end of the arrow for letter *f* through letter *g* and past cone 1 in the diagram).

Coaching Tips

The drill can be set up to be performed so that the first 90-degree cut goes to the left and the last 90-degree cut goes to the right. In either case, student-athletes should stay low and hug the cones as they navigate their way around the various patterns. Also, student-athletes should face cone 3 as they approach it, because cuts will be made off both feet. It is important to use the arms to accelerate out of the cuts around the cones.

Variations

This drill has many variations other than the basic "L" drill pattern, such as the backpedal "L" drill in which the student-athlete begins the first segment using a backpedal movement rather than running forward. The strength and conditioning professional can also vary the drill by having the student-athlete backpedal after reaching cone 3 rather than looping around it. Then, when the student-athlete returns to cone 2, they have to open the hips, meaning that at the point where the student-athlete reaches the cone, they will open the leg closest to the cone and point that foot in the new direction in which they are going to move. This movement pattern applies to student-athletes in many respective sports, but it is especially good for defensive backs in football.

Read and React

True agility is reactive. If two student-athletes are the same size and have the same talent, the one fastest to react and change direction is the more agile student-athlete. In a soccer game, a defender who can perfectly mirror an opposing forward dribbling the ball will prevent the forward from advancing efficiently. In a basketball game, perfectly mirroring an opponent's move can prevent the opponent from making a pass or driving down the lane for an easy score.

Once a strength and conditioning professional has properly trained student-athletes on the fundamentals of change-of-direction speed, it is now time to take the student-athletes to the field and simulate game situations. Many drills use reading and reacting to changes on the field; for example, a drill can involve a left and right shuffle or a 45-degree run up field with eye contact with the strength and conditioning professional. An up or down hand motion can indicate backpedaling and forward sprinting with a start command familiar and appropriate to the sport, and the student-athletes will begin in a backpedal. The strength and conditioning professional can point left, right, up, or down, and the student-athlete is required to plant a foot in the ground and change direction. A stop signal can communicate to the student-athlete to break down as quickly as possible to stop momentum and then chop the feet in place in an athletic stance while waiting for the next command.

Type of Drill

Change of direction

Beginning Position

- Line up one to four student-athletes on the field.
- Inform the student-athletes of the hand motions that will be used and what type of movement will be required.

Movement Phases

1. Read and react patterns can include the following:
   - Backpedal, then sprint forward
   - Backpedal, then sprint at a 45-degree angle down the field
   - Backpedal, sprint at a 45-degree angle up the field, then sprint forward
   - Backpedal, shuffle, then sprint forward
   - Backpedal, side sprint to the left and to the right, then sprint forward
   - Sprint forward, sprint at a 45-degree angle up the field, then sprint forward
   - Sprint forward, then side sprint to the left and right
   - Sprint left, sprint right, then sprint forward

Coaching Tips

The most important coaching point is to emphasize to the student-athletes that they should not anticipate the cue for a direction change; instead, they should move at full speed and use proper breakdown and change of direction technique. Also, the length of each drill should replicate the time of an actual play or sequence on the field. Anything longer can help with anomalies during an actual game and with conditioning, but student-athletes should not be so fatigued as to compromise their form in their lateral movement, backpedal, running, and breakdown. Perfect technique for each repetition is needed for best results.

Sample Programs

Many sport programs will allow a strength and conditioning professional to develop speed and agility for student-athletes regardless of their training level. See table 10.1 for a four-week sample speed and acceleration program and table 10.2 for an example of an agility training session.

Conclusion

This is a general overview of the speed and agility drills a high school sport coach or strength and conditioning professional can immediately implement in a program and build a foundation of knowledge for student-athletes. While many more drills exist, it is far better for student-athletes to master 10 drills and perform them repeatedly than it is to implement 100 drills. Have student-athletes master these drills to the point where they can teach others. At that point, adding and modifying drills based on the program's needs is appropriate.

TABLE 10.1   Four-Week Sample Speed and Acceleration Program (Two Sessions Per Week)

Block and focus	Drills	Frequency, volume, and rest period
"A" block: acceleration development and form	1. "A" march 2. "A" skip 3. Ankling 4. High knee 5. "A" run 6. Sprint	**Maximum velocity series:** Ankling: 5 yd (4.6 m) × 4 High knee: 5 yd (4.6 m) × 4 Ankling and high knee blend: 10 yd (9.1 m) × 4 Ankling and high knee "A" run: 20 yd (18.3 m) × 4 **Acceleration:** 10 yd (9.1 m) × 4 (1.5 min rest) 20 yd (18.3 m) × 4 (2 min rest)
"B" block: acceleration to maximum speed	1. "A" march 2. "A" skip 3. Ankling 4. High knee 5. "A" run 6. Kneeling start[a] 7. Flying 10s[b]	**Maximum velocity series:** Ankling: 5 yd (4.6 m) × 4 High knee: 5 yd (4.6 m) × 4 Ankling and high knee blend: 10 yd (9.1 m) × 4 Ankling and high knee "A" run: 20 yd (18.3 m) × 4 **Kneeling start:** 10 yd (9.1 m) × 4 with right knee down (1.5 min rest) 10 yd (9.1 m) × 4 with left knee down (1.5 min rest) **Acceleration:** Flying 10s: × 4 (2 min rest)
"C" block: maximum velocity	1. "A" march 2. "A" skip 3. Ankling 4. High knee 5. "A" run 6. Push-up start[c] 7. Flying 40s[b]	**Maximum velocity series:** Ankling: 5 yd (4.6 m) × 4 High knee: 5 yd (4.6 m) × 4 Ankling and high knee blend: 10 yd (9.1 m) × 4 Ankling and high knee "A" run: 20 yd (18.3 m) × 4 **Push-up start:** 10 yd (9.1 m) × 4 (2 min rest) **Acceleration:** Flying 40s: × 4 (3.5 min rest)

> *continued*

TABLE 10.1   > *continued*

Block and focus	Drills	Frequency, volume, and rest period
"D" block: maximum velocity and speed endurance	1. "A" march 2. "A" skip 3. Ankling 4. High knee 5. "A" run 6. Kneeling start[a] 7. Push-up start[c] 8. Flying 40s (block start) 9. Gears[d]	**Maximum velocity series:** Ankling: 5 yd (4.6 m) × 4 High knee: 5 yd (4.6 m) × 4 Ankling and high knee blend: 10 yd (9.1 m) × 4 Ankling and high knee "A" run: 20 yd (18.3 m) × 4 **Kneeling starts:** 10 yd (9.1 m) × 2 with right knee down (1.5 min rest) 10 yd (9.1 m) × 2 with left knee down (1.5 min rest) **Push-up start:** 10 yd (9.1 m) × 2 (2 min rest) **Sprints (with block start):** 40 yd (36.6 m) × 2 (3.5 min rest) **Gears:** 80-100 total yd (73.2-91.4 m) × 4 (4 min rest)

Before each session, perform a dynamic warm-up with marches and skips. Where a rest interval is not provided, the rest interval can simply be walking back to the starting line.

[a]Kneeling start: The lead knee should be over the lead toe and should be flexed to approximately 50 degrees; the knee of the back leg should not touch the ground (i.e., the overall body position is like a crouched split stance with a neutral spine).

[b]Flying 10s (or 40s): Build up speed for 10 (or 40) yards or meters behind the starting line to reach maximum speed at the starting line and continue sprinting at maximum speed for 10 (or 40) yards or meters.

[c]Push-up start: Get into a push-up position facing the starting line but with the body slightly raised off the ground, not relaxed. To start, push the body up and forward, and get the foot under the drive leg to accelerate forward.

[d]See the coaching tips section of the gears drill on page 307 for more guidelines.

TABLE 10.2   Example of an Agility Training Session

Drill	Reps	Work-to-rest ratio
Breakdown (sprint 10 yd [9.1 m], then breakdown in 3-5 [2.7-4.6 m] yd)	4	1:12
Lateral walk (10 yd [9.1 m])	2 (1 each direction)	1:1
Lateral lunge (10 yd [9.1 m])	2 (1 each direction)	1:1
Lateral skip (10 yd [9.1 m])	2 (1 each direction)	1:12
Pro agility drill	4	1:12
"L" drill	4	1:12
READ AND REACT (5-15 YD [4.6-13.7 M] PER DIRECTION)		
Backpedal, then sprint forward	2	1:12
Backpedal, then sprint at a 45-degree angle down the field	2	1:12
Backpedal, sprint at a 45-degree angle up the field, then sprint forward	2	1:12
Backpedal, shuffle, then sprint forward	2	1:12
Backpedal, side sprint to the left and to the right, then sprint forward	2	1:12
Sprint forward, sprint at a 45-degree angle up the field, then sprint forward	2	1:12
Sprint forward, then side sprint to the left and right	2	1:12
Sprint left, sprint right, then sprint forward	2	1:12

11

Individual and Group Activities

Daniel Flahie, MSEd, CSCS,*D

Aerobic endurance training is an important component of a well-rounded exercise program for the high school student-athlete. Aerobic endurance training has been shown not only to decrease the risk of coronary artery disease (2, 6), hypertension (10, 28), and heart disease (10), but also has the potential to improve memory (26, 40) and decrease symptoms of depression (39). Less than 7 percent of high school student-athletes will continue on to compete in an NCAA collegiate sport, with even less becoming a professional athlete (34). With this in mind, the strength and conditioning professional should not only work to develop skills that directly contribute to increased performance on the court, field, or ice, but work to develop skills and attributes for a healthy life after high school sports. Upwards of 20 percent of middle and high school student-athletes have been shown to be either overweight or obese, with nearly 15 percent of these student-athletes having stage 1 or stage 2 hypertensive blood pressure readings (27, 45). Along with data that suggest despite playing sports, retired athletes have similar cardiovascular disease risk profiles with that of the general population (33), this is cause for concern. Heart disease, which is still considered the leading cause of death in the United States (21), is a disease that can be influenced positively by cardiovascular health and aerobic endurance exercise (10). With these considerations, this chapter focuses on the program design considerations and exercise selection of aerobic endurance training for the high school student-athlete.

Program Design Guidelines for Aerobic Endurance Training

Program design is one of the most important aspects of creating an efficient and effective aerobic endurance training program. Fortunately, aerobic endurance program design and prescription is very similar to that of other training modalities discussed in chapters 8 through 10. Regardless of the modality of training, the principle of training specificity holds true. This is the concept that physiological

319

adaptation is specific to a given activity, which includes fiber type recruitment, energy system involvement, and muscular involvement (30, 37). When considering aerobic endurance training, some significant physiological adaptations differentiate this modality of training from other methods such as strength, speed, or power training. For example, in terms of aerobic endurance training (also known as *cardiovascular training*), increases in type I muscle fiber size, blood capillary size and density, myoglobin content, and mitochondria volume and efficiency are the primary physiological adaptations (11, 24, 30).

Fiber Types

Human skeletal muscle contains three primary fiber types: type I, type IIx, and type IIa (37). **Type I** fibers are slow-twitch fibers and have a high resistance to fatigue and a high capacity for aerobic energy production; however, they are not responsible for high-intensity, powerful movements (37). Essentially, type I fibers are the endurance fibers and are predominant in events such as distance swimming or any other sustained, low-intensity activities. **Type IIx** fibers are called explosive or fast-twitch fibers. These muscle fibers are almost complete opposites of the type I fibers in that they have high capacities for explosive and powerful movements. They are quickly fatigued (37), which is a major reason near-maximal or maximal levels of intensity cannot be sustained for long periods of time. **Type IIa** fibers are considered intermediate fibers and have blended characteristics of the other two fiber types (37). It is important to note that this is a rudimentary explanation of fiber types; each of the three types have wide-ranging properties that can be influenced or that can influence training.

The concept of fiber types is particularly important to consider when training high school student-athletes, because training and conditioning methods should be designed to meet the demands of an intended sport. For example, if a student-athlete is primarily involved in power sports such as football or basketball, the bulk of their conditioning should involve repeated shorter, explosive bouts of sprinting instead of sustained, longer-duration running. Conversely, if the student-athlete is primarily a cross-country runner, the bulk of their training should consist of a more sustained aerobic endurance approach. This consideration becomes even more difficult when working with student-athletes who are involved in several sports that have differing levels of physical demand.

Energy Systems

Another important consideration that goes hand in hand with fiber types is that of energy system development and use. Three basic energy systems are used while at rest and during exercise: the **ATP** (adenosine triphosphate)-**PC** (phosphocreatine) system, the **glycolytic** system (also known as *glycolysis*), and the **oxidative** (also known as aerobic) energy system (24, 37). The ATP-PC system is an anaerobic energy–producing system, which means oxygen is not required to produce energy. Glycolysis can also create energy without the presence of oxygen, and it is through this system that lactate is formed (24). Lactate has often been attributed to the occurrence of delayed-onset muscle soreness; however, this notion is untrue (37). Although lactate levels in the muscle and blood do accumulate during high-intensity exercise, the levels return to baseline fairly quickly (9). Lastly, the oxidative energy system does require the presence of oxygen to create energy, which takes place within the mitochondria of the cell (24). The energy systems are often misinterpreted as having clearly defined starting and stopping points, which is not accurate. All energy systems are present and working in some capacity at all times, but their contribution to energy production is dictated by the level of intensity of a given exercise. In up to 10 seconds, the ATP-PC contributes the most to energy production, and from 10 seconds to 1 minute glycolysis contributes the majority. Between 1 and 3 minutes, a large combination of glycolysis and the oxidative system contributes to energy production, and anything over 3 minutes in duration is primarily fueled by the oxidative energy system. Two important considerations must be remembered when dealing with the energy systems. First, these duration ranges only apply when student athletes are at their relative maximum intensity for a given duration. For example, sitting and scrolling through the internet for 10 seconds does not primarily use the ATP-PC system, but instead uses the aerobic energy system because the relative intensity is low. Second, there are not clearly defined starting and stopping points as to when each energy system contributes to overall ATP production. Instead, all three continually contribute to energy production, but the degree of the contribution is dependent on the relative intensity of a given activity. Instead of visualizing the energy systems as on-off switches, think of them as a sliding scale (24).

As previously mentioned, a well-designed aerobic endurance training program must be specific and tailored to meet the desired goals of the team or individual student-athlete. For example, if a student-athlete's primary sport is cross-country, the training program should consist primarily of running versus swimming or cycling. However, it is still beneficial to perform activities not directly related to the primary given sport. This concept is known as **cross-training**, and while the training effects have minimal transfer, it can potentially reduce the likelihood of overtraining, overuse injuries, and psychological fatigue (47). Programs also need to occur at a high enough intensity level to elicit the desired change or adaptation. However, this does not mean that student-athletes need to be worked or trained as hard as possible all the time. In fact, rest and recovery are essential components to a well-designed training program. Soreness, fatigue, and exhaustion do happen but should never be sought after as a marker of an effective training session. Student-athletes do not have to be sore and tired after every training session to elicit adaptation.

Apart from ensuring aerobic training is specific and at high enough intensity levels to elicit positive responses, the strength and conditioning professional must be aware of several important factors when designing programs. The first of these factors is **maximal aerobic capacity**, also known as $\dot{V}O_2max$. $\dot{V}O_2max$ is simply the maximal capacity the body has to take in, transport, and use oxygen during maximal exertion and is one of the best indicators of cardiorespiratory endurance capacity (24). Another important consideration is exercise economy, or how much energy is spent at a given intensity level (34). Student-athletes who possess a high level of exercise economy will use less energy and therefore will be more efficient and able to sustain higher levels of intensity, which again points to the importance of individualized training programs. In other words, as a student-athlete becomes more skilled at a given exercise (such as running), the energy demands are reduced for any given pace (24). This means that a student-athlete with a higher exercise economy can sustain a given pace for longer periods of time and with less energy used versus a student-athlete with a lower exercise economy.

The last factor to consider is the **lactate threshold**, which is the level at which blood lactate begins to accumulate above resting levels (24). Typically, in untrained student-athletes, the lactate threshold occurs between 50 and 60 percent of their $\dot{V}O_2$max, and between 70 and 80 percent in highly trained aerobic endurance athletes (24). The physiological mechanisms behind the lactate threshold are beyond the scope of this book, but understanding when the lactate threshold occurs in student-athletes can be an important program design consideration in the high school setting. After the strength and conditioning professional is familiar with the basics of theses physiological concepts, they can begin to formulate a periodization training program for their student-athletes. When designing an aerobic endurance training program, the strength and conditioning professional will follow a five-step process that includes selecting the mode, intensity, frequency, duration, and progression of exercises to ensure safe, effective, and training status–appropriate training programs.

Age and Training Status Considerations

Prior to creating an effective aerobic endurance training program, the strength and conditioning professional must consider the age and training status of the student-athletes they are working with. A benefit of working in the high school setting is that the **chronological age** (i.e., the number of years of being alive) of the student-athletes will, for the most part, be known and consistent. However, what will likely be different within the group of student-athletes are their biological and training ages. Biological age refers to several variables including skeletal age and physical, cognitive, and sexual maturity (22, 29).

Considering student-athletes from a **biological age** perspective rather than a chronological age perspective allows the strength and conditioning professional to better assign groups and individualize programs based on training status rather than age. For example, two athletes may both be 15 years old, but one could be more physically mature and thus would require a different training program. If both student-athletes were given identical programs, it may be too difficult for one and too easy for the other. Both scenarios are disadvantageous to the student-athletes and could potentially cause injury for the less trained and experienced student-athlete and stagnation for the more trained and experienced student-athlete.

Another important training consideration is the concept of **training age**, which is simply the amount of time a student-athlete has followed a structured and supervised training program. Being cognizant of training age status among student-athletes is essential to develop individualized programming that is both safe and effective for every student-athlete. Training ages can vary as drastically as biological ages in a given population; therefore, chronological age is not always the best method of grouping student-athletes for exercise.

Mode

The first step in designing an aerobic endurance training program is to determine the **mode**, or type of exercise to be performed. Many exercise modes, such as running, cycling, swimming, or circuit-type training where student-athletes cycle through a variety of exercises, can be used when designing a program. The implementation of stationary training equipment, such as ellipticals, treadmills, stair climbers, stationary bikes, and rowing machines, can also be a viable option. It is important to recall the concept of specificity when determining the exercise modality. For example, selecting running-based exercises would be advantageous to student-athletes whose primary sport is cross-country. However, for student-athletes who are involved in multiple sports, implementing various exercise modes can be beneficial. By following this cross-training principle, student-athletes are also less likely to experience overuse injuries, and it can be used during rehabilitation from an injury (47). Many high school students do not compete in athletics, in which case exposing them to a wide variety of exercise modalities may be beneficial to their overall health and fitness (47).

Intensity

The **intensity** level of a given exercise must be considered when programming for aerobic endurance exercise. Physiological adaptations will only take place when appropriate levels of intensity are performed by the student-athlete. If intensity levels are too low, little to no change may occur (24, 43); however, intensity levels must be appropriately combined with exercise duration. As the level of intensity of a given exercise increases, the duration of the exercise will decrease. Several methods can be used to both track and assign intensity levels of aerobic endurance exercise. These include rating of perceived exertion (RPE) scales and target heart rate ranges that are calculated using a percentage of the student-athlete's maximum heart rate (MHR) or an equation called the Karvonen formula.

Rating of Perceived Exertion Scales

Rating of perceived exertion (RPE) scales have been heavily researched in the field of sport science and have proven to be a valid and reliable marker of intensity levels during exercise, especially when combined with other intensity testing measures (7, 15). RPE scales are used by the student-athlete to subjectively determine how difficult a given exercise intensity is by providing the strength and conditioning professional with a number that is linked to a description of the level of difficulty. Examples of scales include the Borg 6-20 category scale (4), Borg category-ratio-10 scale (15), and the scale seen in table 11.1.

RPE scales can be used by both the student-athlete and the strength and conditioning professional to individualize the intensity level of exercises for each student-athlete, and such scales allow the student-athlete to self-pace the exercise

TABLE 11.1

Rating	Description
1	Nothing at all (lying down)
2	Extremely little
3	Very easy
4	Easy (could do this all day)
5	Moderate
6	Somewhat hard (starting to feel it)
7	Hard
8	Very hard (making an effort to keep up)
9	Very, very hard
10	Maximum effort (cannot go any further)

Reprinted by permission from Hagerman (2012).

based on training status. It is a simple and effective way to quickly judge the intensity level of a given exercise and provides the strength and conditioning professional instant feedback to determine if intensity levels should be increased or decreased.

Heart Rate Calculations

RPE scales work well when determining intensity levels midexercise; however, if a particular intensity level is desired, heart rate calculations can be used prior to exercise to determine a targeted range. The two primary methods used when determining exercise intensity percentages using heart rates are the **maximum heart rate** (MHR) and **Karvonen** methods (table 11.2). Both methods provide the strength and conditioning professional with a fairly accurate intensity assignment tool; however, it should be noted that estimated heart rate maximums based on age alone can have an error of up to 10 beats per minute or more (1). As access to heart rate monitors and wearable technology have increased, target heart rate

TABLE 11.2   Heart Rate Calculations

MHR method	Karvonen method
FORMULAS (THESE CALCULATIONS WILL BE PERFORMED TWICE TO DETERMINE THE TARGET HEART RATE RANGE [THRR] DESIRED FOR THE GIVEN ACTIVITY.)	
1. Age-predicted maximal heart rate (APMHR): 220 – age 2. Target heart rate (THR): APMHR × desired exercise intensity	1. Age-predicted maximal heart rate (APMHR): 220 – age 2. Heart rate reserve (HRR): APMHR – resting heart rate (RHR) 3. Target heart rate (THR): (HRR × exercise intensity) + RHR
Example: An 18-year-old student-athlete is assigned an exercise intensity range of 65%-75% of their predicted MHR.	Example: An 18-year-old student-athlete is assigned an exercise intensity of 60%-70% of their functional capacity.
1. APMHR: 220 – 18 = 202 beats/minute 2. Low-end THRR: 202 × 0.65 = 131 beats/minute 3. High-end THRR: 202 × 0.75 = 152 beats/minute	1. APMHR: 220 – 18 = 202 beats/minute 2. RHR = 60 beats/minute 3. HRR: 202 – 60 = 142 beats/minute 4. Low-end THRR: (142 × 0.60) + 60 = 145 beats/minute 5. High-end THRR: (142 × 0.70) + 60 = 159 beats/minute
Based on this formula, this student-athlete should train at an intensity level between 131 and 152 beats/minute.	Based on this formula, this student-athlete should train at an intensity level between 145 and 159 beats/minute.
TO EASILY MONITOR HEART RATE DURING EXERCISE, DIVIDE THESE THRR NUMBERS BY 6 TO DETERMINE HOW MANY BEATS/MINUTE SHOULD BE COUNTED WHEN CHECKING THE STUDENT-ATHLETE'S HEART RATE IN 10-SECOND INTERVALS.	
Example: 131 ÷ 6 = 22; 152 ÷ 6 = 25	Example: 145 ÷ 6 = 24; 159 ÷ 6 = 27
In this case, the strength and conditioning professional should count between 22 and 25 heartbeats during a 10-second period.	In this case, the strength and conditioning professional should count between 24 and 27 heartbeats during a 10-second period.

Adapted from Reuter and Dawes (38).

zone training has gained in popularity and can be a useful method of assigning intensities.

Several methods can be used to dictate intensity levels using heart rate reserve, but perhaps the simplest would be to use a percent of MHR as follows (1):

- Very light is below 57 percent MHR
- Light is between 57 and 63 percent MHR
- Moderate is between 64 and 76 percent MHR
- Vigorous is between 77 and 95 percent MHR
- Maximal is greater than or equal to 96 percent MHR

The most accurate way to determine intensity levels is to perform laboratory testing to find a student-athlete's true $\dot{V}O_2max$; however, this is often unavailable, which is why heart rate calculations can be an inexpensive and efficient alternative. It is important to note that MHR, $\dot{V}O_2max$, and the lactate threshold share a close relationship, which becomes important when developing training programs, especially with programs such as pace-tempo training.

Frequency

Frequency is the number of exercise or training sessions performed per day or per week. Frequency is often dictated by other factors; for example, if an exercise program contains higher-intensity or long-duration sessions, the frequency of those sessions should be lower. Also, training age needs to be considered because student-athletes with lower training ages require more recovery days between sessions, especially during the initial phases of a training program. Another consideration is whether the student-athlete is currently competing in a sport or in the off-season. Practice and competitions must be factored into the total volume of the training program, because too much training can increase the risk of illness, injury, or overtraining, especially in running (19), but too little training will provide too little stimulus for improvement. In the high school setting, this problem is even more complex because many student-athletes compete in multiple sports for the duration of the school year. A typical off-season program could have up to five training days per week, with the potential for multiple sessions per day, whereas an in-season training program may only have one to three days depending on the demands of the sport.

Duration

Exercise **duration** is the length of time it takes to complete a given exercise or training session. As stated earlier, the duration of an exercise is largely dictated by the intensity of the session. As intensity increases, duration must decrease due to physiological constraints such as lactate accumulation. Exercise performed at higher intensities, such as levels at or above 80 percent of a student-athlete's $\dot{V}O_2max$ or heart rate reserve (HRR), may last for only 30 minutes due to lactate accumulation, whereas exercise at 70 percent or lower $\dot{V}O_2max$ or HRR may be sustained for hours depending on training status (38).

Progression

Progression is key in maintaining and increasing physiological improvements related to aerobic endurance training. The concept of progressive overload states that for physiological adaptation to occur, demands must be placed on the body that are progressively higher than normal, otherwise improvements will stagnate (23). A commonly used model in the strength and conditioning community is the **general adaptation syndrome** (GAS). The GAS has three phases: alarm, resistance, and fatigue (physiological exhaustion) (43). In the first phase, the student-athlete encounters a new stimulus, such as a 30-minute run at 75 percent $\dot{V}O_2$max or HRR. Initially, the student-athlete may experience soreness or a small dip in performance, but with adequate rest the student-athlete will be better able to handle the demands of that run. This is known as the resistance phase. Ideally, a strength and conditioning professional never wants a student-athlete to reach the physiological exhaustion phase, because this is the result of overtraining and may increase the likelihood of injury or illness. It is important to note that this does not mean student-athletes cannot be tired after training. The exhaustion phase refers to continual demands above the student-athlete's ability to recover.

A useful acronym that can be employed when developing an aerobic endurance training program that encompasses all the variables listed above is the principle of **FITT-VP**, which stands for frequency, intensity, time, type, volume, and progression (5). All these variables must be considered when developing an aerobic endurance training program to help avoid injuries and overtraining, and to continually improve the performance of the student-athletes. Regardless of the type of training program or the method of training used, these variables can and should be used.

Common Types of Programs

Some commonly used training methods for developing cardiovascular improvements are long, slow distance training, pace-tempo training, high-intensity interval training, sprint-interval training, and fartlek training. These sample programs are by no means an exhaustive list, and the actual variables should be individually adjusted for each student-athlete based on training status and sport season.

Long, Slow Distance Training

Long, slow, distance training (LSD) is a commonly used method of training for aerobic endurance student-athletes such as those in cycling, marathon runners, and triathlon athletes. LSD training is characterized by being slower than race speed and lasting at least the same amount of time and often much longer than what the student-athlete would encounter in competition. It can be seen how the intensity and duration variables are manipulated here: an increase in duration means a decrease in level of intensity. If employing an RPE scale to monitor intensity, this would register between a 2 and 4 on the Borg CR-10 scale or the scale in table 11.1, and between an 8 and 12 on the Borg 6-20 scale (38). In other words, the student-athlete should be able to carry on a conversation with little difficulty (38). Long, slow, distance training is a key component for an endurance student-athlete; however, its use should be limited when working with many team sport student-athletes who rely on power and strength, because prolonged, low-intensity aerobic exercise has been shown to have negative effects on power and strength gains (14, 16). A growing body of evidence suggests that combining low-intensity training and high-intensity interval training is an effective way to develop aerobic endurance performance (31). Table 11.3 provides a sample week-long program using an LSD-style training program for a high school cross-country student-athlete.

Pace-Tempo Training

Pace-tempo training employs intensity levels that are higher than LSD training but still significantly lower than those used in high-intensity interval training or sprint-interval training. Pace-tempo training is also known as threshold training because it is performed at or near the lactate threshold (3). Traditionally, pace-tempo training is performed either continuously, known as steady pace-tempo training, or in intermittent bouts. Both steady pace-tempo training and intermittent pace-tempo training are performed at a student-athlete's lactate threshold. The differences between the two is that steady pace-tempo training is performed continuously for typically 20 to 30 minutes, whereas intermittent pace-tempo training is performed in multiple series of shorter intervals, with short recovery periods in between. As a strength and conditioning professional, it is important to follow the prescribed intensity and not allow student-athletes to train at higher intensity levels. If a student-athlete feels the intensity is too low, opt for longer distances instead of higher intensity levels. If higher intensity levels are desired, a high-intensity interval training or sprint-interval training protocol should be implemented. See table 11.4 for a sample week-long training program using the concepts of pace-tempo training.

TABLE 11.3 Sample LSD Training Program for a High School Cross-Country Runner

Sunday	Monday	Tuesday	Wednesday	Thursday	Friday	Saturday
Rest day	45-min fartlek run	**60-min LSD run below race pace at a distance longer than the race**	45-min interval run	3.2-mile run at race pace over hills and flats	**60-min LSD run below race pace at a distance longer than the race**	Rest day

Adapted from Reuter and Dawes (38).

Comments:
- *Frequency:* Because LSD-style training runs are typically longer than race distance, sessions should be spread out during the week to allow for adequate recovery time and to help reduce the likelihood of overtraining or overuse injuries.
- *Duration:* The goal of LSD-style training runs is to run for a longer distance than the competition distance.
- *Intensity:* To be able to run for a longer distance than typical competition distance, the student-athlete should run at a lower intensity (slower pace) than they would run for competition. Unlike pace-tempo training, high respiratory stress is not needed to acquire the full benefits of LSD training.

TABLE 11.4 Sample Pace-Tempo Training Program for a High School Cross-Country Runner

Sunday	Monday	Tuesday	Wednesday	Thursday	Friday	Saturday
Rest day	60-min LSD run	**30-min pace-tempo run**	45-min fartlek run	45-min easy run	**30-min pace-tempo run**	90-min LSD run

Adapted from Reuter and Dawes (38).

Comments:
- *Frequency:* Pace-tempo runs are typically more physically stressful than LSD training on the student-athlete; therefore, the two pace-tempo-style training days should be spread out during the week to allow for more recovery between sessions.
- *Duration:* Due to the higher training intensity of pace-tempo training runs, exercise duration is typically shorter than race distance to accommodate for the higher intensity.
- *Intensity:* To acquire the full benefits of this method of training, the student-athlete should run at a high intensity or training pace (minutes per mile or per kilometer); high respiratory stress is required to simulate race pace, especially since the duration is often shorter than race length.

High-Intensity Interval Training

High-intensity interval training (HIIT) has gained in popularity and has shown to have similar physiological adaptations to more traditional aerobic endurance programs such as LSD and pace training but with considerably less invested time (31, 41). There are some conflicting definitions of what constitutes HIIT training, but typically a HIIT protocol requires the student-athlete's heart rate to reach between 80 and 95 percent of MHR (31). HIIT work-to-rest-rest ratios can be programmed in a variety of ways, but a common protocol is 4 to 6 rounds of 30 seconds with 1 to 3 minutes of rest between rounds (24). However, HIIT sessions can be performed up to 4 minutes or longer (24, 38) with the caveat that with an increase in duration, intensity inevitably must be decreased.

Since 1996, **Tabata training** has been a formalized example of HIIT that consists of repeated bouts of 20 seconds of supramaximal exercise at roughly 170 percent of a student-athlete's $\dot{V}O_2$max followed by 10 seconds of rest (24, 46).

Sprint-Interval Training

Sprint-interval training (SIT; also known as *supramaximal training* or *SMIT*) is another method of short, intense interval training similar to HIIT training. A key difference between SIT and HIIT training is that SIT training is performed at levels higher than a student-athlete's $\dot{V}O_2$max for shorter durations and longer recovery periods (31, 41). As with HIIT, SIT protocols offer much variety (31, 41), but a common version consists of 4 to 12 repeated 30-second rounds at levels above $\dot{V}O_2$max with 4 minutes of rest between rounds (41).

As stated earlier in the chapter, it is likely that the strength and conditioning professional will work with many multisport student-athletes or student-athletes that only play sprint- and power-based sports. These athletes still need to develop an aerobic base but often cannot afford to lose muscle mass, strength, or power as can happen in traditional aerobic endurance programs (14, 16). A potential benefit of HIIT and SIT training is that student-athletes will still improve physiological variables related to the cardiovascular system (31) while better maintaining muscular size, strength, and power capabilities versus traditional LSD-type training methods (42). Recall the principles of specificity, fiber types, and energy system development. A student-athlete will adapt to the types of training they are exposed to, and it is the job of the strength and conditioning professional to understand and apply these concepts to better equip student-athletes for their given sport or sports. The student-athletes who play a primarily power-driven sport such as football or basketball would benefit less from LSD-type training than would lacrosse or distance swimming student-athletes. That is not to say a football player could potentially benefit from the occasional LSD-style training, but the bulk of training should not consist of this method.

Fartlek Training

Fartlek training is a combination of many of the aforementioned methods of training and can be used to break up the monotony of aerobic endurance training as well as provide the student-athlete with more autonomy in dictating a given training session. Fartlek training is a very laissez-faire style of training and allows student-athletes to run at any distance, speed, or intensity level they desire (13).

Student-athletes performing a fartlek training session simply select a desired time or distance and combine LSD and interval-type training intermittently throughout the duration of the session. A major benefit of this style of training is that it works on both the aerobic and anaerobic energy systems (13), providing the student-athlete with a well-rounded training session. This style of training can be implemented in running, cycling, or swimming or on a variety of stationary exercise machines, and has proven to be an effective training modality to increase $\dot{V}O_2$max in athletes (13). Table 11.5 provides a sample week-long training program focused on the fartlek training principle.

TABLE 11.5 Sample Fartlek Training Program for a High School Cross-Country Runner

Sunday	Monday	Tuesday	Wednesday	Thursday	Friday	Saturday
Rest or easy run	60-min LSD run	**45-min fartlek run of hard and easy work on hills and flats**	25-min pace-tempo run	45-min LSD run	25-min LSD run	Race

Adapted from Reuter and Dawes (38).

Comments:

- *Frequency:* Fartlek training can be particularly stressful on the student-athlete. Due to the typical intensity of this method of training, only one fartlek training day should occur during the week.
- *Duration:* The total distance or duration of the training portion of the interval work bouts should be at or near the competition distance as the student-athlete becomes more highly trained.
- *Intensity:* To acquire the full benefits of the fartlek training session, the student-athlete should run at an intensity (pace) close to $\dot{V}O_2$max when completing the work bout portions of the fartlek training sessions.

Aerobic Endurance Exercises

The strength and conditioning professional should employ the concept of specificity whenever possible and conduct the bulk of aerobic endurance training as close to the demands of a student-athlete's given sport. However, situations will arise when alternative methods are warranted such as when implementing cross-training principles, during injury rehabilitation, or when inclement or seasonal weather prevents student-athletes from training outdoors. During these instances, several aerobic endurance training machines can be used following the training methods and concepts discussed in this chapter. The following section provides basic setup, movement guidelines, and safety considerations, and features five of the most common machines available.

Exercise Finder

Elliptical Trainer

Initial Setup

• Ellipticals are typically preset to a standard position, so no initial setup is required beyond properly standing on the machine.

• A resistance level may be selected to determine difficulty, and this can be adjusted at any point during the activity.

Beginning Position

• Face the center of the elliptical and place one foot on each pedal.

• Stand upright, face forward, and grab the handrails. The torso should be upright over the hips with body weight evenly distributed on each foot. Keep the head up and look forward, with the shoulders relaxed in a neutral but not rounded position.

Movement Guidelines

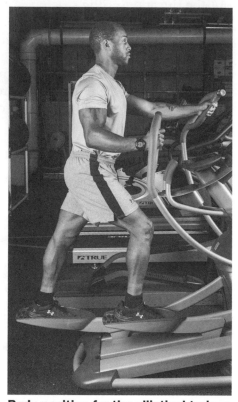

Body position for the elliptical trainer.

1. Pedal forward, using both the legs and arms in an alternating, reciprocal fashion. Note that some ellipticals may require movement to be initiated before intensity settings can be adjusted.

2. The feet should remain in contact with the pedals at all times. Avoid the knees moving excessively over the toes.

3. The handrails can be held at all times to maintain balance, which is suggested for higher speeds; however, if holding the handrails is deemed unnecessary, remove the hands and perform arm pumping actions similar to that of walking or running.

4. Quadriceps activity may be emphasized by focusing on the forward motion of the exercise, or hamstring and gluteal activity may be emphasized by focusing on the backward motion of the exercise.

5. Upon completion of the exercise, gradually slow to a complete stop and then step backward off of the pedals.

Safety Guidelines

The elliptical is a relatively safe exercise machine and is excellent for untrained and inexperienced student-athletes to use. Some ellipticals are designed without a back on the foot pedal, which can lead to a student-athlete's foot slipping off the back. While this is a rare occurrence, this design should be noted prior to use. Student-athletes should avoid removing their hands from the handrails at high speeds or if they are unfamiliar with the machine, because this may cause a loss of balance, which increases the risk of falling.

Treadmill

Initial Setup

• Prior to starting the treadmill, locate the red emergency stop button in case a sudden need to stop the treadmill arises.

• Fully read the instructions on the treadmill console to understand how to adjust the speed and incline of the treadmill. Because a multitude of treadmills are on the market, these first two familiarization steps are crucial for the safety of all users.

Beginning Position

• Begin by facing the treadmill and climbing onto the machine, making sure to straddle the belt by placing the feet on the platforms that run parallel to the belt.

• When the belt begins motion, hold onto the rails on either side of the treadmill, and bring both feet onto the belt. Maintain hand contact with the rails to ensure balance until accustomed to the speed of the treadmill.

Movement Guidelines

1. After locating the emergency stop button and carefully reading the instructions, turn on the treadmill, and adjust the speed to the desired warm-up speed.

2. It is important to hold onto the handrails until comfortable with the speed of the belt.

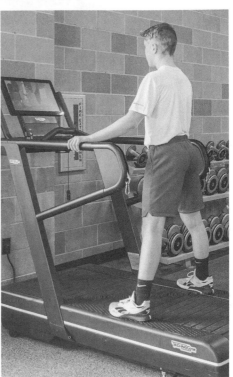

Safe straddling beginning position for the treadmill.

3. Once comfortable with the desired speed, remove the hands from the rails, and perform a normal walking or running gait pattern, with alternating leg and arm swinging actions.

4. Adjust to the desired speed or incline if a predesigned program was not chosen by using the buttons on the monitor. (Another option is to have the strength and conditioning professional adjust the speed and incline for the student-athlete.)

5. When the desired exercise duration is complete, reduce the speed of the treadmill to a comfortable walking pace and perform a 3- to 5-minute cooldown.

6. When all desired activity is complete, press the red stop button, hold onto the handrails, and step onto the platforms parallel to the belt.

7. Once the belt has come to a complete stop, step off the back or side of the treadmill.

Safety Guidelines

Stepping or falling off the back of the treadmill is the number one safety concern for treadmill exercise. To reduce the likelihood of stepping or falling of the back of the treadmill, the student-athlete should walk or run toward the front of the treadmill but not too close to the front to avoid stepping on the front of the machine. Another safety concern is unintentionally stepping on the platform on either side of the belt while walking or running. To reduce the likelihood of this occurring, the student-athlete should focus on remaining in the middle of the belt while exercising. Avoid holding onto the front portion of the treadmill or leaning back, because this creates poor movement technique and a loss of balance. If a student-athlete must grab onto the rails during the exercise, the speed is too great and must be reduced to ensure the student-athlete can perform the exercise under control.

Stair Climber

Initial Setup

• Locate the red stop button, and carefully read the instructions regarding starting, stopping, and adjusting the speed of movement on the exercise.

• Once familiar with the machine, start the exercise.

Beginning Position

• Face the center of the stair climber, and place one foot on each pedal. If the stair climber has stairs rather than pedals, place one foot on a separate stair, in the typical position in which one would climb stairs.

• Stand upright, face forward, and grab the handrails. The torso should be upright over the hips with body weight evenly distributed on each foot and with the whole foot in contact with the pedal or stair. Keep the head up and look forward, with shoulders relaxed in a neutral but not rounded position.

Movement Guidelines

1. To begin movement, initiate stepping while still holding the handrails for balance and support.

2. Take deep steps (roughly 4-8 inches [10-20 cm]), while focusing on maintaining an upright posture and forward gaze. It is important to step as if on a real set of stairs. If operating a pedal machine, do not step at the upper limit of the machine. Instead, step where a traditional step would be. If operating a machine with revolving stairs, do not attempt to step up multiple steps.

3. Hold onto the handrails, but do not lean on them for support. Maintain an upright posture with the shoulders relaxed and not rounded. Maintain a torso position over the hips, and keep the toes pointed forward with knees aligned over the top of the feet. If excessively hunching forward or relying on handrail support, reduce the speed of the exercise until proper technique is maintained.

4. When the exercise is complete, stop the machine and hold onto the handrails for support while stepping backward off the machine one leg at a time.

Safety Guidelines

The stair climber is a relatively safe exercise machine and is excellent for untrained and inexperienced student-athletes to use. The most common safety concern is tripping on the stairs and risking falling backward off the machine due to fast speeds. To ensure this from happening, the strength and conditioning professional should closely monitor technique as the student-athlete increases speed. When technique begins to falter, the strength and conditioning professional should direct the student-athlete to reduce speed or cease the exercise.

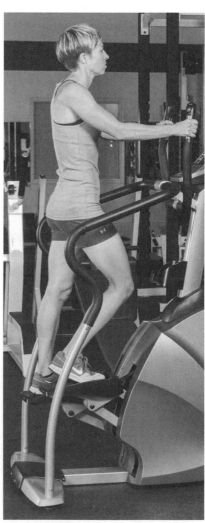

Body position for the stair climber.

Stationary Bike

Initial Setup

• The seat height should be adjusted so that the knee flexes between 25 and 30 degrees at the bottom portion of the cycling phase and so that the knee is directly over the center of the pedal to avoid a forward and backward rocking motion of the hips during exercise.

• The foot straps should be adjusted to ensure a snug fit so the feet do not come loose during pedaling and to ensure the ball of the foot is in contact with the pedals at all times.

• The handlebars should be adjusted to ensure the arms are extended at a slight downward angle that allows a slight elbow flexion of 10 to 15 degrees. Note that with "bullhorn" handlebars, several hand positions can be used including a pronated grip with the palms facing down (creating an upright posture); a neutral grip with the palms facing each other (creating more forward lean); or a racing position with forearms placed on the handlebars (creating an even greater forward lean).

• A variety of resistance settings are available on the stationary bike, which allow greater levels of intensity without risking wildly erratic upper and lower body movements.

Beginning Position

• Sit on the seat at a comfortable height to allow 25 to 30 degrees of knee flexion at the bottom portion of the cycling phase and the knee to come approximately even with the hips and parallel to the floor at the top portion of the cycling phase.

• The arms should be at a slight downward angle with 10 to 15 degrees of flexion at the elbow.

• The torso should be fully upright with shoulders relaxed and not rounded, with the head facing forward.

• Feet should be firmly planted on the pedals, which are in contact with the balls of the feet.

Movement Guidelines

1. Begin pedaling forward, maintaining contact of the pedals with the balls of the feet.

2. Maintain a neutral posture, and avoid rounding the shoulders, even when assuming a forward-leaning position.

3. When the exercise is complete, gradually slow down the cycle speed until the pedals have come to a complete stop.

4. Remove the feet from the straps one at a time and step off the bike.

Safety Guidelines

The stationary bike is a very safe exercise machine and is excellent for untrained and inexperienced student-athletes to use. The most common safety concern is the student-athlete hitting the knees on the handlebars during the top portion of the cycle or hyperextending the knees at the bottom portion of the cycle. To reduce the likelihood of this occurring, follow the setup guidelines. Another concern is the potential for a foot to dislodge from the pedal, which would risk the pedal hitting the student-athlete's leg. To avoid this, make sure the foot is firmly strapped down and secure prior to exercise. The last major safety concern is the potential for the student-athlete to tip over the stationary bike due to a loss of balance from erratic pedaling motions. However rare, the strength and conditioning professional should ensure a proper resistance level is set on the bike to avoid excessive and erratic pedaling.

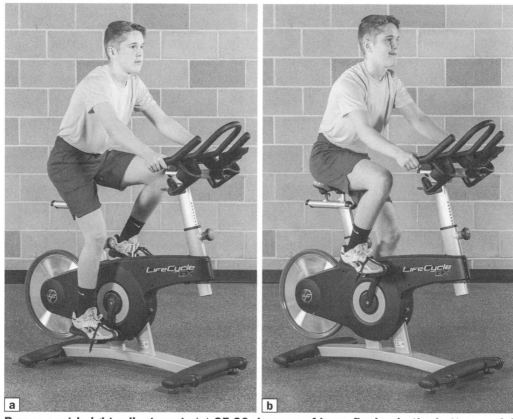

Proper seat height adjustment: *(a)* 25-30 degrees of knee flexion in the bottom pedal position and *(b)* the knee to be approximately even with the hips and parallel to the floor in the top pedal position.

Rowing Machine

Initial Setup

- The rowing machine requires no setup beyond adjusting the foot strap and turning it on to record time or distance.

Beginning Position

- Sit at the front of the machine with the legs flexed at or near a 90-degree angle and with a slight forward lean of the hips.
- The torso should be upright, and the shoulders should be down and unrounded.
- Securely strap the feet into the foot pedals and face the toes forward.
- Extend the arms forward and place the hands on the handle with a pronated grip.

Movement Guidelines

1. Assume the beginning position.
2. Extend the hips and knees while simultaneously pulling the handle toward the body, just below the chest. This is the *drive* phase.
3. At the *finish* of the movement, the hips and legs should be fully extended and the arms fully flexed in a row position, with a moderate backward lean of the torso.
4. During the *recovery* phase, once again extend the arms and flex the knees and hips to return to the beginning position.
5. It is important to maintain a neutral torso and forward head position throughout the duration of this exercise. A common technique flaw is to allow the shoulders and upper back to round, especially during the drive and recovery phases of the exercise.

Safety Guidelines

The rowing machine is relatively safe and is excellent for untrained and inexperienced student-athletes to use. The most common safety concern is the student-athlete rounding the shoulders and back forward during the recovery portion of the exercise, which could put excessive stress on the lower back. Another safety concern is excessive hyperextension of the knees during the finish portion of the exercise. To avoid this, the strength and conditioning professional should ensure proper technique has been thoroughly discussed and that the student-athletes have practiced the rowing motion at low speeds.

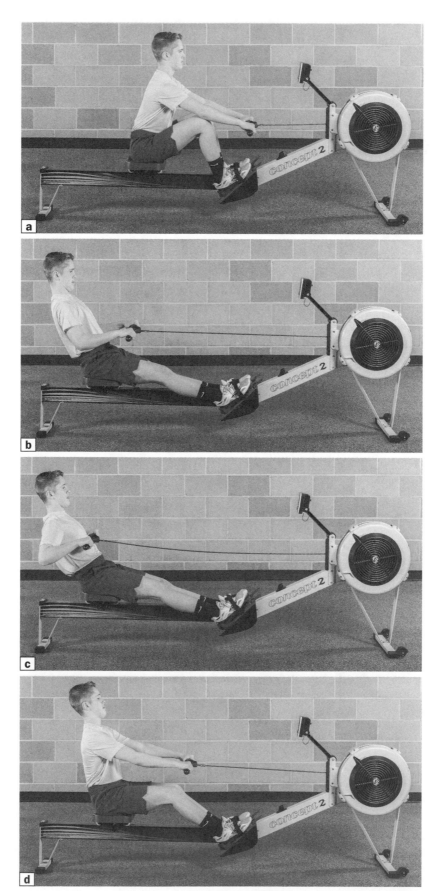

Proper rowing phases: *(a)* **beginning,** *(b)* **drive,** *(c)* **finish,** and *(d)* **middle of the recovery.**

Program Design Guidelines for Circuit Training

Program design for circuit training features the same underlying principles as it does for the conventional aerobic endurance training methods discussed earlier in this chapter. As with other endurance exercise activities, using the FITT-VP principle will ensure continued progression as well as the safety and well-being of the student-athletes being a top priority. However, some important differences must be considered when implementing circuit training programs as opposed to the more traditional training methods with high school student-athletes. Two important considerations are space availability equipment access and availability. The type of available equipment makes up the bulk of the mode considerations for circuit training, but space availability or lack thereof will also influence the decision-making process as to the mode of exercise.

Circuit training often resembles a hybrid between resistance training and aerobic endurance training, which is advantageous when time availability is an issue. Circuit training has shown to be an effective method for increasing and maintaining muscular strength (8), muscular endurance (25, 32), muscular power (8, 17), and aerobic endurance (25, 32). However, due to its blended nature, circuit training lacks specificity compared to standalone resistance or aerobic training programs, and while circuit training can be an efficient way to increase muscular and aerobic endurance simultaneously, it is not as effective as programs done specifically targeting the aforementioned variables (25).

Age and Training Status Considerations

Because circuit training may encompass components of resistance and plyometric training, additional training age considerations must be addressed. It is important to note that an individual student-athlete may have different training ages for aerobic endurance, resistance, and plyometric training, so the prescribed circuit training program should reflect those individual considerations. Along with determining previous experience with structured resistance and plyometric training, a strength and conditioning professional should also determine previous intensity levels, length of recent participation in a structured program, and the knowledge and ability to execute proper technique in all the exercises programmed in the circuit training program (44).

Mode

Determining the mode for circuit training can be accomplished in a variety of ways. As mentioned earlier, equipment availability and space availability will play a large role in determining the type of circuit training implemented. Another way to determine the mode of a circuit training program is to use the training age concept. For example, a circuit training program based on training age could initially focus on bodyweight movements for untrained and inexperienced student-athletes and gradually add in resistance implements such as dumbbells, kettlebells, weight machines, bands, or medicine balls, and more advanced plyometric movements as student-athletes progress in their training status. Circuit training exercises can also be determined by body region, such as upper and lower body (36), or by movement such as pushing versus pulling exercises (44) or quad-dominant versus hamstring- and gluteal-dominant. Lastly, a focus on muscular strength and muscular endurance or a focus on aerobic endurance could dictate the types of exercises implemented into a circuit training program.

Intensity

When determining the intensity of circuit training programs, RPE, MHR, and the Karvonen method can once again be used to assign desired intensity levels and to monitor intensity during the session. However, because circuit training often encompasses components of resistance and plyometric training, intensity considerations from those two modalities must be considered as well. Resistance training intensity considerations for circuit training can be accomplished by determining the weight of resistance implements used. Factors that affect plyometric intensity are single- versus double-leg landing, single- versus double-arm throws, speed of movement, height or distance of jumps, and how much a student-athlete weighs (36), because greater body weight will place more stress on muscles, joints, and connective tissues.

Lastly, sets, repetitions, exercise selection, exercise order, individual exercise time, rest between sets and repetitions, and the total exercise time can all be manipulated to produce more or less intensity. For example, regarding exercise order, placing all lower body exercises together will add intensity, whereas spreading lower body exercises throughout the session will allow for more recovery for similar muscle groups. Another way to manipulate exercise order to increase intensity is to place all compound, multijoint exercises together. Exercise selection can also be manipulated to increase or decrease the intensity of the circuit. For example, adding more compound, multijoint exercises and exercises that require more movement such as squats, lunges, skier jumps, jumping jacks, or box jumps will increase the intensity of the circuit. In contrast, adding more single-joint or stationary exercises such as glute bridges, bird dogs, planks, or stability ball leg curls will decrease the intensity of the circuit.

Frequency

Due to the relatively high demands of circuit training, the frequency of training sessions must be carefully considered. It should be remembered that as intensity increases, frequency should decrease. A recent meta-analysis of several circuit training programs found the average sessions per week to be between two and four (41); however, it should be noted that in these studies the circuit training program was the only means of exercise the participants were performing. Given the nature of the high school population, it is likely that most student-athletes participate in one or more other physically demanding activities such as a sport, so a high volume of circuit training sessions is not advisable. Referring to the sample programs of traditional aerobic endurance programs, a circuit training program could be substituted for a HIIT or SIT training day as part of a well-rounded training program.

Duration

The duration of circuit training programs is highly variable and depends heavily on the training status of the student-athletes and the level of intensity of a given program. Duration protocols include a range for both effort and rest, such as short bursts at percentages well above $\dot{V}O_2$max levels, typically lasting for 20 to 30 seconds, similar to a Tabata protocol, with varying rest times from 10 seconds to 2 minutes between exercises and up to 4 minutes of rest between rounds (8, 41). Many protocols use a repetition and set scheme with either multiple repetitions, ranging from 4 to 12, of the same exercise (41), or various exercises in a similar repetition range (25). Duration can be further increased in protocols with multiple exercises by performing multiple rounds or adding another round with different exercises.

Progression

Progression for circuit training can be dictated by using the GAS method to ensure a student-athlete will continually be exposed to progressive overload but not risk entering the exhaustion phase of the GAS. Progression can be dictated by increasing the difficulty level of the exercise by increasing resistance or duration, or by adding more exercises or additional rounds. Because the nature of circuit training is not highly specific, it should be used as a strength and conditioning tool or a cross-training method rather than as a goal for a student-athlete to improve time or repetition number in circuit training for its own sake.

Safety Guidelines

Circuit training programs should be tailored to specifically meet the needs and training status of the individual student-athlete, and the following guidelines should be conducted prior to creating a program. Previous experience with structured resistance and plyometric training should be noted prior to developing a circuit training program. The strength and conditioning professional should determine previously exposed intensity levels, length of recent participation in a structured program, and the knowledge and ability to execute proper technique in all the exercises programmed in the circuit training. The student-athlete should first clearly demonstrate proper form and technique for all prescribed exercises within the circuit training program prior to the beginning of the program to ensure proper movement literacy and to reduce the likelihood of injury.

Common Types of Programs

This section provides an initial guide and template that can be used either by following the examples listed here or by creating new circuits based on the three options (body weight, dumbbell and medicine ball, and running). As discussed, circuit training has been shown to improve a wide range of physiological variables including muscular strength, muscular endurance, power, and aerobic endurance (8, 17, 25, 32). Due to the lack of specificity, circuit training can be a great addition to any student-athlete's aerobic endurance program, and it provides the strength and conditioning professional with an immense amount of flexibility, allowing for easy exercise substitution to increase or decrease the intensity of the circuits based on the individual needs and training status of the student-athlete.

Bodyweight Circuit

Table 11.6 uses a bodyweight-only protocol, which can be advantageous for individuals who have a low training age in resistance, plyometric, or aerobic endurance. Bodyweight training protocols can also be convenient when no training equipment is available or when programming circuit training for at-home training. This sample program features a combination of resistance, plyometric, and aerobic endurance–style exercises. The protocol is as follows: 10 exercises performed for 15 to 30 seconds with 10 to 20 seconds of rest between exercises, and 2 to 4 minutes rest between rounds. Based on the student-athlete's training status, 1 to 5 rounds should be performed.

Dumbbell and Medicine Ball Circuit

A more advanced circuit can be performed with the addition of dumbbells and medicine balls. The addition of these implements allows for a more well-rounded training session and multiple movement variations. Table 11.7 depicts a sample protocol consisting of 14 exercises performed for 15 to 30 seconds with 10 to 20 seconds of rest between exercises, and 2 to 4 minutes of rest between rounds. Based on the student-athlete's training status, 1 to 5 rounds should be performed.

Running-Based Circuit

If the coach desires a greater emphasis on the cardiovascular system, a running-based circuit training program can be implemented. This is another great alternative when access to exercise equipment is limited or for student-athletes who participate in more aerobic endurance–based sports such as cross-country or swimming. Table 11.8 depicts a sample training program consisting of 8 exercises performed for 30 to 90 seconds with a 1:1 work-to-rest ratio recovery

TABLE 11.6 Sample Bodyweight Circuit Training Program

Perform exercises in order after a 5- to 10-minute warm-up.	Protocol: 1-5 rounds; 15-30 seconds per exercise; 10-20 seconds of rest between exercises; 2-4 minutes of rest between rounds
1. Bilateral squat	2. Bodyweight row
3. Push-up or modified push-up	4. Bird dog
5. Mountain climbers	6. Forward walking lunge
7. Right side plank	8. Left side plank
9. Step-up	10. Pull-up

TABLE 11.7 Sample Dumbbell and Medicine Ball Circuit

Perform exercises in order after a 5- to 10-minute warm-up.	Protocol: 1-5 rounds; 15-30 seconds per exercise; 10-20 seconds of rest between exercises; 2-4 minutes of rest between rounds
1. Dumbbell squat and press	2. Medicine ball jump-slam
3. Farmer carry	4. Weighted split squat
5. Floor dumbbell chest press	6. Two-arm dumbbell row
7. Standing medicine ball side-to-side rotations*	8. Walking dumbbell lunge
9. Skater jump	10. Standing dumbbell biceps curl
11. Standing dumbbell triceps extension	12. Dumbbell jump squat
13. Dumbbell swing (can use a kettlebell if available)	14. Jumping jack

*Stand with feet shoulder-width apart and arms extended with elbows slightly flexed, and rotate side to side.

TABLE 11.8 Sample Running-Based Circuit

Perform exercises in order after a 5- to 10-minute warm-up.	Protocol: 1-3 rounds; 30-90 seconds per exercise; 1:1 work-to-rest ratio following each exercise; 2-4 minutes of rest between rounds
1. Sprint or run	2. Bodyweight squat
3. Side shuffle	4. High plank
5. Sprint or run	6. Push-up
7. Side shuffle	8. Walking lunge

period between exercises and 2 to 4 minutes of rest between rounds. Based on the student-athlete's training status, 1 to 3 rounds should be performed.

Guidelines for Group Play and Activities

Group-style exercise simply takes the concepts of circuit training and applies them in a large group setting. A major benefit to this style of training is that it creates a team-like atmosphere, which could increase student-athletes' exercise motivation. A limiting factor to implementing this type of program is space availability and student-athlete maturity level. However, by using the bodyweight or running-based circuits, a strength and conditioning professional can bring a large group of student-athletes into a gymnasium or onto a football field and conduct a large group training session with relative ease. In order for a group training session to be successful, student-athletes must possess the maturity level to stay on task during the session. With larger or younger groups, the chance of student-athletes not staying on task will likely increase.

Recommendations for Organizing and Leading Groups

The psychological and psychophysiological responses to group exercise training should be considered by the strength and conditioning professional prior to the implementation of this type of training. According to the self-determination theory, student-athletes must meet three basic psychological needs to experience a high degree of exercise motivation (35):

- *Autonomy:* actions match personal goals
- *Relatedness:* connection to others
- *Competence:* feeling that they can meet and complete the challenges they are facing

To meet these needs, programming can be done with scaled options based on each student-athlete's training status for each given exercise, careful instruction and exercise demonstration prior to training, and continuous verbal communication and motivation given by the strength and conditioning professional.

Another consideration is how to effectively create and organize groups. Common options include placing student-athletes in groups based on:

- biological or training age (preferred),
- chronological age,

- sex, or
- sport played.

Alternatively, student-athletes can be purposely placed in a mixed group of varying training statuses.

The strength and conditioning professional must also decide whether to participate in the group training session or simply demonstrate the exercise technique and then watch for technique flaws during the training session. If only one strength and conditioning professional is present, it is recommended to only demonstrate exercise technique and then watch for technique flaws or issues. This allows for the strength and conditioning professional to spot technique flaws and correct movement patterns more easily without having to stop the session. If more than one strength and conditioning professional is present, one may lead the group exercise while the other monitors the student-athletes for technique flaws and provides movement instruction. Research has shown that the psychophysiological responses to exercise are intensity dependent (48). In other words, having a strength and conditioning professional participate may aid in participant motivation. This is especially true when exercises are performed appropriately to meet levels of participants' training status (48).

Safety Guidelines

Group training programs should have scaled exercise options to meet the needs and training status of the individual student-athletes. Previous experience with structured resistance and plyometric training should be noted prior to developing a group training program in order to create appropriate exercise variations for differing levels of training status. Additionally, the strength and conditioning professional should determine previously exposed intensity levels, length of recent participation in a structured program, and the knowledge and ability to execute proper technique in all the exercises programmed in the group training program.

Common Types of Programs

Of the many types of group play and related activities, the most common are versions of circuit training or small-sided games.

Group Circuit Training

The circuit training programs provided in tables 11.6 through 11.8 easily can be turned into group training programs, but a few important considerations should be noted:

- Group training programs can be conducted by having every student-athlete perform the same exercise at the same time before moving on to the next exercise. For example, in the sample program in table 11.6, all the participants perform the bilateral bodyweight squat exercise together, and then proceed to the bodyweight row, and so on until the round is completed. A benefit of using this style is that the strength and conditioning professional can demonstrate each exercise prior to the start of the round and monitor technique because each person will be performing the same exercise.

- Group training can also be conducted by creating stations in which each participant rotates in a designated order. Using the sample program in 11.6 again, each participant would start at one of the 10 exercise stations. The participant would perform the given exercise and then rotate to the next station. The participant at station 1 would move to station 2 and so on, with the participant at station 10 rotating to station 1. A return to the starting station would signal the end of the round. If there are more than 10 participants, the strength and conditioning professional either can create multiple sections of the exercises or multiple participants can perform the same exercise and rotate as a group.

Small-Sided Games

Another alternative to traditional group circuit training-based exercises is the use of **small-sided games** (SSGs) to increase aerobic endurance fitness in high school student-athletes. Some SSG options include ultimate frisbee; 4v4 or 3v3 basketball, soccer, and lacrosse; football; and volleyball. Apart from being a valid conditioning method for aerobic endurance improvements (12, 18), SSGs offer the benefit of providing a fun and competitive experience, and they use the concept of cross-training, which has been shown to decrease the risk of overuse injuries that result from only using one type of training method (47). Intensity levels in SSGs can be monitored based on heart rate calculations (20) like other methods of aerobic endurance training. The intensity levels can be manipulated by changing the number of participants, the duration of the activity, or both, with fewer participants and shorter durations showing increases in intensity levels (12). This type of training is excellent for team sport or multisport athletes because it exposes them to a wide variety of skills and game-like scenarios along with using the concepts of HIIT and SIT training, while abiding by the concepts of sport specificity, fiber types, and energy system demands. See table 11.9 for sample soccer, flag football, and lacrosse SSGs.

TABLE 11.9   Sample Small-Sided Games

Game and positions	Game play	Description
Soccer: 1 goalie and 2-3 free players per side	Set up two goals 25 yds (23 m) apart and play a 4v4 or 3v3 game.	Duration can be manipulated by having a time limit.
Flag football: 4-7 players per side	Teams can set up on their 25-yd (23 m) line and play within a smaller area than using the entire length of the field.	By shortening the field, the games will be faster paced and allow for more engagement among the participants.
Lacrosse: 1 goalie and 3 free players per side	One team plays offense for a given duration, and the other team plays defense. After a certain time, teams can switch.	Duration can be manipulated by having one team remain on offense or defense until a certain number of goals have been made.

Additional options: Three or more teams can be used with one or more teams resting while the other two teams play; they rotate after a certain length of time. Additionally, if the strength and conditioning professional uses the offense-defense only strategy, teams can rotate between playing offense, defense, and sitting out.

Conclusion

Aerobic endurance training is an important component of a well-rounded training program for the high school student-athlete, not only for athletic improvement, but for the mitigation of risks from a plethora of cardiovascular conditions as well as other issues such as depression. Student-athletes will only compete in athletics for a small portion of their lives, with many never competing beyond the high school level (34). Therefore, it is paramount that student-athletes are given the tools to lead a healthy and active lifestyle for the remainder of their lives beyond high school.

Programs should be specific and individualized to meet the needs of the student-athlete, with special considerations given to sport participation. Programs must be considerate of training age and sport season and should be designed to improve performance in a structured, periodized manner. This chapter featured a wide variety of training modalities and considerations, and a thoughtful combination of all training types should be used so that all physiological variables may be developed and improved upon.

NSCA Strength and Conditioning Professional Standards and Guidelines

ABSTRACT

THIS IS THE UPDATED VERSION OF THE NSCA STRENGTH AND CONDITIONING PROFESSIONAL STANDARDS AND GUIDELINES. THE LAST UPDATE WAS PERFORMED IN 2009.

The Strength and Conditioning profession involves the combined competencies of sport/exercise science, administration, management, teaching, and coaching. Practitioners must also comply with various laws and regulations while responding to instances of potential injury and related claims and suits. This creates remarkable challenges and requires substantial experience, expertise, and other resources to effectively address them, especially in multisport (e.g., collegiate and scholastic) settings.

Ample resources are available in some of these settings but in many others, however, they are not. Budgets, equipment, facilities, and staff are often limited (or lacking altogether), with a resulting mismatch between the participants' demand for safe and effective programs and services, and the institution's provision of them. It is important for Strength and Conditioning practitioners and their employers to

Address correspondence to the NSCA National Office at nsca@nsca.com.

understand that this standard of care is a shared duty; the institution and individual are thus jointly responsible for fulfilling it. Collectively, these issues are the driving forces behind this project.

The purpose of the NSCA Strength and Conditioning Professional Standards and Guidelines document is to help identify areas of liability exposure, increase safety, and decrease the likelihood of injuries that might lead to legal claims and suits, and ultimately improve the standard of care being offered. This document is intended to be neither rigid nor static and will be updated periodically to reflect the industry's best practices. It is hoped that Strength and Conditioning practitioners and the institutions employing them will mutually benefit from applying this information, and in turn significantly enhance the quality of services and programs provided to their participants.

NOTICE

This document is intended to provide relevant practice parameters for Strength and Conditioning professionals to use when carrying out their responsibilities in providing services to athletes or other participants. The standards and guidelines presented here are based on published scientific studies, pertinent statements from other associations, analysis of claims and litigation, and a consensus of expert views. However, this information is not a substitute for individualized judgment or independent professional advice.

Neither the NSCA nor the contributors to this project assume any duty owed to third parties by those reading, interpreting, or implementing this information. When rendering services to third parties, these standards and guidelines cannot be adopted for use with all participants without exercising independent judgment and decision-making based on the Strength and Conditioning professional's individual training, education, and experience. Furthermore, Strength and Conditioning practitioners must stay abreast of new developments in the profession so that these standards and guidelines may evolve to meet particular service needs.

Neither the NSCA nor the contributors to this project, by reason of authorship or publication of this document, shall be deemed to be engaged in practice of any branch of professional discipline (e.g., medicine, physical therapy, law) reserved for those licensed under state law. Strength and Conditioning practitioners using

KEY WORDS:
principles of practice

this information are encouraged to seek and obtain such advice, if needed or desired, from those licensed professionals.

INTRODUCTION

SCOPE OF PRACTICE

The legal responsibilities and professional scope of practice for Strength and Conditioning professionals can be subdivided into 2 domains: (42) "Scientific Foundations" and "Practical/Applied". Each of these involves corresponding activities, responsibilities, and knowledge requirements (refer to Appendices 1 and 2):

Scientific foundations.
- Exercise Sciences (e.g., Anatomy, Exercise Physiology, Biomechanics, Sport Psychology)
- Nutrition

Practical/Applied.
- Exercise Technique
- Program Design
- Organization and Administration
- Testing and Evaluation

LEGAL DUTIES AND CONCEPTS

Strength and Conditioning practitioners have legal duties to provide an appropriate level of supervision and instruction to meet a reasonable standard of care and to provide and maintain a safe environment for the participants under their supervision. These duties also involve informing users of risks inherent in and related to their activities, and preventing unreasonable risk or harm resulting from "negligent instruction or supervision (16,17,21)." Statler and Brown (56) summarize the following key liability concepts for the Strength and Conditioning professional:
- Assumption of risk: voluntary participation in activity with knowledge of the inherent risk(s). Athletic activities, including strength and conditioning, involve certain risks. Participants must be thoroughly informed of the risks of activity, and required to sign a statement to that effect.

- Liability: a legal responsibility, duty, or obligation. Strength and Conditioning professionals have a duty to the participants they serve to take reasonable steps to prevent injury and to act prudently when an injury occurs (5).
- Negligence: failure to act as a reasonable and prudent person would under similar circumstances. Four elements must exist for a Strength and Conditioning professional to be found liable for negligence: duty, breach of duty, proximate cause, and damages (47). Simply stated, a Strength and Conditioning professional is negligent if he/she is proven to have a duty to act and to have failed to act with the appropriate standard of care, proximately causing injury or damages to another person.
- Standard of care: what a prudent and reasonable person would do under similar circumstances. A Strength and Conditioning professional is expected to act according to his/her education, training, and certification status (e.g., CSCS, NSCA-CPT, EMT, cardiopulmonary resuscitation [CPR], automated external defibrillator [AED], First Aid).

Standards versus guidelines. It is important to distinguish between "standards" and "guidelines" because each term has different legal implications (9,60):
- Standard: a required procedure that probably reflects a legal duty or obligation for standard of care (note that the standard statements in this document use the word "must"). The standards set forth in this document may ultimately be recognized as a legal standard of care to be implemented into the daily operations of strength and conditioning programs and facilities.
- Guideline: a recommended operating procedure formulated and developed to further enhance the quality of services provided (note that the guideline statements in this document use the word "should"). Guidelines are not intended to be

standards of practice or to give rise to legally defined duties of care, but in certain circumstances they could assist in evaluating and improving services rendered.

While the publication of this document does not amount to a judicial determination of the standard of care to be applied in a particular case, it is presumed that the standards stated herein will likely be given authoritative weight in actual litigations.

Published standards of practice = potential legal duties. Proof of duty or standard of care in a negligence case can be determined in various ways, one of which is from standards of practice published by professional associations and organizations. In actual litigation, published standards of practice can be introduced through expert testimony or in the discovery phase of pretrial to help determine whether a defendant was negligent in carrying out his/her legal duties (9). The current trend in most jurisdictions is to allow such standards as admissible evidence, where they are generally recognized as being indicative of widely accepted practices. Furthermore, courts examining these issues in negligence cases have ruled that violations of such professional standards often constitute a breach of duty.

If properly adopted and applied, published standards of practice can minimize liability exposures associated with negligence, and thereby serve as a potential shield for those who comply with them. They can also be used as a sword against those who do not comply, potentially increasing liability risks associated with negligence (9). The key issue in this regard seems to be the practitioner's consistent application of established standards of practice in the provision of daily service. For example, if his/her conduct is proven to be consistent with accepted standard(s), it will be difficult to show breach of duty, thereby providing protection against negligence. If his/her conduct is not proven to be consistent with accepted standard(s), however, it may be easier for the injured party to show breach of duty due to failure to follow such standards, which can lead to a ruling of negligence.

TYPES OF STANDARDS

In addition to standards for desired operational practices published by professional organizations such as the NSCA, there are also standards for technical/physical specifications published by independent organizations such as the American Society for Testing and Materials (ASTM) or U.S. Consumer Product Safety Commission (CPSC). These are briefly described below:

Operational practices. In a negligence lawsuit, established standards of care can be used to gauge a practitioner's professional competence by comparing his/her actual conduct with written benchmarks of expected behavior. In addition to the standards and guidelines from allied professional organizations such as the American College of Sports Medicine (ACSM) (3,12,60), American Heart Association (AHA) (3,35,36), and National Athletic Trainers' Association (NATA) (39) referenced in this document, the following associations have also published standards of practice:

- Aerobics and Fitness Association of America. Exercise Standards and Guidelines (4th ed). Ventura, CA: AFAA, 2002.
- American Academy of Pediatrics. Strength training by children and adolescents. Pediatrics 121: 835–840, 2008. Available at: http://pediatrics.aappublications.org/content/121/4/835. Accessed 11/5/2017.
- American Physical Therapy Association. Guide to Physical Therapist Practice (2nd ed). Alexandria, VA: APTA, 2003.
- National Association for Sport and Physical Education. Moving Into the Future: National Standards for Physical Education (2nd edition). Reston, VA: NASPE, 2004.
- National Athletic Trainers' Association Board of Certification. Standards of Professional Practice. Dallas,

TX: NATA, 2016. Available at: http://www.bocatc.org/public-protection#standards-discipline Accessed 11/5/2017.
- President's Council on Fitness, Sports and Nutrition. The Role of Resistance Training for Children and Adolescents. Available at: http://www.fitness.gov/blog-posts/role_resistance_training.html. Accessed 11/5/2017.
- Society of Health and Physical Educators. Quality Coaches, Quality Sports: National Standards for Sport Coaches (2nd ed). Champaign, IL: Human Kinetics, 2006.
- US Center for SafeSport. Available at: https://safesport.org/ Accessed 11/5/2017.

Technical and physical specifications. Technical and physical specifications of equipment and facilities relevant to the Strength and Conditioning profession have been published by the ASTM and CPSC. The CPSC also operates the National Electronic Injury Surveillance System (NEISS), a surveillance and follow-back system that gathers data from hospital emergency departments to provide timely information on consumer injuries associated with certain products or activities. Some of these data have been used to research weight training injuries, as will be addressed in the Injury Trends, Litigations, and Standard of Care Load section.

STANDARDS OF PRACTICE AS THEY APPLY TO RISK MANAGEMENT

Risk management is a proactive administrative process that helps minimize legal liability, as well as decrease the frequency and severity of injuries and subsequent claims and lawsuits (8). It may not be possible to eliminate all risks of injury and liability exposure in strength and conditioning settings; however, it can be effectively minimized and mitigated by implementing sound risk management strategies. The Strength and Conditioning practitioner is ultimately responsible for risk management, but all facility staff should be involved in

the various aspects of the process. Eickhoff-Shemek (10) proposes a 4-step procedure for applying standards of practice to the risk management process:

1. *Identify and select standards of practice, as well as all applicable laws.* Because so many standards of practice are published by various organizations, it is challenging for the Strength and Conditioning professional to be aware of all of them, and determine which ones are appropriate when implementing the risk management plan. In terms of participant safety, the most conservative or stringent standards in a given industry should generally be used.

2. *Develop risk management strategies reflecting standards of practice and all applicable laws.* This step involves writing procedures describing specific responsibilities and/or duties that staff would carry out in particular situations. The procedures should be written clearly, succinctly, and without excessive detail (too much detail may not allow the flexibility practitioners need in particular situations and make implementation of those strategies difficult or impractical). Once the written procedures are finalized, they should be included in the staff policies and procedures manual.

3. *Implement the risk management plan.* Implementation of the risk management plan primarily involves staff training to ensure that the practitioner's daily conduct will be consistent with written policies and procedures and selected laws and standards of practice. The policies and procedures manual should be used in conjunction with the initial training of new employees, as well as during regular in-service training, where all employees practice a particular (e.g., emergency) procedure. From a legal perspective, it is also important to explain to staff why it is essential to carry out such duties appropriately.

4. *Evaluate the risk management plan.* Like the law, standards of practice are not static and need to be updated periodically to reflect change. The risk management plan should

be formally evaluated at least annually, as well as after each incidence of accident or injury to determine whether emergency procedures were performed correctly and what could be done to prevent a similar incident in the future.

LIABILITY EXPOSURE IN THE STRENGTH AND CONDITIONING PROFESSION

While each strength and conditioning program and facility is unique, the NSCA Professional Standards and Guidelines Task Force has identified 9 areas of potential liability exposure, as delineated below. It is important to note that they are interrelated. For example, proper instruction and supervision is associated with personnel qualifications, as well as facility layout and scheduling issues. Noncompliance in any area can therefore affect others, and in turn compound the risk of liability exposure and potential litigation. Furthermore, the Strength and Conditioning practitioner and his/her employer share the corresponding duties and responsibilities.

Collectively within these liability exposure areas, 11 standards and 14 guidelines for Strength and Conditioning practitioners have further been identified (these are presented in the next section of this document). These standards and guidelines are intended to serve as an authoritative and unbiased source for professional guidance. The rationale for each is summarized below.

Preparticipation screening and clearance. A physical examination is imperative for all participants before participating in a strength and conditioning program and should be performed by a properly qualified health care provider with the requisite training, medical skills, and background to reliably perform a physical examination. This should include a comprehensive health and immunization history (as defined by current guidelines from the Centers for Disease Control and Prevention (CDC)), as well as a relevant physical examination, part of

which includes an orthopedic evaluation. Some type of cardiovascular screening, as discussed below, is also recommended. The Strength and Conditioning staff should receive documentation about any condition that would potentially require special training considerations (e.g., sickle-cell disease), even if the participant has been given medical clearance to participate. Participants who are returning from an injury or illness must also be required to provide documentation of medical clearance before returning to a strength and conditioning program. Therefore, communication between the Sports Medicine/Athletic Training staff and the Strength and Conditioning staff must be clear and timely.

Currently, there are no universally accepted standards for screening participants nor are there approved certification procedures for health care professionals who perform such examinations. However, a joint Pre-Participation Physical Evaluation Task Force of 6 organizations (American Academy of Family Physicians, American Academy of Pediatrics, American College of Sports Medicine, American Medical Society for Sports Medicine, American Orthopaedic Society for Sports Medicine, and American Osteopathic Academy of Sports Medicine) has published a widely accepted monograph including detailed instructions on performing a preparticipation history and physical examination, determining clearance for participation, and a medical evaluation form to copy and use for each examination (46). In addition, the American Heart Association and American College of Sports Medicine have published statements on preparticipation screening for those involved in fitness-related activities (3,35,36). Relevant points are summarized as follows:

- *Educational institutions have an ethical, medical, and possible legal obligation to implement cost-efficient preparticipation screening strategies (including a complete medical history and physical examination), and thereby ensure that high school and college*

athletes are not subject to unacceptable risks. Support for such efforts, especially in large athletic populations, is mitigated by cost-efficiency considerations, practical limitations, and an awareness that it is not possible to achieve zero risk in competitive sports.

- *Preparticipation athletic screening should be performed by a properly qualified health care provider with the requisite training, medical skills, and background to reliably perform a physical examination, obtain a detailed cardiovascular history, and recognize heart disease.* A licensed physician is preferred, but an appropriately trained registered nurse or physician assistant may be acceptable under certain circumstances in states where non-physician health care workers are permitted to perform preparticipation screening. In the latter situation, however, a formal certification process should be established to demonstrate expertise in performing cardiovascular examinations.

- *A complete and careful personal and family medical history and physical examination designed to identify (or raise suspicion of) cardiovascular risk factors known to cause sudden death or disease progression is the best available and most practical approach to screening populations of competitive sports participants.* Such screening is an obtainable objective, and should be mandatory for all participants. Initially a complete medical history and physical examination should be performed before participation in organized high school athletics (grades 9–12). An interim history should be obtained in intervening years. For collegiate athletes, a comprehensive personal/family history and physical examination should be performed by a qualified examiner initially on entering the institution, before beginning training and competition. Screening should be repeated every 2 years thereafter unless more frequent examinations are indicated; and an interim history and blood pressure measurement should be obtained each subsequent year to determine whether another physical examination, and possible further testing, is required (e.g., due to abnormalities or changes in medical status).

- *Health appraisal questionnaires should be used before exercise testing and/or training to initially classify participants by risk for triage and preliminary decision-making.* After the initial health appraisal (and medical consultation and/or supervised exercise test, if indicated), participants can be further classified for exercise training on the basis of individual characteristics. When a medical evaluation/recommendation is advised or required, written and active communication between facility staff and the participant's personal physician or health care provider is strongly recommended. Furthermore, participants should be educated about the importance of obtaining a preparticipation health appraisal and medical evaluation/recommendation (if indicated), as well as the potential risks incurred without obtaining them.

Personnel qualifications. Qualified and knowledgeable personnel must be hired to properly supervise and instruct participants using Strength and Conditioning facilities and equipment. A three-pronged approach is recommended.

First, the Strength and Conditioning practitioner should acquire expertise, and have a degree from an accredited college/university in one or more of the topics comprising the "Scientific Foundations" domain identified in the Certified Strength and Conditioning Specialist (CSCS) Examination Content Description (42) (i.e., anatomy, exercise/sport physiology, biomechanics, sport psychology, nutrition; see Appendix 1), or in a related subject (e.g., exercise/sport pedagogy, psychology, motor learning, training methodology, kinesiology). Note that the NSCA's Education Recognition Program (ERP) has been developed to recognize institutions of higher learning that meet such requirements,

and also helps to identify an educational career path for the Strength and Conditioning profession. Likewise, practitioners should make an ongoing effort to acquire knowledge and competence in the content areas outside their primary area of expertise. In 2004, the Commission on Accreditation of Allied Health Education Programs (CAAHEP) began accrediting programs in exercise science and exercise physiology (https://www.caahep.org/ Accessed 11/5/2017), so if the practitioner is unable to attend an NSCA-ERP institution, training in an accredited program in exercise science or exercise physiology will ensure that the "Scientific Foundations" are thoroughly covered.

High school settings are unique in that most teaching positions require a teacher certification from an accredited program, typically in Physical Education, for an individual who will be working with students in an athletic setting. The Society of Health and Physical Educators (SHAPE), formerly known as AAHPERD, has also created national standards and guidelines for physical education teacher education that address the unique issues pertinent to exercise and sport in the high school environment (https://www.shapeamerica.org/ Accessed 11/5/2017).

Second, accredited certifications offered through professional organizations with continuing education requirements and a code of ethics (e.g., the CSCS credential; see Appendix 2) are available to Strength and Conditioning practitioners interested in acquiring the necessary competencies. Depending on the practitioner's specific duties, responsibilities, and interests, relevant certifications offered by other governing bodies may also be appropriate, depending on the requirements for obtaining and maintaining certification.

Third, a Strength and Conditioning practitioner's knowledge and skill development can be enhanced by applying the "performance team" concept (i.e., aligning a staff comprised of

qualified professionals with interdependent expertise and shared leadership roles; see Appendix 3) (27,28). The scope of practice for the Strength and Conditioning profession has expanded and diversified to the point where it is very challenging, and often unrealistic, for each individual to acquire proficiency in all areas. Therefore, specific roles and responsibilities must be outlined and understood by all members of the Strength and Conditioning staff and matched with each person's training and experience. The productivity of a hierarchical (single-leader) work group can be significantly improved by applying the team model to staffing; the same team dynamics that augment the group's effectiveness also tend to enhance individual members' learning and skill acquisition (27).

Program supervision and instruction. Although serious accidents are rare in supervised exercise programs, the liability costs associated with inadequate or lax supervision are very expensive, and the plaintiff's recovery rate in such negligence lawsuits can be high. The main causes of these incidents are poor facility maintenance, defective equipment, and inadequate instruction or supervision. The importance of staffing is readily apparent in each circumstance. For example, Rabinoff (48) reviewed 32 litigations arising from negligent weight training supervision and found that 3 issues were raised by the plaintiff's attorneys in each case: poor instruction (or instructor qualifications); lax/poor supervision; and failure to warn of inherent dangers (in the equipment, facility, or exercise). The standard of care used in each case was based on statements established by the NSCA, ACSM, or SHAPE. A prevalent trend in such litigations is the issue of "professional instructor qualifications," such as appropriate degrees, recognized certifications, training, experience, and continuing education (refer to guideline 2, and Appendices 1 and 2).

Participants in a Strength and Conditioning facility must be properly supervised and instructed at all times to ensure maximum safety, especially because of the athletic, skillful nature of many activities implemented in strength and conditioning programs, in accordance with the dynamic correspondence (54) and practice specificity (49,50) principles. Bucher and Krotee (5) recommend the following cardinal principles of supervision:

- Always be there (mentally and physically).
- Be active and hands-on.
- Be prudent, careful, and prepared (e.g., knowledgeable of proper technique/spotting, program design).
- Be qualified (e.g., accredited degree, CSCS/NSCA-CPT, CPR/AED, First Aid).
- Be vigilant.
- Inform participants of safety and emergency procedures.
- Know participants' health status.
- Monitor and enforce rules and regulations.
- Monitor and scrutinize the environment.

In addition to the physical and mental presence of qualified professionals during strength and conditioning activities, effective instruction and supervision involves a range of practical considerations (2,4,19,21,23,56,59):

- A clear view of all areas of the facility, or at least the zone being supervised by each practitioner and the participants in it. This issue is related to facility design and layout, encompassing equipment placement with respect to visibility, versatility, and accessibility. (refer to standard 4)
- The practitioner's proximity to the group of participants under his/her supervision. This includes the ability to see and communicate clearly with one another, and quick access to participants in need of immediate assistance or spotting.
- The number and grouping of participants to make optimal use of available equipment, space, and time.
- The participants' age(s), experience level(s), and need(s).
- The type of program being conducted (e.g., skillful/explosive free-weight movements versus machine or guided-resistance exercises) and the corresponding need for coaching and spotting.

In an ideal world, strength and conditioning activities should be scheduled to distribute activity throughout the day, and thereby promote an optimal training environment (refer to Appendix 4 for basic guidelines on calculating space needs). Even with careful planning, however, most facilities have times of peak usage (e.g., as a result of team practices and participants' class schedules). Beyond a certain point, it is impractical to simply spread strength and conditioning activities over a wider range of times to maintain an acceptable professional-to-participant ratio. The central issue is to accommodate peak usage times by providing adequate facilities and qualified staff, such that all participants are properly instructed and supervised (refer to guideline 2) (23,31,60). Furthermore, proper techniques, movement mechanics, and safety should be emphasized to minimize injury risk and liability exposure (7,14,25) (also see the NSCA position statements summarized in Appendix 5). Likewise, instructional methods, procedures, and progressions that are consistent with accepted professional practices should be used (45,49,50,54,57,58).

While reasonable steps should be taken to make optimal use of the Strength and Conditioning facility and staff, a potential mismatch between available resources and demand for programs and services exists in many institutions during times of peak usage. As explained below in the Injury Trends, Litigations, and Standard of Care Load section, the combined effects of exponential growth in collegiate/scholastic athlete participation, corresponding liability exposures, and equal opportunity/access laws create a remarkable standard of care load and liability challenge for Strength and Conditioning practitioners and their employers. A 2-pronged approach can thus be recommended.

First, strength and conditioning activities should be planned, and the required number of qualified staff should be present, such that recommended guidelines for minimum average floor space allowance per participant (100 ft^2), minimum professional-to-participant ratios (1:10 junior high school, 1:15 high school, 1:20 college), and number of participants per barbell or training station (up to 3) are applied during peak usage times (2,23,56). In general circumstances, this corresponds to 1 Strength and Conditioning practitioner per 3–4 training stations and/or 1,000 ft^2 area (junior high school); 5 training stations and/or 1,500 ft^2 area (high school); or 6–7 training stations and/or 2,000 ft^2 area (college), respectively. It is extremely important to note that these ratios do not take into account the use of complex lifts such as the weightlifting movements and their derivations, or the use of the primary structural (multijoint) free-weight exercises. Therefore, a much smaller supervision ratio is warranted in these circumstances (e.g., 1:12 instead of 1:20 for college-level). In addition, there are no data regarding how the ratios should differ with training status. Therefore, professional discretion should be used to adjust these guidelines with respect to the practical considerations discussed above.

Second, Strength and Conditioning practitioners and their employers should work together toward a long-term (e.g., 3–5 years) goal of matching the professional-to-participant ratio in the Strength and Conditioning facility to each sport's respective coach-to-athlete ratio. This is relatively straightforward in collegiate settings where the NCAA limits the number of coaches per sport in Division I (NCAA Division I Manual, Bylaw 11.7; updated annually) and also provides sports participation data (refer to Appendix 6; note that coach-to-athlete ratios for individual-event sports are lower than those for team sports) (40). In the absence of similar information in other (e.g., scholastic) settings, such determinations can be made on an individual institution basis; or possibly according to trends within a district, division, or state.

Facility and equipment set-up, inspection, maintenance, repair, and signage. In some cases, Strength and Conditioning professionals are involved in all phases of facility design and layout. Perhaps more commonly, however, they assume responsibility for an existing facility, in which case the opportunities to plan or modify it may be limited. In either case, the Strength and Conditioning practitioner and his/her employer are jointly responsible for maximizing the safety, effectiveness, and efficiency of the facility, such that the allotted space and time can be put to optimal use (24) (also see Appendix 4).

The Strength and Conditioning professional should establish written policies and procedures for equipment/facility selection, purchase, installation, set-up, inspection, cleaning, maintenance, and repair. Safety audits and periodic inspections of equipment, maintenance, repair, and status reports should all be included. Manufacturer-provided user manuals, warranties, and operating guides, and other relevant records (e.g., pertaining to equipment selection, purchase, installation, set-up, inspection, cleaning, maintenance and repair; refer to guideline 6), should be kept on file and followed regarding equipment operation and maintenance (5).

The Strength and Conditioning professional should understand the concept of "product liability," which refers to the legal responsibilities of a product manufacturer and/or vendor if a person sustains injury or damage due primarily to a defect or deficiency in design or manufacturing (56). While this issue applies to manufacturers and vendors, there are actions and/or behaviors that can increase the Strength and Conditioning professional's responsibility, consequently putting him/her at risk for claims or suits (16). The following steps should be taken to minimize liability exposures caused by strength and conditioning equipment (5,11,30):

- Buy the equipment exclusively from reputable manufacturers, and be certain that it meets existing standards and guidelines for professional/commercial (not home) use.
- Use the equipment only for the purpose intended by the manufacturer; do not modify it from the condition in which it was originally sold unless such adaptations are clearly designated and instructions for doing so are included in the product information.
- Post any signage provided by the manufacturer on (or in close proximity to) the equipment.
- Do not allow unsupervised participants to use the equipment.
- Regularly inspect the equipment for damage and wear that may place participants at risk for injury.

Emergency planning and response. An emergency response plan is a written document that details the proper procedures for caring for participants who incur injuries during activity as well as lightning safety (refer to Appendix 7 for sample guidelines). While all Strength and Conditioning facilities should have such a document, it is important to appreciate that the document itself does not save lives. Indeed, it may offer a false sense of security if it is not backed up with appropriate training and preparedness by qualified, professional staff. Therefore, all personnel in Strength and Conditioning facilities must:

- Know the emergency response plan and the proper procedures for dealing with an emergency (e.g., location of phones, activating emergency medical services, designated personnel to care for injured participants, ambulance access, and location of emergency supplies).
- Review and practice emergency policies and procedures regularly (e.g., at least quarterly).
- Maintain current certification in guidelines for cardiopulmonary resuscitation and automated external defibrillators (CPR-AED) as established by the American Heart

Association and International Liaison Committee on Resuscitation (1). Several organizations, such as the American Heart Association, Red Cross, National Safety Council, and St. John Ambulance, offer acceptable certifications. First Aid training and certification may also be necessary if Sports Medicine personnel such as an MD, PA, or ATC are not immediately available.

- Adhere to universal precautions for preventing exposure to and transmission of bloodborne pathogens, as established by the CDC (51), Occupational Safety and Health Administration (OSHA) (43), and the NCAA Sports Medicine Handbook (44). Bloodborne and Airborne Pathogens Training by the National Safety Council may be necessary if personnel are not immediately available to properly respond to exposure to blood or other potentially infectious materials.

Records and record keeping. Documentation is fundamental to the management of strength and conditioning programs and facilities. In addition to developing and maintaining a policies and procedures manual (56), a variety of records should be kept on file (5):

- Personnel credentials
- Professional standards and guidelines
- Policies and procedures for operation and safety, including a written emergency response plan (refer to standard 5; Appendix 7)
- Manufacturer-provided user's manuals, warranties, and operating guides; and equipment selection, purchase, installation, set-up, inspection, cleaning, maintenance, and repair records
- Injury/incident reports, preparticipation medical clearance, and return to participation clearance documents (after the occurrence of an injury, illness, change in health status or an extended period of absence) for each participant under their supervision
- In collegiate and scholastic settings, athletes are required to sign

protective legal documents (e.g., informed consent, agreement to participate, waiver, personal contract; refer to Appendix 8) covering all athletically related activities, including strength and conditioning; however, in other settings, the Strength and Conditioning professional should consider having participants sign such legal documents

- Training logs, progress entries and/ or activity instruction/supervision notes

Legal and medical records should be kept on file as long as possible in the event of an injury claim or suit. Statutes of limitations (i.e., the time in which individuals may file a lawsuit) vary from state to state, so it is good practice to maintain files indefinitely or consult with a legal authority (22). All records should be kept as securely as possible, with limited access by anyone not on staff. Examples of securing records include locked filing cabinets and password-protected computers and computer files. As is the case with other organizational and administrative tasks, it is necessary to have adequately and appropriately trained staff to properly keep and maintain such records.

Equal opportunity and access. Federal, state, and possibly local laws and regulations prohibit discrimination or unequal treatment (e.g., according to race, color, national origin, religion, sex, gender identity and expression, political affiliation, age, disability, veteran status, genetic information, or sexual orientation or other such legal classifications) in most organizations, institutions, and professions. For example, practitioners employed in federally funded educational (i.e., collegiate or scholastic) settings must comply with civil rights statutes including Title IX of the Education Amendments of 1972, which mandates gender equity in providing opportunity and access to athletic facilities, programs, and services. The Strength and Conditioning professional must obey the letter and spirit of these laws when working with participants as well as with staff. If

a Strength and Conditioning professional witnesses any discriminatory or unequal treatment of individuals or teams while performing duties in the scope of employment, the illegal conduct must be immediately reported to a supervisor, compliance department, and/or the general counsel for the employment entity. To protect the interests of the Strength and Conditioning professional, it is also recommended to consult with a private legal entity when the foregoing situation is encountered.

Participation in strength and conditioning activities by children. Resistance training can be an important component of youth fitness, health promotion, and injury prevention. Such programs are safe when properly designed and supervised, and can increase children's strength, motor fitness skills, sports performance, psychosocial well-being, and overall health (12,32,33). Indeed, many of the benefits associated with adult strength and conditioning activities are attainable by prepubescent and adolescent participants who participate in age-specific training (12,32,33). However, it is important for the Strength and Conditioning practitioner to take certain precautions with children (13).

In a 20-year retrospective review of weight training injuries that were evaluated and/or treated in U.S. hospital emergency departments (based on NEISS data), Jones (26) found an alarming incidence of injuries to young children. Children <7 years of age are almost 6 times more likely to be injured than those >15 years of age, with the majority (80%) resulting from playing with or around weight training equipment in the home. The CPSC estimated in 2015 that approximately 8,850 children younger than 5 years are injured each year with exercise equipment (e.g., include stationary bicycles, treadmills, and stair climbers), with an additional 45,725 injuries per year to children 5–14 years of age (https://origin.prod.cpsc.gov/ s3fs-public/2015%20Neiss%20data%

20highlights.pdf Accessed 11/5/ 2017). This has clear implications regarding the importance of supervising children in these age groups, and their exposure to such equipment or facilities. In support of this, Malina (34) reported that estimated injury rates in resistance training programs were 0.176, 0.053, and 0.055 per 100 participant-hours in pre- and early-pubertal youth, respectively, in the programs examined. Twenty-two studies were examined and all used high levels of supervision and low instructor to participant ratios, which was believed to be the reason for the extremely low injury rates.

Another area of potential injury concern for children and pubescents/adolescents is the use of maximum (max) testing (one repitition maximum [1RM]). While Faigenbaum and others (12,13,32,33) have shown max testing to be safe in these age groups, it is emphasized that maintaining proper technique is critical. As an alternative, simple field-based measures such as vertical jump, long jump, and handgrip strength, which have been correlated to 1RM strength may be used (32). Attention to NSCA-prescribed guidelines (7,14,25) for lifting technique should always be followed.

Supplements, ergogenic aids and drugs. The issue of using ergogenic aids, including nutritional supplements and drugs, is complicated by several factors. First, dietary supplements are regulated as foods rather than drugs according to the Dietary Supplement Health and Education Act of 1994. Consequently, concerns exist regarding quality control/assurance and possible consequences for consumers can exist. Strength and Conditioning practitioners are often approached for advice on nutrition and supplementation but may be limited through state laws in what advice can be administered. Spano (55) outlines the roles and responsibilities of the Sport Nutritionist and other professionals who may give nutrition advice. However, the Strength and Conditioning practitioner should be aware of the following:

- The Federal Trade Commission has primary responsibility for advertising claims. Simply stated, advertising for any product, including dietary supplements, must be truthful, substantiated, and not misleading.
- The U.S. Food and Drug Administration has primary responsibility for product labeling claims. The legislation enforced by this agency includes current good manufacturing practice regulations and selected portions of the Federal Food, Drug and Cosmetic Act related to dietary supplements. Note that the U.S. Pharmacopeia and National Formulary, which establishes manufacturing practices for nutritional supplements (i.e., standards for identity, strength, quality, purity, packaging, labeling, and storage), is cited as a primary resource in this legislation.

A second complicating factor is that the boundaries between dietary supplements, drugs, and conventional foods are unclear. This is especially problematic for competitive athletes and coaches, because such products may contain substances that are banned by 1 or more sport governing bodies despite the manufacturer's or vendor's use of terms such as "herbal", "legal", "natural", "organic", "safe and effective", etc. Furthermore, supplement manufacturers are constantly developing new products with different combinations of ingredients, making it more challenging to identify those that may be problematic.

A third factor is that banned substance policies and procedures, testing protocols, and related rules and regulations differ among sport governing bodies at all levels (e.g., USOC, MLB, NBA, NFL, NHL, NCAA, NAIA, NFHS). Therefore, a compound that is permissible according to 1 governing body may be impermissible according to another. The US Anti-Doping Agency (USADA; https://www.usada.org/about/ Accessed 11/5/2017) and the World Anti-Doping Agency (WADA; https://www.wada-ama.org/ Accessed 11/5/2017) have many resources including lists, handbooks, overviews, guides, and FAQ web pages to assist coaches and athletes in ensuring they are avoiding all banned substances, in addition to those provided by a specific sport governing body.

The National Federation of State High School Associations' Sports Medicine Advisory Committee is opposed to the use of dietary supplements to obtain a competitive advantage and has created a position statement to that effect (http://www.nfhs.org/media/1015652/dietary-supplements-position-statement-2015.pdf Accessed 11/5/2017). Furthermore, Strength and Conditioning practitioners at NCAA member institutions need to be aware of NCAA Division I Bylaw 16.5.2.g: "An institution may provide permissible nutritional supplements to a student-athlete for the purpose of providing additional calories and electrolytes. Permissible nutritional supplements do not contain any NCAA banned substances and are identified according to the following classes: carbohydrate/electrolyte drinks, energy bars, carbohydrate boosters, and vitamins and minerals." The NCAA Committee on Competitive Safeguards and Medical Aspects of Sports has subsequently developed lists of permissible versus nonpermissible nutritional supplements, although these will probably change as the market continues to evolve and new products are evaluated.

INJURY TRENDS, LITIGATIONS, AND STANDARD OF CARE LOAD: EFFECTS OF RISING ATHLETIC PARTICIPATION

The lack of qualified instruction and supervision can be identified, either directly or indirectly, as a causative factor in the available information on injuries and litigations associated with weight training. In some cases, this is clearly documented (26,29), while in others it can be inferred. For example, the relatively high coach-to-athlete ratio (and corresponding standard of care) in Olympic-style weightlifting is a likely reason for the low incidence of injury in this sport despite its technical and athletic nature (18,29). Based on the collective information summarized below, it is difficult to overemphasize the fundamental importance of qualified staffing in fulfilling the institution's and Strength and Conditioning professional's shared legal duties for safety, supervision, and standard of care.

Collegiate settings. Year-round strength and conditioning activities are now the rule rather than the exception in collegiate athletic programs. According to NCAA data on student-athlete participation (40), the overall number of participants increased 108% (from 231,445 to 482,533) between 1981–82 and 2014–15. Of special interest are the changes in female participation during this period. The increase in women's participation was 186% (from 74,239 to 212,474) as compared with 63% for men (from 169,800 to 276,599).

The total number of, and time of participation in, athletically related activities has also expanded accordingly. While desirable in terms of preparation, the allowance of nontraditional seasons, off-season skill instruction, and year-round strength and conditioning activities increases each student-athlete's potential for injury and liability exposure, as well as the corresponding standard of care load placed on support staff. The NATA recently published a detailed overview of injury incidence in collegiate athletics, and found that it has risen sharply and consistently with the increase in participants and exposures (39). The potential liability issues for Strength and Conditioning professionals and their employers are further compounded by the exponential rise in female participation and laws mandating equal opportunity and access to athletic programs, services, and facilities (refer to standard 7).

Scholastic settings. The sheer number of high school athletes, and growing emphasis on year-round strength and conditioning activities in scholastic settings, presents a tremendous challenge in terms of demand for standard of care, and accompanying liability exposure. Student-athlete participation in organized high school sports increased 100% (from approximately 4 million to approximately 8 million) between 1971 and 2016 (41). Of special interest are the changes in female participation during this period. The relative increase in girls' participation was 1,000% (from about 0.3 million to 3.3 million) as compared with 24% for boys (from approximately 3.7 million to 4.5 million).

As is the case in collegiate settings, the combination of increasing participation in athletic activities, a corresponding rise in liability exposures, and laws mandating equal opportunity and access creates a remarkable standard of care load and challenge in terms of legal duties for Strength and Conditioning practitioners and their employers (refer to standard 7).

Other populations. Studies examining the incidence and types of weight training injury report varying injury rates, but similar distributions of injury types. Weight training injuries seem to be associated with various training methods (e.g., bodybuilding, powerlifting, Olympic-style weightlifting, fitness/recreational weight training) and equipment (e.g., free weights, machines). Of these, explosive types of training and free-weight apparatus are often incorrectly believed to be inherently more dangerous than other methods. In some of the earliest investigations, Hamill (18) conducted a survey of sport injury rates in 13–16-year-old school children and found that the injury rate in Olympic-style weightlifting (0.0017 per 100 hours) is even lower than that for weight training (0.0035 per 100 hours) and that each of these injury rates were much lower than those observed for other, more popular sports (e.g., basketball 0.03; football 0.10; gymnastics 0.044; athletics 0.57). Calhoon and Fry (6) analyzed weightlifting injury reports at the U.S. Olympic Training Centers over a 6-year period and found that elite weightlifters' injuries were strains, tendinitis, or sprains typical of acute (59.6%) or chronic (30.4%) overuse or

inflammation. Injury rates were calculated to be 0.33 per 100 hours of weightlifting exposure, and the recommended number of training days missed for most (90.5%) injuries was 1 day. These authors concluded that weightlifting injury patterns and rates are similar to those reported for other sports and activities. More recently, Keogh and Winwood (29) compiled data from several investigations and found that bodybuilding had the lowest injury rates (0.024 injuries per 100 hours), with strongman (0.53 injuries per 100 hours) and Highland Games (0.75 injuries per 100 hours) reporting the highest rates. The shoulder, lower back, knee, elbow, and wrist/hand were generally the most commonly injured anatomical locations; strains, tendinitis, and sprains were the most common injury type (29,38). Very few significant differences in any of the injury outcomes were observed as a function of age, sex, competitive standard, or bodyweight class, although Myer (38) found a higher incidence of "accidental" injuries in youth versus adults.

Although risk-factor studies of acute weight training injuries are lacking, recognized contributing factors include poor technique, lack of supervision, skeletal immaturity, and steroid abuse (37). Some of these factors are confirmed in the NSCA (33) and ACSM (12) published statements on youth resistance training. Chronic weight training injuries, however, have been attributed to excessive weight training and improper training techniques (52,53,61). Each of these factors can be positively influenced with qualified instruction and supervision.

PREPARTICIPATION SCREENING AND CLEARANCE

STANDARD 1.1
Strength and Conditioning professionals can only work with participants who have undergone health care provider screening and clearance before participation, in accordance with instructions specified by the AAFP-AAP-ACSM-AMSSM-AOSSM-

AOASM Pre-participation Physical Evaluation Task Force (46), the AHA and ACSM (3,35,36), as well as relevant governing bodies and/or their constituent members (e.g., NCAA/NAIA (44) for collegiate athletes; state legislatures, or individual state high school athletic associations/districts for scholastic athletes). In the collegiate athletics environment, the Athletic Training staff is involved in this process in accordance with NATA guidelines. In recreational activity programs, Strength and Conditioning professionals must require participants to undergo preparticipation screening and clearance in accordance with AHA and ACSM recommendations (3,35,36). For children, the clearance decision must include a determination or certification than the child has reached a level of maturity allowing participation in such activities as addressed in the "Participation in Strength and Conditioning Activities by Children" standards statement (refer to guideline 8).

GUIDELINE 1.1
Strength and Conditioning professionals should cooperate and communicate with each of a training participant's health care providers and provide service in the participant's best interest according to instructions specified by such providers.

PERSONNEL QUALIFICATIONS

GUIDELINE 2.1
The Strength and Conditioning practitioner should acquire a minimum of a bachelor's or master's degree from an accredited college or university (verification by transcript or degree copy) in one or more of the topics comprising the "Scientific Foundations" domain identified in the Certified Strength and Conditioning Specialist (CSCS) Examination Content Description (42) (see Appendix 1), or in a related subject area. An ongoing effort should also be made to acquire knowledge and skills in the other content areas.

GUIDELINE 2.2
The Strength and Conditioning practitioner should achieve and maintain

professional certification(s) with continuing education requirements and a code of ethics, such as the CSCS credential offered through the NSCA (see Appendix 2). Depending on the practitioner's scope of activities, responsibilities, and knowledge requirements, related certifications offered by other governing bodies may also be appropriate.

GUIDELINE 2.3

The productivity of a Strength and Conditioning staff member, as well as learning and skill development of individual members, should be enhanced by aligning a performance team composed of qualified practitioners with interdependent expertise and shared leadership roles (see Appendix 3). Once the team is assembled, respective activities and responsibilities from the domains identified in the Certified Strength and Conditioning Specialist (CSCS) Examination Content Description (42) (see Appendix 1), as well as appropriate liaison assignments, should be delegated according to each member's particular expertise.

PROGRAM SUPERVISION AND INSTRUCTION

STANDARD 3.1

Strength and conditioning programs must provide adequate and appropriate supervision by well-qualified and trained personnel, especially during peak usage times. To ensure maximum health, safety, and instruction, Strength and Conditioning professionals must be physically and mentally present during strength and conditioning activities, have a clear view of the entire facility (or at least the zone being supervised by each practitioner) and the participants in it, be physically close enough to the participants under their supervision to be able to see and clearly communicate with them, and have quick access to those in need of spotting or assistance.

STANDARD 3.2

In conjunction with appropriate safety equipment (e.g., power racks), attentive spotting must be provided for participants performing activities in which free weights are supported on the trunk or moved over the head/face (7,14).

GUIDELINE 3.1

Strength and conditioning activities should be planned, and the requisite number of qualified staff (refer to guideline 2) should be available such that recommended guidelines for minimum average floor space allowance per participant (100 ft^2), minimum professional-to-participant ratios (1:10 or lower junior high school, 1:15 or lower high school, 1:20 or lower college), and number of participants per barbell or training station (3) are achieved during peak usage times (23,56). Younger participants, novices, special populations, or participants engaged in complex-movement strength and conditioning activities should be provided with greater supervision (e.g., 1:12 instead of 1:20; refer to guideline 8). Strength and Conditioning practitioners and their employers should work together toward a long-term goal of matching the professional-to-participant ratio in the Strength and Conditioning facility to each sport's respective coach-to-athlete ratio (refer to Appendix 6).

FACILITY AND EQUIPMENT SET-UP, INSPECTION, MAINTENANCE, REPAIR AND SIGNAGE

STANDARD 4.1

Exercise devices, machines, and equipment, including free weights, must be assembled, set up, and placed in activity areas in full accordance with manufacturer's instructions, tolerances, and recommendations and with accompanying safety signage, instruction placards, notices, and warnings posted or placed according to ASTM standards so as to be noticed by users before use. In the absence of such information, professionals must complete these tasks in accordance with authoritative information available from other sources.

STANDARD 4.2

Before being put into service, all exercise devices, machines, and free weights must be thoroughly inspected and tested by Strength and Conditioning professionals to ensure they are working and performing properly and as intended by the manufacturer.

STANDARD 4.3

Exercise machines, equipment, and free weights must be inspected and maintained at intervals specified by manufacturers. In the absence of such specifications, these items must be regularly inspected and maintained according to a schedule determined by the Strength and Conditioning practitioner based on their knowledge and experience.

STANDARD 4.4

Exercise devices, machines, equipment, and free weights that are in need of repair, as determined by regular inspection or as reported by users, must be immediately removed from use until serviced and repaired and be re-inspected and tested to ensure that they are working properly before being returned to service. If such devices are involved in incidents of injury, legal advisors or risk managers must be consulted for advice before service/repair or destruction.

GUIDELINE 4.1

Strength and Conditioning professionals and their employers should ensure that facilities are appropriate for strength and conditioning activities. Factors to be reviewed and approved before activity include, but are not limited to, floor surface, lighting, room temperature and air exchange (24).

GUIDELINE 4.2

Manufacturer-provided user's manuals, warranties, and operating guides should be preserved and followed (refer to guideline 6).

GUIDELINE 4.3

All equipment, including free weights, should be cleaned and/or disinfected as recommended by the manufacturer and/or OSHA. Users should be directed to wipe down skin-contact surfaces after each use.

EMERGENCY PLANNING AND RESPONSE

STANDARD 5.1

Strength and Conditioning professionals must be trained and certified in current guidelines for CPR established by AHA/ILCOR (1). Training in universal precautions for preventing disease transmission established by the CDC (51) and OSHA (43) is required if personnel are not immediately available to properly respond to exposure to blood or other potentially infectious materials. First Aid training/certification is also necessary if Sports Medicine personnel (e.g., MD or ATC) are not immediately available during strength and conditioning activities. New staff engaged in strength and conditioning activities must comply with this standard within 6 months of employment.

STANDARD 5.2

Strength and Conditioning professionals must develop a written, venue-specific emergency response plan to deal with incidents such as injuries, lightning strikes, and reasonably foreseeable untoward events within each facility. The plan must be posted at strategic areas within each facility and practiced at least quarterly. The emergency response plan must be initially evaluated (e.g., by facility risk managers, legal advisors, medical providers, and/or off-premise emergency response agencies) and modified as necessary at regular intervals. As part of the plan, a readily accessible and working telephone must be immediately available to summon on-premise and/or off-premise emergency response resources.

GUIDELINE 5.1

The components of a written and posted emergency response plan should include access to a physician and/or emergency medical facility when warranted; communication and transportation between the venue and the medical facility; appropriate and necessary emergency care equipment on-site that is quickly accessible; and a thorough understanding of the personnel and procedures associated with the plan by all individuals (refer to Appendix 7).

RECORDS AND RECORD KEEPING

GUIDELINE 6.1

In conjunction with written policies and procedures, Strength and Conditioning professionals should develop and maintain various records including manufacturer-provided user's manuals, warranties, and operating guides; equipment selection, purchase, installation, set-up, inspection, cleaning, maintenance, and repair records; personnel credentials; professional standards and guidelines; safety policies and procedures, including a written emergency response plan (refer to standard 5); training logs, progress entries, and/or activity instruction/supervision notes; and injury/incident reports, preparticipation medical clearance, and return to participation clearance documents. All records should be kept as securely as possible, with limited access by anyone not on staff. Examples of securing records include locked filing cabinets and password-protected computers and computer files. In settings where participants are not otherwise required to sign protective legal documents (e.g., informed consent, agreement to participate, waiver; refer to Appendix 8) covering all athletically related activities, the Strength and Conditioning professional should have such legal documents prepared by an appropriate professional, for participants under his/her supervision. These records should be preserved and maintained for a period determined by the institution where the facility is housed or professional legal advice and consultation.

EQUAL OPPORTUNITY AND ACCESS

STANDARD 7.1

Strength and Conditioning professionals and their employers must provide facilities, training, programs, services, and related opportunities in accordance with all laws, regulations, and requirements, mandating equal opportunity, access, and non-discrimination. Such federal, state, and possibly local laws and regulations apply to most organizations, institutions, and professionals. Discrimination or unequal treatment based on race, color, national origin, religion, sex, gender identity and expression, political affiliation, age, disability, veteran status, genetic information or sexual orientation, or other such legal classifications is generally prohibited.

GUIDELINE 7.1

If a Strength and Conditioning professional witnesses any discriminatory or unequal treatment of individuals while performing duties in the scope of employment, the illegal conduct must be immediately reported to a supervisor, compliance department, and/or the general counsel for the employment entity. To protect the interests of the Strength and Conditioning professional, it is also recommended to consult with a private legal counsel when the foregoing situation is encountered.

PARTICIPATION IN STRENGTH AND CONDITIONING ACTIVITIES BY CHILDREN

GUIDELINE 8.1

Children younger than 7 years should not be permitted to engage in strength and conditioning activities with free weights or exercise devices/machines in facilities designed for use by adults and adolescents and should be denied access to such training areas. Other forms of strength and conditioning activities may be beneficial for such children, and should be recommended according to the established guidelines (12,32,33), and with a greater degree of instruction and supervision than that supplied to adolescents and adults. Children participating in such activities should be cleared as specified in the NSCA's "Standard for Preparticipation Screening and Clearance" (refer to standard 1).

GUIDELINE 8.2

Children between 7 and 14 years of age who have reached a level of physical, emotional, and intellectual maturity allowing participation in specified strength and conditioning activities, as determined and certified by their medical care provider (or by the Strength and Conditioning professional acting in concert with a child's medical care provider), and after clearance for participation as specified in the NSCA's "Standard for Pre-participation Screening and Clearance" (refer to standard 1), should be individually assessed by the Strength and Conditioning professional in conjunction with the child's parent(s)/guardian(s)/custodian(s) to determine whether such children may engage in such activities in areas containing free weights and exercise devices/machines generally used by adults and older children. If so permitted, such activities should be developed and implemented according to established guidelines (12,32,33) and with a greater degree of instruction and supervision than that supplied to adolescents and adults.

GUIDELINE 8.3

Children who are 14 years of age and older, according to the Strength and Conditioning practitioner's professional judgment, have reached a level of physical, emotional, and intellectual maturity, allowing them to engage in specified Strength and Conditioning activities (provided they have been granted parental consent and been cleared for participation as specified in the NSCA's "Standard for Pre-participation Screening and Clearance"; refer to standard 1), may engage in such activities in areas containing free weights and exercise devices/machines generally used by adults and with a greater degree of instruction and supervision than that supplied to adult populations while training.

SUPPLEMENTS, ERGOGENIC AIDS, AND DRUGS

STANDARD 9.1

Strength and Conditioning professionals must not prescribe, recommend, or provide drugs, controlled substances or supplements that are illegal, prohibited, or harmful to participants for any purpose including enhancing athletic performance, conditioning, or physique. Only those substances that are lawful (via third-party testing) and have been scientifically proven to be beneficial, or at least not harmful, may be recommended to participants by Strength and Conditioning professionals, and only to individuals age 18 or above and not in an individualized manner.

APPENDIX 1. STRENGTH AND CONDITIONING PRACTITIONER DEFINITION

In 1996, 2004, and again in 2012, the NSCA Certification Commission (changed to Certification Committee in 2008) and its examination service conducted a Job Analysis study with the purpose of surveying the activities, responsibilities, and knowledge requirements of a Certified Strength and Conditioning Specialist (CSCS). The results were used to describe the job activities of the CSCS in sufficient detail to provide a basis for the development of a professional, job-related certification examination that will certify strength and conditioning specialists as competent professionals. An early step in the process was to create a "practitioner" definition. Essentially, this definition is a job description that establishes the legal and professional scope of practice of the appropriate activities of a CSCS (refer to Appendix 2):

Certified Strength and Conditioning Specialists are professionals who apply foundational knowledge in a practical setting to assess, motivate, educate, and train athletes for the primary goal of improving sport performance. They conduct general physical and sport-specific testing sessions, design and implement safe and effective strength training and conditioning programs, and provide guidance for athletes in nutrition and injury prevention. Recognizing their area of expertise is separate and distinct from the medical, dietetic, athletic training, and sport coaching fields; Certified Strength and Conditioning Specialists consult with and refer athletes to these professionals when appropriate.

The 1996 CSCS Job Analysis study evaluated the results of a questionnaire sent to randomly selected NSCA members who were CSCS-certified as of October 1996. Respondents were asked to assign an importance to 112 tasks that a CSCS typically performs on the job. From these data, the NSCA Certification Commission's CSCS Job Analysis Committee determined the inclusion criteria of the tasks (5 of the original 112 were excluded), the distribution of tasks within each CSCS examination domain and its subcategories, as well as distribution of the examination question type (i.e., recall, application, and analysis) within each domain and its subcategories. The document resulting from the CSCS Job Analysis study is the "CSCS Examination Content Outline," which forms the basis for the Certified Strength and Conditioning Specialist (CSCS) Examination Content Description (42), an examination preparation resource available through the NSCA. The 2004 questionnaire was sent to certified individuals and the new results were used to change the format of the examination, with more emphasis placed on the practical/applied section. In 2012, survey data results were reviewed by the CSCS Job Analysis Committee and decision rules were established. These rules were used to determine which tasks were appropriate for assessment and inclusion in the final test content outline.

CSCS EXAMINATION CONTENT OUTLINE

Adapted from: Certified Strength and Conditioning Specialist (CSCS) Examination Content Description (42)

Scientific foundations

I. Exercise Sciences (59 questions)
   A. Apply knowledge of muscle anatomy and physiology.
   B. Apply knowledge of neuromuscular anatomy and physiology.
   C. Apply knowledge of basic principles of biomechanics regarding exercise selection, execution, and sport performance.

D. Apply knowledge of bone and connective tissue (tendons and ligaments) anatomy and physiology.

E. Apply knowledge of bioenergetics and metabolism.

F. Apply knowledge of neuroendocrine physiology.

G. Apply knowledge of cardiopulmonary anatomy and physiology.

H. Apply knowledge of physiological adaptations to exercise and training.

I. Apply knowledge of the anatomical, physiological, and biomechanical differences of athletes (e.g., age, sex, training status, specific sport or activity).

J. Apply knowledge of psychological techniques used to enhance the training and performance.

II. Nutrition (21 questions)

A. Apply basic knowledge of nutritional factors affecting health and performance.

B. Apply basic strategies for manipulating food choices and training methods to maximize performance.

C. Recognize signs, symptoms, and behaviors associated with eating disorders and altered eating habits.

D. Apply basic knowledge of the effects, risks, and alternatives of common performance-enhancing substances and methods.

III. New "untried" questions (15 non-scored questions)

Practical/applied

I. Exercise Technique (38 questions)

A. Teach and evaluate resistance training exercise technique.

B. Teach and evaluate plyometric exercise technique.

C. Teach and evaluate speed/sprint technique (e.g., resisted and assisted sprinting, speed-strength).

D. Teach and evaluate agility technique (e.g., forward, backward, and lateral movements; turn, transition, acceleration, and deceleration maneuvers).

E. Teach and evaluate metabolic conditioning/energy systems development.

F. Teach and evaluate flexibility exercise technique.

G. Teach spotting procedures and techniques.

II. Program Design (39 questions)

Based on an athlete's health status, training age, capabilities, and training goals, design training programs that maximize performance and minimize injury potential by

A. Incorporating various training methods and modes.

B. Selecting exercises.

C. Applying the principles of exercise order.

D. Determining and assigning exercise intensities (e.g., load, resistance, heart rate).

E. Determining and assigning training volumes (defined as sets × reps).

F. Determining and assigning work/rest periods, recovery and unloading, and training.

G. Determining and assigning exercise progression (e.g., mode, intensity, duration, frequency).

H. Applying the principles of periodization.

I. Designing programs for an injured athlete during the reconditioning period (e.g., assigning exercises for a given injury or condition in collaboration with sport medicine professionals).

III. Organization and Administration (13 questions)

A. Determine the design, layout, and organization of the strength and conditioning facility (e.g., flooring, ceiling height, mirror placement, ventilation, lighting, characteristics of the equipment) based on athletic needs and industry standards.

B. Determine the primary duties and responsibilities of the members of the strength and conditioning staff.

C. Determine the policies and procedures associated with the operation of the strength and conditioning facility (e.g., facility/equipment cleaning and maintenance, rules, scheduling, emergency procedures).

D. Create a safe training environment within the strength and conditioning facility.

IV. Testing and Evaluation (20 questions)

A. Select and administer tests to maximize test reliability and validity.

B. Administer test protocols and procedures to ensure reliable data collection.

C. Evaluate and interpret test results.

V. New "untried" questions (15 non-scored questions)

APPENDIX 2. CERTIFIED STRENGTH AND CONDITIONING SPECIALIST (CSCS) PROGRAM

The CSCS program was initiated in 1985 to identify individuals who possess the knowledge and skills to design and implement safe and effective strength and conditioning programs. This certification program encourages a higher level of competence among practitioners, which ultimately raises the quality of strength training and conditioning programs for athletes by those who are CSCS-certified.

A CSCS educates and trains primarily athletes in proper strength training and conditioning practices. Strength and Conditioning CSCS professionals work in a variety of environments, including high school, college, university, and professional institutions, sports medicine clinics, health, and fitness clubs, corporate wellness centers, and in professional sports. Competencies assessed in the CSCS examination are determined through a Job Analysis conducted by an independent professional examination service based on input from current Strength and Conditioning professionals. Every step in the process leading to the development of valid certification examinations meets the stringent guidelines of the National Commission for Certifying Agencies (NCCA). Pass/fail rates and reliability statistics are published annually.

Writers of the examinations include renowned practitioners, researchers, educators, and psychometricians. Although there are many certification programs associated with physical training, the CSCS certification examination program is 1 of only 2 that have been specifically designed to assess the competencies of those who strength train and condition athletes.

ACCREDITATION

In 1993 the NSCA Certification Commission certification program became the first fitness-related certification accredited by the esteemed NCCA*. The rigorous CSCS and NSCA-Certified Personal Trainer (NSCA-CPT) examinations are among the most challenging in the industry.

*Note: The NCCA is the accreditation body of the Institute for Credentialing Excellence, a nonprofit nongovernment agency that promotes excellence in competency assurance for practitioners in all occupations and professions. The NCCA measures the ability of certifying organizations in any industry to accurately discriminate between qualified and unqualified professionals. To earn NCCA recognition, a credentialing body must demonstrate an ability to develop and administer psychometrically sound examinations that effectively differentiate qualification level through a series of criteria, including:

- The certifying organization is responsible for all decisions pertaining to certification and recertification (including, but not limited to, examination content, eligibility requirements, grievance and disciplinary policies, setting fees, program operation, etc.) without being subject to approval by any other body.
- The examination is developed from a Job Analysis study.
- Pass/fail rates and reliability statistics are a matter of public record.
- Examination development involves qualified professionals, such as content experts and psychometricians with expertise in examination development.

Accreditation for professional or personnel certification programs provides impartial, third-party validation that the program has met recognized national and international credentialing industry standards for development, implementation, and maintenance of certification programs.

CSCS EXAMINATION FORMAT

To earn the CSCS credential, candidates must pass a rigorous examination that consists of 2 sections. A candidate must pass both sections to be CSCS-certified (and may retake any section not passed). The first section, called "Scientific Foundations", consists of 80 scored multiple-choice questions in the areas of:

- Exercise Sciences (Anatomy, Exercise Physiology, Biomechanics, Sport Psychology)
- Nutrition

The second section, "Practical/Applied", consists of 110 scored multiple-choice questions, 30–40 of which contain video and/or images that assess competencies in exercise techniques, functional anatomy, and testing procedures with the exercises, muscles, and/or joints shown. The areas covered include:

- Exercise Technique
- Program Design
- Organization and Administration
- Testing and Evaluation

CONTINUING EDUCATION PROGRAM

The purpose of having continuing education as part of a certification program is to encourage certificants to stay abreast of evolving knowledge and skills in the profession, and, in doing so, to promote the ongoing competency of those who are certified. The NSCA requires each certificant to do the following to remain certified:

- Complete 6 continuing education units (CEUs) or a prorated amount of CEUs if certified within the 3-year reporting period.
- Maintain current CPR certification.
- Submit a completed CEU Reporting Form and recertification fee.
- Maintain documentation of activities listed on the CEU Reporting Form.

The NSCA is committed to certifying individuals who demonstrate the knowledge and skills necessary to design and implement safe and effective strength training and conditioning and personal training practices. With the credibility possessed by the CSCS and NSCA-CPT examinations comes the responsibility to ensure the integrity of the credentials awarded. This philosophy implies that the responsibility of its certificants is not limited to the well-being of the athletes and/or clients, and the reputation of others in their field; with the overall goal being an improvement of health and well-being for all.

The NSCA is dedicated to maintaining a high standard for its members and certificants. The following Code of Ethics assures that CSCS and NSCA-CPT certificants are aware of the standards of ethical behavior that should be followed in the practice of their profession.

Principle 1: Certificants shall respect the rights, welfare, and dignity of all individuals.

1.1. Certificants shall not discriminate on the basis of race, color, national origin, religion, sex, gender identity and expression, political affiliation, age, disability, veteran status, genetic information or sexual orientation, or other such legal classifications.

1.2. Certificants shall provide competent, fair, and equal treatment to all individuals.

1.3. Certificants shall preserve the confidentiality of personal and privileged information of the athlete, client, or the NSCA.

1.4. Certificants shall not release any information to a third party not involved with the athlete's or client's care without a written release unless required by law.

Principle 2: Certificants shall comply with all applicable state, local and federal laws, and NSCA Bylaws, policies, and procedures.

2.1. Certificants shall comply with all institutional guidelines.

2.2. Certificants shall comply with all copyright laws.

2.3. Certificants shall be familiar with and follow the NSCA Bylaws and all applicable policies, procedures, rules, standards and guidelines.

2.4. Certificants shall not condone or engage in any illegal or unethical behavior.

Principle 3: Certificants shall maintain and promote high standards.

3.1. Certificants shall not misrepresent, either directly or indirectly, their skills, training, professional credentials, identity, or services.

3.2. Certificants shall only provide services they are qualified to provide through education or experience and which are allowed by practice acts and other pertinent regulations.

3.3. Certificants shall refer athlete or client to more qualified fitness, medical, or health care professional when appropriate.

3.4. Certificants who are researchers or educators shall maintain and promote ethical conduct in research and educational activities.

3.5. Certificants should strive to continuously improve knowledge, skills, and techniques to protect the athlete or client from injury.

Principle 4: Certificants shall not engage in any behavior or form of conduct that adversely reflects on the NSCA.

4.1. Certificants should conduct themselves personally and professionally in a manner that does not compromise their professional responsibility.

4.2. Certificants shall not place financial gain above the welfare of the NCSA, athlete's or client's and shall not in any arrangement exploit the NSCA, athlete or client.

4.3. Certificants shall avoid substance abuse and, if necessary, seek rehabilitation for chemical dependency.

Certificants should also strive to safeguard the public by reporting violations of this Code of Ethics.

APPENDIX 3. STRENGTH AND CONDITIONING PERFORMANCE TEAM DEVELOPMENT

Teams are preferable to single-leader groups when there is a need for collective work products (i.e., multiple skills, judgments, and experiences) by members working together in real time, shifting leadership roles, and mutual as well as individual accountability (27,28). By contrast, single-leader/hierarchical work groups are appropriate when the sum of independent workers' contributions is adequate, singular rather than shared leadership is effective, task(s) and corresponding solution(s) are familiar, workers' skills can be applied productively without interaction (other than sharing information), and speed and efficiency have priority over extra performance results (27,28).

Extraordinarily demanding challenges are the driving forces behind high-performance teams. Common features of such teams include (27,28):

- Members are committed to a clear mission, common approach, collaboration, and mutual accountability and responsibility.

- Expectations and goals are high but achievable, and performance evaluation is based on results.
- Roles are interdependent; leadership is shared; abilities, experiences, expertise, knowledge, skills, and talents are complementary; contribution, participation, and influence are balanced.
- Effective task performance is facilitated by encouraging and rewarding creativity, innovation, and risk taking in all decision making or problem solving activities.

The strength and conditioning staff can be aligned through hiring of practitioners with formal education and specialization in specific scientific foundations (e.g., anatomy, exercise physiology, biomechanics, sport psychology) (42). An assembled team allows for cooperative expertise by practitioners with complementary skills and provides an educational opportunity for staff members to gain knowledge outside their specialization by working with outside liaisons. The table below provides a practical example of a strength and conditioning performance team. The director of strength and conditioning is responsible for delineating the appropriate duties and responsibilities to the rest of the strength and conditioning staff for program design, exercise technique, organization and administration, and testing and evaluation (56).

Scientific foundations education/Expertise	Practical and applied activities/Responsibilities	Liaison assignment(s)
Exercise/sport anatomy; biomechanics	Exercise technique; testing and evaluation; rehabilitation and reconditioning	Exercise/sport scientist; team coaches; sports medicine team
Exercise/sport physiology	Program design; testing and evaluation	Exercise/sport scientist; team coaches
Exercise/sport nutrition	Nutrition	Exercise/sport scientist; sport nutritionist/dietitian
Exercise/sport pedagogy	Program design; exercise technique; organization and administration	Exercise/sport scientist; team coaches; athletic administration
Exercise/sport psychology; motor learning	Exercise technique; rehabilitation and reconditioning	Exercise/scientist; sports medicine team; team coaches
Training methodology	Program design; organization and administration	Exercise/sport scientist; team coaches; athletic administration
Kinesiology; physiotherapy; sports medicine	Rehabilitation and reconditioning	Sports medicine team

Area	Examples	Formula
Prone and supine exercises	Bench press; lying triceps extension	Actual weight bench length (6–8 ft) + safety space cushion of 3 ft multiplied by suggested user space for weight bench width of 7 ft + safety space cushion of 3 ft. Example: If using a 6 ft long weight bench for the bench press exercise (6 ft + 3 ft) × (7 ft + 3 ft) = 90 ft (2)
Standing exercises	Biceps curl; upright row	Actual bar length (4–7 ft) + double-wide safety space cushion of 6 ft multiplied by suggested user space for standing exercise width of 4 ft. Example: If using a 4 ft curl bar for the biceps curl exercise (4 ft + 6 ft) × (4 ft) = 40 ft (2)
Standing exercises in a rack	Back squat; shoulder press	Actual bar length (5–7 ft) + double-wide safety space cushion of 6 ft multiplied by suggested user space for standing exercise in a rack width of 8–10 ft. Example: If using a 7 ft. Olympic bar for the back squat exercise (7 ft + 6 ft) × (10 ft) = 130 ft (2)
Olympic lifting area	Power clean	Lifting platform length (typically 8 ft) + perimeter walkway safety space cushion of 4 ft multiplied by lifting platform width (typically 8 ft) + perimeter walkway safety space cushion of 4 ft. Example: (8 ft + 4 ft) × (8 ft + 4 ft) = 144 ft (2)

APPENDIX 4. STRENGTH AND CONDITIONING FACILITY SCHEDULING

TABLE D1. CALCULATIONS FOR SPACE NEEDS (24)

Note: Many facilities use combination platforms and racks (multi-purpose training stations) as a way to save space and allow participants to complete several exercises in 1 location. Accordingly, the standing rack and Olympic lifting area calculations above should be combined.

APPENDIX 5. STRENGTH AND CONDITIONING TRAINING PLAN DEVELOPMENT

A detailed discussion of developing a Strength and Conditioning training plan is beyond the scope of this project. For more specific information on program design, the Strength and Conditioning practitioner should refer to Chapters 17–21 of Essentials of Strength Training and Conditioning, 4th edition (15) as well as the NSCA position statements listed below.

NSCA Position Statements (https://www.nsca.com/nsca-tools-and-resources/); PDF files (Accessed 11/5/2017).

Long-Term Athletic Development–2016

Androgen and Human Growth Hormone Use–2009

Youth Resistance Training–2009

APPENDIX 6. NCAA DIVISION I ATHLETE-TO-COACH RATIOS

TABLE F1: NCAA DIVISION I OVERALL CHAMPIONSHIP SPORTS PARTICIPATION (2014–15) AND RESULTING ATHLETE-TO-COACH RATIOS, AS THE ONLY DIVISION WITH LIMITATIONS ON NUMBER OF COACHES (NCAA DIVISION I MANUAL, BYLAW 11.7) (40)

TABLE F2: NCAA DIVISION I MEN'S CHAMPIONSHIP SPORTS PARTICIPATION (2014–15) AND RESULTING ATHLETE-TO-COACH RATIOS, BY SPORT (40)

TABLE F3: NCAA DIVISION I WOMEN'S CHAMPIONSHIP SPORTS PARTICIPATION (2014–15) AND RESULTING ATHLETE-TO-COACH RATIOS, BY SPORT (40)

APPENDIX 7. EMERGENCY CARE AND PLANNING

Source: NCAA Sports Medicine Handbook (44)

EMERGENCY CARE AND COVERAGE

Reasonable attention to all possible preventive measures will not eliminate sports injuries. Each scheduled practice or contest of an institution-sponsored intercollegiate athletics event, as well as out-of-season practices and skills sessions, should include an emergency plan. Like student-athlete welfare in general, a plan is a shared responsibility of the athletics department; administrators, coaches; and medical personnel should all play a role in the establishment of the plan, procurement of resources; and understanding by all parties. Components of such a plan should include

1. The presence of a person qualified and delegated to render emergency care to a stricken participant;
2. The presence or planned access to a physician for prompt medical evaluation of the situation, when warranted;
3. Planned access to early defibrillation;
4. Planned access to a medical facility, including a plan for communication and transportation between the athletics site and the medical facility for prompt medical services, when warranted. Access to a working telephone

Sport	Teams	Athletes	Average squad size	Limit on no. of coaches	Athletes per coach
Total (men + women)	6,475	175,952		112	
Average (39 sports)			27.2	2.9	9.5

Sport	Teams	Athletes	Average squad size	Limit on no. of coaches	Athletes per coach
Baseball	295	10,396	35.2	3	11.8
Basketball	345	5,432	15.7	4	3.9
Cross country	311	4,845	15.6	2	7.8
Fencing	20	383	19.2	2	9.6
Football	250	27,873	111.5	11	10.1
Golf	297	2,947	9.9	2	5.0
Gymnastics	15	304	20.3	3	6.8
Ice hockey	59	1,638	27.8	3	9.3
Lacrosse	68	3,109	45.7	3	15.2
Rifle	17	131	7.7	2	3.9
Skiing	11	155	14.1	2	7.0
Soccer	200	5,738	28.7	3	9.6
Swimming/diving	134	3,839	28.6	3	9.5
Tennis	258	2,678	10.4	2	5.2
Track (indoor)	257	10,174	39.6	3	13.2
Track (outdoor)	278	11,067	39.8	3	13.3
Volleyball	21	405	19.3	3	6.4
Water polo	22	566	25.7	2	12.9
Wrestling	76	2,520	33.2	3	11.1
Total	2,934	94,200		59	
Average (19 sports)			32.1	3.1	10.4

or other telecommunications device, whether fixed or mobile, should be assured;

5. All necessary emergency equipment should be at the site or quickly accessible. Equipment should be in good operating condition, and personnel must be trained in advance to use it properly. This equipment should include but is not limited to, an AED, a bag-valve mask, advanced airway tools, a spine board, and other stabilization supplies for the head and neck, splints, and bleeding control materials, such as a tourniquet and large sterile dressings. Sports medicine providers should be trained to use emergency equipment before deployment. In addition, emergency information about the student-athlete should be available both on campus and while traveling for use by medical personnel;

6. An inclement weather policy that includes provisions for decision making and evacuation plans (See NCAA Guideline 1E);

7. A thorough understanding by all parties, including the leadership of visiting teams, of the personnel and procedures associated with the emergency care plan;

8. Certification in CPR techniques, first aid, and prevention of disease transmission (as outlined by OSHA guidelines) should be required for all athletics personnel associated with practices, competitions, skill instruction, and strength and conditioning. New staff engaged in these activities should comply with these rules within 6 months of employment;

9. A member of the institution's sports medicine staff should be empowered to have the unchallengeable authority to cancel or modify a workout for health and safety (i.e., environmental changes), as he or she deems appropriate;

10. Institutions should ensure that the emergency action plan incorporates roles and responsibilities of coaching staff, medical staff, spectators, and others during injury evaluation/response on the field, to ensure appropriate first response and medical evaluation. The emergency action plan should provide that appropriate medical staff have access to the injured athlete without interference; and

11. Institutions should have on file and annually update an emergency action plan for each athletics venue

Sport	Teams	Athletes	Average squad size	Limit on no. of coaches	Athletes per coach
Basketball	343	4,984	14.5	4	3.6
Bowling	34	299	8.8	2	4.4
Cross country	342	6,031	17.6	2	8.8
Fencing	24	397	16.5	2	8.3
Field hockey	77	1,732	22.5	3	7.5
Golf	259	2,170	8.4	2	4.2
Gymnastics	61	1,085	17.8	3	5.9
Ice hockey	35	846	24.2	3	8.4
Lacrosse	106	3,172	29.9	3	10.0
Rifle	24	151	6.3	2	3.2
Rowing	88	5,668	64.4	3	21.5
Skiing	12	175	14.6	2	7.3
Soccer	326	8,963	27.5	3	9.2
Softball	289	6,044	20.9	3	7.0
Swimming/diving	195	5,393	27.7	3	9.2
Tennis	318	2,912	9.2	2	4.6
Track (indoor)	319	12,816	40.2	3	13.4
Track (outdoor)	329	13,075	39.7	3	13.2
Volleyball	328	5,165	15.7	3	5.2
Water polo	32	674	21.1	2	10.5
TOTAL	3,541	81,752		53	
Average (20 sports)			23.1	2.7	8.7

to respond to student-athlete catastrophic injuries and illnesses, including but not limited to, concussions, heat illness, spine injury, cardiac arrest respiratory distress (e.g., asthma), bleeding and sickle-cell trait collapses. All athletics health care providers and coaches, including strength and conditioning coaches, sport coaches and all athletics personnel conducting activities with student-athletes, should review and practice the plan at least annually.

LIGHTNING SAFETY

Lightning is the most consistent and significant weather hazard that may affect intercollegiate athletics. Within the United States, the National Oceanic and Atmospheric Administration (NOOA) estimates that 40 fatalities and about 10 times that many injuries occur from lightning strikes every year. NOAA estimates that as many as 62 percent of lightning strike fatalities occur during outdoor organized sport activities. Although the probability of being struck by lightning is low, the odds are significantly greater when a storm is in the area and proper safety precautions are not followed.

Education and prevention are the keys to lightning safety. Prevention should begin long before any intercollegiate athletics event or practice occurs by being proactive and having a lightning safety plan in place. The following steps are recommended to mitigate the lightning hazard:

A. Develop a lightning safety plan for each outdoor venue. At a minimum, the plan should include the following:
  1. The use of lightning safety slogans to simplify and summarize essential information and knowledge. For example, the following slogan from the National Lightning Safety Institute is an effective guide: "If you see it, flee it; if you can hear it, clear it." This slogan reflects the fact that on the first sound of thunder, lightning is likely within 8 to 10 miles and capable of striking your location. No punishment or retribution should be applied to someone who chooses to evacuate if perceiving that his or her

life is in danger because of severe weather.

2. Designation of a person to monitor threatening weather and to notify the chain of command who can make the decision to remove a team, game personnel, television crews, and spectators from an athletics site or event. That person must have recognized and unchallengeable authority to suspend activity.

3. Planned instructions/announcements for participants and spectators, designation of warning and all clear signals, proper signage, and designation of safer places from the lightning hazard.

4. Daily monitoring of local weather reports before any practice or event, and a reliable and accurate source of information about severe weather that may form during scheduled intercollegiate athletics events or practices. Of special note should be National Weather Service-issued thunderstorm "watches" or "warnings" and the warning signs of developing thunderstorms in the area, such as high winds or darkening skies. A "watch" means that conditions are favorable for severe weather to develop in an area; a "warning" means that severe weather has been reported in an area and for everyone to take the proper precautions. It should be noted that neither watches nor warnings are issued for lightning. An NOAA weather radio is particularly helpful in providing this information.

5. Identification of, and a mechanism for ensuring access to, the closest safer buildings, vehicles, and locations to the field or playing area, and an estimate of how long it takes to evacuate to that location for all personnel at the event. A safer building or location is defined as:a. Any fully enclosed building normally occupied or frequently used by people, with plumbing and/or electrical wiring that acts to electrically ground the structure. Avoid using the shower, plumbing facilities, and electrical appliances, and stay away from open windows and doorways during a thunderstorm.b. In the absence of a sturdy, frequently inhabited building, any vehicle with a hard metal roof (neither a convertible nor a golf cart) with the windows shut provides a measure of safety. The hard metal frame and roof, not the rubber tires, are what protects occupants by dissipating lightning current around the vehicle and not through the occupants. It is important not to touch the metal framework of the vehicle. Some athletics events rent school buses as safer locations to place around open courses or fields.

B. For large-scale events, continuous monitoring of the weather should occur from the time pre-event activities begin throughout the event.

C. Venue-specific activity-suspension, venue evacuation, and activity-resumption plans:

1. On the first sound of thunder, lightning is likely within 8 to 10 miles and capable of striking your location. Please note that thunder may be hard to hear if there is an athletics event going on, particularly in stadia with large crowds. Lightning can strike from blue sky and in the absence of rain. At least 10 percent of lightning occurs when there is no rainfall and when blue sky is often visible somewhere in the sky, especially with summer thunderstorms. Lightning can, and does, strike 10 (or more) miles away from the rain shaft. Be aware of local weather patterns and review local weather forecasts before an outdoor practice or event.

2. Ensure a safe and orderly evacuation from the venue with announcements, signage, safety information in programs, and entrances that can also serve as mass exits. Planning should account for the time it takes to move a team and crowd to their designated safer locations. Individuals should not be allowed to enter the outdoor venue and should be directed to the safer location.

3. Avoid using landline telephones except in emergency situations. People have been killed while using a landline telephone during a thunderstorm. Cellular or cordless phones are safe alternatives to a landline phone, particularly if the person and the antenna are located within a safer structure or location, and if all other precautions are followed.

4. To resume athletics activities, lightning safety experts recommend waiting 30 minutes after both the last sound of thunder and last flash of lightning. A useful slogan is "half an hour since thunder roars, now it's safe to go outdoors." At night, be aware that lightning can be visible at a much greater distance than during the day as clouds are being lit from the inside by lightning. This greater distance may mean that the lightning is no longer a significant threat. At night, use both the sound of thunder and seeing the lightning channel itself to decide on resetting the 30-minute "return-to-play" clock before resuming outdoor athletics activities.

D. Emergency care protocols: People who have been struck by lightning do not carry an electrical charge. Therefore, CPR is safe for the responder. If possible, an injured person should be moved to a safer location before starting CPR. Lightning-strike victims who show signs of cardiac or respiratory arrest need prompt emergency help. If you are in a 911 community, call for help. Prompt, aggressive CPR has been highly effective for the survival of victims of lightning strike. Automatic external defibrillators are a safe and effective means of reviving persons in cardiac arrest. Planned access to early defibrillation should be part of your emergency plan. However, CPR should never be delayed while searching for an AED.

Note: Weather watchers, real-time weather forecasts and commercial weather-warning, and lightning monitoring devices or services are all tools that can be used to aid in the monitoring, notification, and decision-making regarding stoppage of play, evacuation, and return to play.

APPENDIX 8. PROTECTIVE LEGAL DOCUMENTS

Notes: This appendix provides general legal information. Protective legal documents should not be adopted or used in any context without individualized legal advice. The information in this appendix has been adapted with permission from an article by JoAnn Eickhoff-Shemek, entitled "Distinguishing Protective Legal Documents", published in the ACSM's Journal of Health and Fitness (8).

TYPES OF PROTECTIVE LEGAL DOCUMENTS

Institutions such as universities/colleges and high schools often require athletes to read and comprehend, and sign some type of protective legal document(s) before participation in athletically related activities, including strength and conditioning. These documents can help protect the institution and its employees from potentially costly legal claims and lawsuits. The law involving protective legal documents is quite complex, and understanding their function and the specific legal protection they provide is often confusing.

Several types of protective legal documents exist. Three that are commonly used in the health/fitness field may be applicable in Strength and Conditioning settings: informed consent, agreement to participate, and waiver. Each provides protection from lawsuits arising from certain types of injuries that can occur while participating in activities, as explained below.

CAUSES OF INJURY ASSOCIATED WITH PHYSICAL ACTIVITY

There are 3 causes of injury associated with physical activity: inherent risks, negligence, and extreme forms of conduct (10).

Inherent risks

As the term implies, these risks are inherent in the activity. Generally, injuries caused by inherent risks are accidental in nature, not preventable, and no one's fault. The informed consent and agreement to participate documents provide the best legal protection for lawsuits arising from such injuries. Although actual sections and content of protective documents vary (and depend upon state law), the following are generally included in informed consent and agreement to participate documents:

Informed consent.
- Purpose of the activity
- Risks of the activity*
- Benefits of the activity
- Confidentiality
- Inquiries
- Signatures

Agreement to participate.
- Nature of the activity
- Possible consequences of injury*
- Behavioral expectations of the participant
- Condition of the participant
- Concluding statement
- Signatures

*Note: "assumption of risk" language.

A section within each of these documents is devoted to informing the participant of the potential risks, including those inherent in the activity. It is important that this section carefully describes these risks (e.g., types of accidents that might occur and the consequences of these accidents), and that the language used is understandable to the person who will be signing it. This provides an "assumption of risk" defense, meaning the participant knew and fully understood the risks, appreciated the risks, and voluntarily assumed them. In general, the law does not allow individuals to recover compensation for injuries resulting from assumed risks.

Negligence

Injuries can be caused by negligence, which is a failure to act as a reasonable and prudent professional would act under the circumstances. Participants can

be injured by negligent acts of the Strength and Conditioning staff (e.g., failure to inspect/maintain exercise equipment, failure to provide CPR or First Aid when needed). A waiver document, also called a prospective release, provides the best legal protection for lawsuits arising from injuries caused by negligence. Once again, while the actual sections and content of such documents vary depending on state law, waiver documents generally include exculpatory clause; description of risks ("assumption of risk" language); indemnification language (may not be valid); severability clause; affirmation of legal capacity; and signatures.

The "exculpatory clause" is a key section within the waiver explicitly stating that the participant releases the Strength and Conditioning facility for any liability associated with negligence by the facility or its employees. This clause, which must be written very carefully to be enforceable, provides evidence that the participant gave up (waived) his/her right to file a negligence lawsuit against the facility. However, the exculpatory clause does not provide protection from lawsuits arising from injuries because of inherent risks, and an "assumption of risk" section is often added to the waiver for this purpose.

Extreme forms of conduct

Injuries can also be caused by extreme forms of conduct (often called gross negligence, willful and wanton conduct, or reckless conduct). For example, if the Strength and Conditioning staff had previous knowledge of an existing danger or risk but took no corrective action to help prevent resulting injuries, this failure to act would most likely constitute an extreme form of conduct. Generally, no documents can provide legal protection for grossly negligent or reckless conduct. A few states may allow the use of a waiver to protect from such conduct, but most do not (11).

MAKING PROTECTIVE LEGAL DOCUMENTS ENFORCEABLE

Protective legal documents, signed by participants before their participation in strength and conditioning programs and services, can provide a good defense for the Strength and Conditioning facility after an injured participant files a claim or lawsuit. A variety of factors should be considered for these forms to be legally enforceable (8,20):

- A lawyer who is knowledgeable about the law regarding protective documents must review your protective legal documents to help ensure they are written properly and reflect the law in your state.

- Informed consent and waiver documents are contracts, and can only be signed by adults because minors cannot enter into a contract. "Agreement to participate" documents are not contracts, and therefore can be signed by adults as well as minors.

- The exculpatory clause used in a waiver is not allowed in an informed consent or agreement to participate. If an exculpatory clause is added to an agreement to participate for adults, it then becomes a waiver.

- The exculpatory clause used in a waiver is not enforceable in medical or research settings, or in certain states where they are against public policy. In educational settings such as a college/university, the general rule is that waivers are against public policy for required activities but may be enforceable for voluntary activities.

- Informed consent documents used in medical settings must be provided before a patient has any kind of medical procedure. If the informed consent is not written or administered properly, the health care provider (and medical facility) could be found negligent for not informing the patient of particular risks. This also applies in research settings because subjects must be properly informed of risks through informed consent (note that this point is applicable in Strength and Conditioning settings, where athletes participate as human subjects in research studies).

- All documents must be administered properly. For example, participants should have ample time to read them and a well-trained employee should verbally explain the document to each participant.

- Protective documents must be stored in a secure place for the amount of time consistent with the statute of limitations, which may be up to 4 years in some states.

The choice of document or combination of documents to use is a very important decision. In situations where strength and conditioning activities are not covered in the employing institution's legal documentation, Strength and Conditioning professionals should consult with a qualified lawyer to assist with these decisions and to review or write the documents before implementation. Because legal advice and consultation can be quite expensive, Strength and Conditioning professionals may reduce costs by "drafting" their own legal documents using information from applicable resources (e.g., most university research protection offices have examples of agreement to participate and waiver documents, and examples of informed consent documents). These resources should be shared with your lawyer when he/she reviews the drafts and makes the final document revisions.

Written protective documents provide important evidence when a lawsuit occurs. For example, if a Strength and Conditioning facility is sued for negligence, but has evidence that the injured party signed a properly written and administered waiver, this document provides the evidence needed to seek summary judgment (i.e., a pretrial motion in which the judge can dismiss the case because, as a matter of law, there is no issue to be tried in a court of law). In this situation, the legal document protects the facility from a potentially costly negligence lawsuit.

APPENDIX 9. NSCA PROFESSIONAL STANDARDS AND GUIDELINES TASK FORCE CONTRIBUTORS

N. Travis Triplett, PhD, CSCS*D, FNSCA (Chair); Vic Brown, MS, CSCS, RSCC*D, ATC; Scott Caulfield, MA, CSCS*D, RSCC*D; Michael Doscher, MS, MSCC, SCCC, CSCS, RSCC*D; Patrick McHenry, MA, CSCS*D, RSCC; Traci Statler, PhD, CC-AASP, CSCS; Reed Wainwright, JD, CSCS, RSCC*D.

Reviewers: Bob Alejo, CSCS, RSCC*E; Brian Gearity, PhD, CSCS, RSCC, FNSCA, ATC; Jon Jost, CSCS, RSCC*E; Teena Murray, MS, RSCC*D, MSCC; and Mike Nitka, MS, CSCS*D, RSCC*E, FNSCA. 2009 version: N. Travis Triplett, PhD, CSCS*D, FNSCA (Chair); Michael Doscher, MS, CSCS*D, CP; Patrick McHenry, MS, CSCS*D, CP; Mack Rubley, PhD, CSCS*D; and Chat Williams, MS, CSCS*D, NSCA-CPT*D. 2001 version: Steven Plisk, MS, CSCS (Chair); Mike Brass, MS, CSCS; JoAnn Eickhoff-Shemek, PhD; Boyd Epley, MEd, CSCS, FNSCA; David Herbert, JD; Joe Owens, MS, CSCS*D; David Pearson, PhD, CSCS*D; and Dan Wathen, MS, ATC, CSCS*D, NSCACPT*D.

This document was reviewed and approved by the National Strength and Conditioning Association Board of Directors.

Conflicts of Interest and Source of Funding: The authors report no conflicts of interest and no source of funding.

REFERENCES

1. American Heart Association guidelines update for cardiopulmonary resuscitation and emergency cardiovascular care. *Circulation* 132(Suppl 2): 315–367, 2015.

2. Armitage-Johnson S. Providing a safe training environment: Parts I and II. *Strength Cond* 16: 64–65, 1994; 16(2): 34.

3. Balady GJ, Chaitman B, Driscoll D, Foster C, Froelicher E, Gordon N, Pate R, Rippe J, and Bazzarre T; AHA and ACSM. Recommendations for cardiovascular screening, staffing and emergency policies at health/fitness facilities. *Circulation* 97: 2283–2293, 1998; Medicine and Science in Sports and Exercise 30(6): 1009–1018, 1998.

4. Borkowski RP. *A Weight Room Safety Checklist. The Free Library.* Scholastic, Inc, 2007. Available at: https://www.thefreelibrary.com/A+weight+room+safety+checklist.-a0167512284. Accessed 11/5/2017.

5. Bucher CA and Krotee ML. *Management of Physical Education and Sport* (11th ed). Boston MA: McGraw-Hill, 1998.

6. Calhoon G and Fry AC. Injury rates and profiles of elite competitive weightlifters. *J Athletic Train* 34: 232–238, 1999.

7. Caulfield S and Berninger D. Exercise technique for free weight and machine training. In: *NSCA's Essentials of Strength Training and Conditioning* (4th ed). Haff GG and Triplett NT, eds. Champaign IL: Human Kinetics, 2016. pp. 350–408.

8. Eickhoff-Shemek J. Distinguishing protective legal documents. *ACSMs Health Fitness J* 5: 27–29, 2001.

9. Eickhoff-Shemek J. Standards of practice. In: *Law for Recreation and Sport Managers* (2nd ed). Cotten D, Wilde J, and Wlohan J, eds. Dubuque, IA: Kendall/Hunt Publishing, 2001. pp. 293–302.

10. Eickhoff-Shemek J and Deja K. 4 steps to minimize legal liability in exercise programs. *ACSMs Health Fitness J* 4: 13–18, 2000.

11. Eickhoff-Shemek JM, Herbert DL, and Connaughton DP. Introducing the risk management pyramid. *ACSMs Health Fitness J* 12: 37–39, 2008.

12. Faigenbaum AD and Micheli LJ; ACSM. *Current Comment from the American College of Sports Medicine: Youth Strength Training*. Indianapolis, IN: ACSM, 1998. Available at: http://www.acsm.org/public-information/sportsmedicinebasics/youth-strength-training. Accessed 11/5/2017.

13. Faigenbaum AD, Myer GD, Naclerio F, and Casas AA. Injury trends and prevention in youth resistance training. *Strength Conditioning J* 33: 36–41, 2011.

14. Haff GG, Berninger D, and Caulfield S. Exercise technique for alternative modes and nontraditional implement training. In: *NSCA's Essentials of Strength Training and Conditioning* (4th ed). Haff GG and Triplett NT, eds. Champaign, IL: Human Kinetics, 2016. pp. 409–438.

15. Haff GG and Triplett NT, eds. *NSCA's Essentials of Strength Training and Conditioning* (4th ed). Champaign, IL: Human Kinetics, 2016.

16. Halling DH. Liability considerations of the strength and conditioning specialist. *Natl Strength Cond Assoc J* 12: 57–60, 1990.

17. Halling DH. Legal terminology for the strength and conditioning specialist. *Natl Strength Cond Assoc J* 13: 59–61, 1991.

18. Hamill BP. Relative safety of weightlifting and weight training. *J Strength Cond Res* 8: 53–57, 1994.

19. Herbert DL. Legal aspects of strength and conditioning. *Natl Strength Cond Assoc J* 15: 79, 1993.

20. Herbert DL and Herbert WG. *Legal Aspects of Preventive, Rehabilitative and Recreational Exercise Programs* (3rd ed). Canton, OH: PRC Publishing, 1993.

21. Herbert DL. Supervision for strength and conditioning activities. *Strength Cond* 16: 32–33, 1994.

22. Herbert DL. A good reason for keeping records. *Strength Cond* 16: 64, 1994.

23. Hillmann A and Pearson DR. Supervision: The key to strength training success. *Strength Cond* 17: 67–71, 1995.

24. Hudy A. Facility design, layout, and organization. In: *NSCA's Essentials of Strength Training and Conditioning* (4th ed). Haff GG and Triplett NT, eds. Champaign, IL: Human Kinetics, 2016. pp. 623–639.

25. Jeffreys I. Warm-up and flexibility training. In: *NSCA's Essentials of Strength Training and Conditioning* (4th ed). Haff GG and Triplett NT, eds. Champaign, IL: Human Kinetics, 2016. pp. 317–350.

26. Jones CS, Christensen C, and Young M. Weight training injury trends: A 20-year survey. *Phys Sportsmed* 28: 61–72, 2000.

27. Katzenbach JR and Smith DK. *The Wisdom of Teams*. Boston, MA: Harvard Business School, 1993.

28. Katzenbach JR. *Real Change Leaders*. New York, NY: Times Books/Random House, 1997.

29. Keogh JWL and Winwood PW. The epidemiology of injuries across the weight-training sports. *Sports Med* 47: 479–501, 2017.

30. Kroll W. Selecting strength training equipment. *Natl Strength Cond J* 12: 65–70, 1990.

31. Kroll B. Liability considerations for strength training facilities. *Strength Cond* 17: 16–17, 1995.

32. Lloyd RS, Faigenbaum AD, Stone MH, Oliver JL, Jeffreys I, Moody JA, Brewer C, Pierce KC, McCambridge TM, Howard R, Herrington L, Hainline B, Micheli LJ, Jaques R, Kraemer WJ, McBride MG, Best TM, Chu DA, Alvar BA, and Myer GD. Position statement on youth resistance training: The 2014 International Consensus. *Br J Sports Med* 48: 498–505, 2014.

33. Lloyd RS, Cronin JB, Faigenbaum AD, Haff GG, Howard R, Kraemer WJ, Micheli LJ, Myer GD, and Oliver JL. National strength and conditioning association position statement on long-term athletic development. *J Strength Cond Res* 30: 1491–1509, 2016.

34. Malina RM. Weight training in youth-growth, maturation and safety: An evidence-based review. *Clin J Sports Med* 16: 478–487, 2006.

35. Maron BJ, Thompson PD, Puffer JC, McGrew CA, Strong WB, Douglas PS, Clark LT, Mitten MJ, Crawford MH, Atkins DL, Driscoll DJ, and Epstein AE; AHA and ACSM. Cardiovascular preparticipation screening of competitive athletes. *Circulation* 94: 850–856, 1996; Medicine and Science in Sports and Exercise 28 (12): 1445–1452, 1996.

36. Maron BJ, Thompson PD, Puffer JC, McGrew CA, Strong WB, Douglas PS, Clark LT, Mitten MJ, Crawford MH, Atkins DL, Driscoll DJ, and Epstein AE; AHA. Cardiovascular preparticipation screening of competitive athletes: Addendum. *Circulation* 97: 2294, 1998.

37. Mazur LJ, Yetman RJ, and Risser WL. Weight-training injuries: Common injuries and preventative methods. *Sports Med* 16: 57–63, 1993,

38. Myer GD, Quatman CE, Khoury J, Wall EJ, and Hewett TE. Youth versus adult "weightlifting" injuries presenting to United States emergency rooms: Accidental versus nonaccidental injury mechanisms. *J Strength Cond Res* 23: 2054–2060, 2009.

39. National Athletic Trainers' Association. *Recommendations and Guidelines for Appropriate Medical Coverage of Intercollegiate Athletics*. Dallas, TX: NATA, 2007. Available at: http://www.nata.org/sites/default/files/amciarecsandguides.pdf. Accessed 11/5/2017.

40. National Collegiate Athletic Association. *NCAA Sports Sponsorship and Participation Rates Report*. Indianapolis, IN: NCAA, 2015. Available at: http://www.ncaapublications.com/productdownloads/PR1516.pdf. Accessed 11/5/2017.

41. National Federation of State High School Associations. *NFHS Participation Survey: 2015-2016*. Indianapolis, IN: NFHS, 2016. Available at: http://www.nfhs.org/ParticipationStatistics/ParticipationStatistics/ Accessed 11/5/2017.

42. CSCS Exam Content Description. Colorado Springs, CO: NSCA, 2016.

43. Occupational Safety and Health Administration, U.S. Department of Labor. OSHA Regulations (Training Requirements in OSHA Standards; 1910.1030: Blood-Borne Pathogens). Washington, DC: OSHA, 2015. Available at: https://www.osha.gov/Publications/osha2254.pdf. Accessed 11/5/2017.

44. Parsons JT, ed; National Collegiate Athletic Association. *2014–15 NCAA Sports Medicine Handbook* (25th ed). Indianapolis, IN: NCAA, 2014. pp. 15–18.

45. Pearson D, Faigenbaum A, Conley M, and Kraemer WJ. Basic guidelines for the resistance training of athletes. *Strength Cond J* 22: 14–27, 2000.

46. Preparticipation Physical Evaluation Task Force, American Academy of Family Physicians, American Academy of Pediatrics, American College of Sports Medicine, American Medical Society for Sports Medicine, American Orthopaedic Society for Sports Medicine and American Osteopathic Academy of Sports Medicine. *Preparticipation Physical Evaluation* (4th ed). Elk Grove Village, IL: American Academy of Pediatrics, 2010.

47. Rabinoff MA. Weight room litigation: What's it all about? *Strength Cond* 16: 10–12, 1994.

48. Rabinoff MA. 32 reasons for the strength, conditioning, and exercise professional to understand the litigation process. *Strength Cond* 16: 20–25, 1994.

49. Schmidt RA and Lee TD. *Motor Control and Learning* (3rd ed). Champaign, IL: Human Kinetics, 1999.

50. Schmidt RA and Wrisberg CA. *Motor Learning and Performance* (2nd ed). Champaign, IL: Human Kinetics, 1999.

51. Siegel JD, Rhinehart E, Jackson M, and Chiarello L; the Healthcare Infection Control Practices Advisory Committee. 2007 guideline for isolation precautions: Preventing transmission of infectious agents in healthcare settings. Available at: https://www.cdc.gov/infectioncontrol/guidelines/isolation/index.html. Accessed 11/5/2017.

52. Siewe J, Rudat J, Rollinghoff M, Schlegel UJ, Eysel P, and Michael JW. Injuries and overuse syndromes in powerlifting. *Int J Sports Med* 32: 703–711, 2011.

53. Siewe J, Marx G, Knoll P, Eysel P, Zarghooni K, Graf M, Herren C, Sobottke R, and Michael J. Injuries and overuse syndromes in competitive and elite bodybuilding. *Int J Sports Med* 35: 943–948, 2014.

54. Siff MC. *Supertraining* (6th ed). Denver, CO: Supertraining Institute, 2003.

55. Spano M. Basic nutrition factors in health. In: *NSCA's Essentials of Strength Training and Conditioning* (4th ed). Haff GG and Triplett NT, eds. Champaign, IL: Human Kinetics, 2016. pp. 175–200.

56. Statler T and Brown V. Facility policies, procedures, and legal issues. In: *NSCA's Essentials of Strength Training and Conditioning* (4th ed). Haff GG and Triplett NT, eds. Champaign, IL: Human Kinetics, 2016. pp. 641–656.

57. Stone MH, O'Bryant HS, Schilling BK, and Koch A. Periodization: Effects of manipulating volume and intensity, parts 1 and 2. *Strength Cond J* 21: 56–62, 1999; 21: 54–60.

58. Stone MH, Plisk S, and Collins D. Training principles: Evaluation of modes and methods of resistance training. *Strength Cond J* 22: 65–76, 2000.

59. Strange D and Nitka M. Who gets a key-Is supervision in the weight room really necessary? *Strength Cond J* 26: 23–24, 2004.

60. Tharrett SJ and Peterson JA, eds; ACSM. *ACSM's Health/Fitness Facility Standards and Guidelines* (4th ed). Champaign, IL: Human Kinetics, 2012.

61. Weisenthal BM, Beck CA, Maloney MD, DeHaven KE, and Giordano BD. Injury rate and patterns among crossFit athletes. *Orthop J Sports Med* 2: 2325967114531177, 2014.

References

Preface

1. Aspen Institute. *Youth sports facts: Challenges to physical activity*. www.aspenprojectplay.org/youth-sports-facts/challenges. Accessed November 6, 2020.

2. Balyi, I. Sport system building and long-term athlete development in British Columbia. *Coaches Report* 8(1):22-28, 2001.

3. Casa, DJ, Anderson, SA, Baker, L, Bennett, S, Bergeron, MF, Connolly, D, Courson, R, Drezner, JA, Eichner, ER, Epley, B, Fleck, S, Franks, R, Guskiewicz, KM, Harmon, KG, Hoffman, J, Holschen, JC, Jost, J, Kinniburgh, A, Klossner, D, Lopez, RM, Martin, G, McDermott, BP, Mihalik, JP, Myslinski, T, Pagnotta, K, Poddar, S, Rodgers, G, Russell, A, Sales, L, Sandler, D, Stearns, RL, Stiggins, C, Thompson, C. The inter-association task force for preventing sudden death in collegiate conditioning sessions: Best practices recommendations. *J Athl Train* 47(4):477-480, 2012.

4. Jeffreys, I. Quadrennial planning for the high school athlete. *Strength Cond J* 30(3):74-83, 2008.

5. LaPrade, RF, Agel, J, Baker, J, Brenner, JS, Cordasco, FA, Côté, J, Engebretsen, L, Feeley, BT, Gould, D, Hainline, B, Hewett, T, Jayanthi, N, Kocher, MS, Myer, GD, Nissen, CW, Philippon, MJ, and Provencher, MT. AOSSM early sport specialization consensus statement. *Orthop J Sports Med* 4(4):1-8, 2016.

6. Lloyd, RS, and Oliver, JL. The youth physical development model: A new approach to long-term athletic development. *Strength Cond J* 34(3):61-72, 2012.

7. Lloyd, RS, Cronin, JB, Faigenbaum, AD, Haff, GG, Howard, R, Kraemer, WJ, Micheli, LJ, Myer, GD, and Oliver, JL. National Strength and Conditioning Association position statement on long-term athletic development. *J Strength Cond Res* 30(6):1491-1509, 2016.

8. Martel, K. USA Hockey's American development model: Changing the coaching and player development paradigm. *Int Sport Coach J* 2(1):39-49, 2015.

9. National Strength and Conditioning Association. *Strategic plan*. www.nsca.com/globalassets/about/nsca-strategic-plan-summary.pdf. Accessed November 6, 2020.

10. Triplett, NT, Brown, V, Caulfield, S, Doscher, M, McHenry, P, Statler, T, and Wainwright, R. NSCA strength and conditioning professional standards and guidelines. *Strength Cond J* 39(6):1-24, 2017.

Introduction

1. Bernhardt, DT, Gomez, J, Johnson, MD, Martin, TJ, Rowland, TW, Small, E, LeBlanc, C, Malina, R, Krein, C, Young, JC, and Reed, FE. Strength training by children and adolescents. *J Pediat*, 107(6):1470-1472, 2001.

2. Duehring, MD, Feldmann, CR, and Ebben, WP. Strength and conditioning practices of United States high school strength and conditioning coaches. *J Strength Cond Res* 23(8):2188-2203, 2009.

3. Duehring, MD, and Ebben, WP. Profile of high school strength and conditioning coaches. *J of Strength Cond Res* 24(2):538-547, 2010.

4. Faigenbaum, AD, Kraemer, WJ, Blimkie, CJ, Jeffreys, I, Micheli, LJ, Nitka, M, and Rowland, TW. Youth resistance training: Updated position statement paper from the National Strength and Conditioning Association. *J Strength Cond Res* 23:S60-S79, 2009.

5. Faigenbaum, AD. Strength training for children and adolescents. *Clin Sports Med* 19(4):593-619, 2000.

6. Greener, T, Petersen, D, and Pinske, K. Traits of successful strength and conditioning coaches. *J Strength Cond Res* 35(1):90-93, 2013.

7. Lloyd, RS, and Faigenbaum, AD. Age and sex related differences and their implication for resistance training. In *Essentials of Strength Training and Conditioning*, 4th ed. Haff, GG, and Triplett, NT, eds. Champaign, IL: Human Kinetics, 135-153, 2016.

8. Lloyd, RS, Cronin, JB, Faigenbaum, AD, Haff, GG, Howard, R, Kraemer, WJ, Micheli, LJ, Myer, GD, and Oliver, JL. National Strength and Conditioning Association position statement on long-term athletic development. *J Strength Cond Res* 30(6):1491-1509, 2016.

9. Lubans, DR, Plotnikoff, RC, and Lubans, NJ. A systematic review of the impact of physical activity programmes on social and emotional well-being in at-risk youth. *Child Adolesc Ment Health* 17(1):2-13, 2012.

10. Lubans, DR, Aguiar, EJ, and Callister, R. The effects of free weights and elastic tubing resistance training on physical self-perception in adolescents. *Psychol Sport Exer* 11(6):497-504, 2010.

11. National Strength and Conditioning Association Secondary School Coaches Working Group. The high school strength and conditioning coach profession.

12. www.nsca.com/education/high-school-coaches-resources/the-high-school-strength-and-conditioning-coach-profession. Accessed March 5, 2020.

13. National Strength and Conditioning Association Secondary School Coaches Working Group. Why your high school needs a qualified strength and conditioning professional. 2016.

14. www.nsca.com/contentassets/323883a707a04775badb00d2fbc9fc2c/why-your-high-school-needs-a-qualified-strength-and-conditioning-professional.pdf. Accessed March 5, 2020.

15. SHAPE America. *National Standards & Grade-Level Outcomes for K-12 Physical Education.* Champaign, IL: Human Kinetics, 2014.

16. Silver, F. What are the benefits of communication skills to teachers? www.work.chron.com/benefits-communication-skills-teachers-4493.html. Accessed August 8, 2018.

17. Triplett, NT, Brown, V, Caufield, S, Doscher, M, McHenry, P, Statler, T, and Wainwright, R. NSCA strength and conditioning professional standards and guidelines. *Strength Cond J* 39(6):1-24, 2017.

18. Vaughn, JM, and Micheli, L. Strength training recommendations for the young athlete. *Phys Med Rehabil Clin N Am* 19(2):235-245, 2008.

19. Velez, A, Golem, DL, and Arent, SM. The impact of a 12-week resistance training program on strength, body composition, and self-concept of Hispanic adolescents. *J Strength Cond Res* 24(4):1065-1073, 2010.

20. Zatsiorsky, VM, and Kraemer, WJ. *Science and Practice of Strength Training,* 2nd ed. Champaign, IL: Human Kinetics, 191-213, 2006.

Chapter 1

1. Barnes, M. Program design. In *NSCA's Strength and Conditioning Manual for High School Coaches.* Monterey, CA: Healthy Learning, 37-38, 2003.

2. Bertelsen, SL, and Thompson, B. High school weight-training curriculum: Course development considerations. *Strategies* 30(3):10-17, 2017.

3. Bucher, CA, and Krotee, MI. *Management of Physical Education and Sport.* 11th ed. Boston: McGraw-Hill, 1998.

4. Centers for Disease Control and Prevention. *Guidelines for school and community programs to promote lifelong physical activity among young people.* www.cdc.gov/mmwr/PDF/rr/rr4606.pdf. Atlanta: U.S. Department of Health and Human Services, 1997.

5. Cheek, C. A reality check for high school strength and conditioning. SimpliFaster. www.simplifaster.com/articles/high-school-strength-conditioning-reality. Accessed December 8, 2020.

6. Collegiate Strength and Conditioning Coaches Association. Strength training facility and policies. www.cscca.org/document/facilityrulesandprocedures. Accessed December 8, 2020.

7. DiPasquale, M. Developing a high school weight training program. January 7, 2020. www.bodybuilding.com/content/developing-a-high-school-weight-training-program.html. Accessed December 8, 2020.

8. Earle, RW. *Staff and Facility Policies and Procedures Manual.* Omaha, NE: Creighton University, 1993.

9. Epley, BD. *Fight Manual.* Lincoln, NE: University of Nebraska Printing 1998.

10. Epley, BD. *Make the Play.* Lincoln, NE: University of Nebraska Printing 1998.

11. Faigenbaum, A, and Hoffman, J. Youth programs. In *Strength Training.* Brown, L, ed. Champaign, IL: Human Kinetics, 319-322, 2007.

12. Faigenbaum, AD, Kraemer, WJ, Blimkie, CJ, Jeffreys, I, Micheli, LI, Nitka, M, and Rowland, TW. Youth resistance training: Updated position statement paper from the National Strength and Conditioning Association. *J Strength Cond Res* 23:S60-S79, 2009.

13. Faigenbaum, AD, McFarland, JE, Herman, R, Naclerio, F, Ratamess, NA, Kang, J, and Myer, GD. Reliability of the one repetition-maximum power clean test in adolescent athletes. *J Strength Cond Res* 26(2):432, 2012.

14. Faigenbaum, AD, and McFarland, JE. Criterion repetition maximum testing. *Strength Cond J* 36(1):88-91, 2014.

15. Hoch, D. Promoting your athletic program to the community. October 1, 2014. www.coachad.com/articles/promoting-your-program-to-the-community/. Accessed December 8, 2020.

16. Kolody, P. *Strength and Conditioning Manual.* Flemington, NJ: Hunterdon Central Regional High School, 1-4. 2011.

17. Lund, J, and Tannehill, D. *Standards-Based Physical Education Curriculum Development.* 3rd ed. Burlington, MA: Jones & Bartlett Publishers, 2014.

18. Metzler, M. *Instructional Models in Physical Education.* 3rd ed. Scottsdale, AZ: Holcomb Hathaway, 2011.

19. National Strength and Conditioning Association. *High School Weight Training: An Instructor's Guide.* Colorado Springs, CO: Palos Verdes Associates, 37-38, 1996.

20. Triplett, NT, Brown, V, Caulfield, S, Doscher, M, McHenry, P, Statler, T, and Wainwright, R. NSCA strength and conditioning professional standards and guidelines. *Strength Cond J* 39(6):1-24, 2017.

21. National Strength and Conditioning Association Secondary School Coaches Working Group. Why your high school needs a qualified strength and conditioning professional. 2016. www.nsca.com/contentassets/323883a707a04775badb00d2fbc9fc2c/why-your-high-school-needs-a-qualified-strength-and-conditioning-professional.pdf. Accessed March 5, 2020.

22. Osborne, T. Components of an effective strength and conditioning program. March 12, 2018. https://nfhs.org/articles/components-of-an-effective-strength-and-conditioning-program. Accessed December 8, 2020.

23. Reggiardo, JP. Structuring your strength & conditioning program: The 5 Phases. July 5, 2017. https://blog.bridgeathletic.com/structuring-your-sc-program. Accessed December 8, 2020.

24. Rink, J. *Designing the Physical Education Curriculum.* New York: McGraw-Hill Higher Education, 2008.

25. SHAPE America. *National standards and grade-level outcomes for K-12 physical education.* Champaign, IL: Human Kinetics, 2014.

26. Statler, T, and Brown, V. Facility procedures, policies, and legal issues. In *Essentials of Strength Training and Conditioning.* 4th ed. Haff, G, and Triplett, NT, eds. Champaign, Il: Human Kinetics, 641-656, 2016.

27. Thompson, WR Worldwide survey of fitness trends for 2019. *ACSMs Health Fit J* 22(6):10-17, 2018.

28. Van Vleet, B. *Developing a school-wide P.E. and strength & conditioning program.* May 20, 2018. https://blog.teambuildr.com/programming-considerations-for-school-wide-program-design. Accessed December 8, 2020.

29. Lloyd, RS, and Faigenbaum, AD. Age- and sex-related differences and their implications for resistance exercise. In *Essentials of Strength Training and Conditioning.* 4th ed. Haff, G, and Triplett, NT, eds. Champaign, IL: Human Kinetics, 135-153, 2016.

30. Vaughn, JM, and Micheli, L. Strength training recommendations for the youth athlete. *Phys Med Rehabil Clin N Am* 19(2):235-245, 2008.

31. Smith, A, Andrish, J, and Micheli, L. The prevention of sport injuries of children and adolescents. *Med Sci Sports Exerc* 25(8 Suppl):1-7, 1993.

32. Quatman, CE, Gregory, DM, Khoury, J, Wall, EJ, and Hewett, TE. Sex differences in "weight-lifting" injuries presenting to United States emergency rooms. *J Strength Cond Res* 23(7):2061-2067, 2009.

33. Duehring, MJ, Feldmann, CR, and Ebben, WP. Strength and conditioning practices of United States high school strength and conditioning coaches. *J Strength Cond Res* 23(8):2188-2203, 2009.

34. Wade, S, Pope, Z, and Simonson, S. How prepared are college freshmen athletes for the rigors of college strength and conditioning? A survey of college strength and conditioning coaches. *J Strength Cond Res* 28(10):2746-2753, 2014.

35. Lloyd, RS, Cronin, JB, Faigenbaum, AD, Haff, GG, Howard, R, Kraemer, WJ, Micheli, LJ, Myer, GD, and Oliver, JL. National Strength and Conditioning Association position statement on long-term athletic development. *J Strength Cond Res* 30(6):1491-1509, 2016.

36. Australia Strength and Conditioning Association. Resistance training for children and youth: A position stand from the Australian Strength and Conditioning Association (ASCA). 2007. www.strengthandconditioning.org/news/692-child-and-youth-resistance-training-position-stand. Accessed July 1, 2020.

37. Mannie, K, and Vorkapich, M. Accent on female strength training. *Coach Athl Dir* 3:8-10, 2007.

38. Zatsiorsky, VM, and Kraemer, WJ. Strength training for young athletes. In *Science and Practice of Strength Training*. 2nd ed. Zatsiorsky, WJ, and Kraemer, VM, eds. Champaign, IL: Human Kinetics, 191-213, 2006.

39. Faigenbaum, A. Strength training for children and adolescents. *Clin J Sport Med* 19(4):593-619, 2000.

40. Granacher, U, Muehlbauer, T, Doerflinger, B, Strohmeier, and Gollhodfer, A. Promoting strength and balance in adolescents during physical education: Effects of a short-term resistance training. *J Strength Cond Res* 25(4):940-949, 2011.

41. Ahmed, C, Hilton, W, and Pituch, K. Relations of strength training to body image among a sample of female university students. *J Strength Cond Res* 16(4):645-648, 2002.

42. Williams, PA, and Cash, TF. Effects of a circuit weight training program on the body images of college students. *Int J Eat Disord* 30(1):75-82, 2001.

43. Radcliffe, JR, Comfort, P, and Fawcett, T. Psychological strategies included by strength and conditioning coaches in applied strength and conditioning. *J Strength Cond Res* 29(9):2641-2654, 2015.

44. National Strength and Conditioning Association. *Strength and Conditioning Professional Standards and Guidelines*. Colorado Springs, CO: National Strength and Conditioning Association, 2009.

45. Aspen Institute Project Play. *State of play 2016: Trends and developments*. Washington, DC: Aspen Institute, 2016.

46. Casa, DJ, et al. The Inter-Association Task Force for Preventing Sudden Death in Secondary School Athletics Programs: Best-practices recommendations. *J Athl Train* 48(4):546-553, 2013.

47. DeMartini, JK and Casa, DJ. Who is responsible for preventable deaths during athletic conditioning sessions? *J Strength Cond Res* 25(7):1781, 2011.

48. Youth Sports Safety Alliance. *National Action Plan for Sports Safety*. 2013.

49. Statler, T, and Brown, V. Facility policies, procedures, and legal issues. In *Essentials of Strength Training and Conditioning* 4th ed. Haff, G, and Triplett, NT, eds. Champaign, IL: Human Kinetics, 623-640, 2016.

50. Wainwright, R. Personal correspondence. Weatherford, TX: Law Office of Reed Wainwright, 2016.

51. McGladrey, B. *High school physical educators' and sport coaches' knowledge of strength training principles and methods*. Doctoral dissertation, University of Utah, 2010.

52. Miller, MG, and Housner, LA. Survey of health-related physical fitness knowledge among preservice and inservice physical educators. *Phys Educ* 55(4):176-186, 1998.

53. Castelli, D, and Williams, L. Health-related fitness and physical education teachers' content knowledge. *J Teach Phys Educ* 26(1):3-19, 2007.

Chapter 2

1. Bayraktar, I. Agility and speed standards for student teenager wrestlers. *Univers J Educ Res* 5(4): 557-560, 2017.

2. Born, DA. *Performance measures and strength evaluation in the high school female athlete*. Doctoral dissertation, University of Georgia, Athens, GA, 2004.

3. Brown, TD, and Vescovi, JD. Comparison of agility and countermovement jump performance among middle school, high school, and college aged female soccer players. In *VTSC*, June 2008. Marlton, NJ: The Sports Performance Essentials, LLC, 2019.

4. Castagna, C, and Castellini, E. Vertical jump performance in Italian male and female national team soccer players. *J Strength Cond Res* 27:1156-1161, 2013.

5. Chelly, MS, Fathloun, M, Cherif, N, Amar, MB, Tabka, Z, and Van Praagh, E. Effects of a back squat training program on leg power, jump, and sprint performances in junior soccer players. *J Strength Cond Res* 23(8):2241-2249, 2009.

6. Chu, DA. *Explosive Power and Strength*. Champaign, IL: Human Kinetics, 167-180, 1996.

7. Cook, G. *Movement: Functional Movement Systems: Screening, Assessment, and Corrective Strategies*. Aptos, CA: On Target, 2010.

8. Faigenbaum, AD, and McFarland, JE. Criterion repetition maximum testing. *J Strength Cond Res* 36(1):88-91, 2014.

9. Faigenbaum, AD, Kang, J, McFarland, J, Bloom, JM, Magnatta, J, Ratamess, NA, and Hoffman, JR. Acute effects of different warm-up protocols on anaerobic performance in teenage athletes. *Pediat Exer Sci* 18(1):64-75, 2006.

10. Faigenbaum, AD, McFarland, JE, Herman, R, Naclerio, F, Ratamess, NA, Kang, J, and Myer, GD. Reliability of the one repetition-maximum power clean test in adolescent athletes. *J Strength Cond Res* 26(2):432, 2012.

11. Faigenbaum, AD, McFarland, JE, Keiper, FB, Tevlin, W, Ratamess, NA, Kang, J, and Hoffman, JR. Effects of a short-term plyometric and resistance training program on fitness performance in boys aged 12 to 15 years. *J Sports Sci Med* 6(4):519, 2007.

12. Fukuda, DH. *Assessments for Sport and Athletic Performance*. Champaign, IL: Human Kinetics, 108, 123, 2018.

13. Gabbett, T, and Georgieff, B. Physiological and anthropometric characteristics of Australian junior national, state, and novice volleyball players. *J Strength Cond Res* 21:902-908, 2007.

14. Greene, JJ, McGuine, TA, Leverson, G, and Best, TM. Anthropometric and performance measures for high school basketball players. *J Athl Train* 33(3):229, 1998.

15. Haff, GG, and Dumke, C. *Laboratory Manual for Exercise Physiology*. Champaign, IL: Human Kinetics, 305-360, 2012.

16. Hoffman, J. *Norms for Fitness, Performance, and Health*. Champaign, IL: Human Kinetics, 27-40, 2006.

17. Hoffman, J. *Physiological Aspects of Sport Training and Performance*, 2nd ed. Champaign, IL: Human Kinetics, 237-267, 2014.

18. Lloyd, RS, Cronin, JB, Faigenbaum, AD, Haff, GG, Howard, R, Kraemer, WJ, Micheli, LJ, Myer, GD and Oliver, JL. National Strength and Conditioning Association position statement on long-term athletic development. *J Strength Cond Res* 30(6):1491-1509, 2016.

19. McGuigan, M. Administration, scoring, and interpretation of selected tests. In *Essentials of Strength Training and Conditioning*, 4th ed. Haff, GG, Triplett, NT, eds. Champaign, IL: Human Kinetics, 259-316, 2016.

20. McKay, BD, Miramonti, AA, Gillen, ZM, Leutzinger, TJ, Mendez, AI, Jenkins, ND, and Cramer, JT. Normative reference values for high school-aged American football players. *J Strength Cond Res* 34(10):2849-2856, 2020.

21. Moraes, E, Fleck, SJ, Dias, MR, and Simão, R. Effects on strength, power, and flexibility in adolescents of nonperiodized vs. daily nonlinear periodized weight training. *J Strength Cond Res* 27(12):3310-3321, 2013.

22. Mujika, I, Santisteban, J, Impellizzeri, FM, and Castagna, C. Fitness determinants of success in men's and women's football. *J Sports Sci* 27:107-114, 2009.

23. National consortium for PE for individuals with disabilities. In *Adapted Physical Education National Standards*, 3rd ed. Kelly, LE, ed. Champaign, IL: Human Kinetics, 2020.

24. National Strength and Conditioning Association Secondary School Coaches Working Group. Why your high School needs a qualified strength and conditioning professional. 2016. www.nsca.com/contentassets/323883a707a04775badb00d2fbc9fc2c/why-your-high-school-needs-a-qualified-strength-and-conditioning-professional.pdf. Accessed March 5, 2020.

25. Schaal, M, Ransdell, LB, Simonson, SR, and Gao, Y. Physiologic performance test differences in female volleyball athletes by competition level and player position. *J Strength Cond Res* 27:1841-1850, 2013.

26. Sheppard, JM, and Triplett, NT. Program design for resistance training. In *Essentials of Strength Training and Conditioning*, 4th ed. Haff, G, Triplett, NT, eds. Champaign, IL: Human Kinetics, 453, 2016.

27. Society of Health and Physical Educators. *National standards and grade-level outcomes for K-12 physical education.* Champaign, IL: Human Kinetics, 2014.

28. Szymanski, DJ, and Vazquez, J. Testing protocols and athlete assessment. In *Strength Training for Baseball.* Coleman, AE, Szymanski, DJ, eds. Champaign, IL: Human Kinetics, 31-64, 2022.

29. Till, K, Cobley, S, O'Hara, J, Brightmore, A, Cooke, C, and Chapman, C. Using anthropometric and performance characteristics to predict selection in junior UK Rugby League players. *J Sci Med Sport* 14:264-269, 2011.

30. Till, K, Tester, E, Jones, B, Emmonds, S, Fahey, J, and Cooke, C. Anthropometric and physical characteristics of English academy rugby league players. *J Strength Cond Res* 28:319-327, 2014.

31. Tomkinson, GR, Carver, KD, Atkinson, F, Daniell, ND, Lewis, LK, Fitzgerald, JS, Lang, JJ, and Ortega, FB. European normative values for physical fitness in children and adolescents aged 9-17 years: Results from 2 779 165 Eurofit performances representing 30 countries. *Br J Sports Med* 52(22):1445-1456, 2018.

32. Triplett, NT, Brown, V, Caulfield, S, Doscher, M, McHenry, P, Statler, T, and Wainwright, R. NSCA strength and conditioning professional standards and guidelines. *Strength Cond J* 39(6):1-24, 2017.

33. Vescovi, JD, and McGuigan, MR. Relationships between sprinting, agility, and jump ability in female athletes. *J Sports Sci* 26:97-107, 2008.

Chapter 3

1. Baechle, TR, and Earle, RW. *Weight Training: Steps to Success*, 5th ed. Champaign, IL: Human Kinetics, 2020.

2. Fleck, SJ, and Kraemer, WJ. *Designing Resistance Training Programs*, 4th ed. Champaign, IL: Human Kinetics, 2014.

3. Half, GG, and Triplett, NT. *Essentials of Strength Training and Conditioning*, 4th ed. Champaign, IL: Human Kinetics, 2016.

4. Hudy, A. Facility design, layout, and organization. In *Essentials of Strength Training and Conditioning*, 4th ed. Haff, GG, and Triplett, NT, eds. Champaign, IL: Human Kinetics, 623, 626, 627, 628, 631, 632, 2016.

5. Mediate, P, and Faigenbaum, AD. *Medicine Ball for All Kids: Medicine Ball Training Concepts and Program-Design Considerations for School-Age Youth.* Monterey, CA: Healthy Learning, 2007.

6. National Strength and Conditioning Association. *Exercise Technique Manual for Resistance Training*, 3rd ed. Champaign, IL: Human Kinetics, 2015.

7. National Strength and Conditioning Association Secondary School Coaches Working Group. Why your high school needs a qualified strength and conditioning professional. 2016.

8. www.nsca.com/contentassets/323883a707a04775badb00d2fbc9fc2c/why-your-high-school-needs-a-qualified-strength-and-conditioning-professional.pdf. Accessed March 5, 2020.

9. Statler, T, and Brown, V. Facility procedures, policies, and legal issues. In *Essentials of Strength Training and Conditioning*, 4th ed. Haff, GG, and Triplett, NT., eds. Champaign, IL: Human Kinetics, 642, 647, 653, 654, 655, 2016.

10. Triplett, NT, Brown, V, Caulfield, S, Doscher, M, McHenry, P, Statler, T, and Wainwright, R. NSCA strength and conditioning professional standards and guidelines. *Strength Cond J* 39(6):1-24, 2017.

Chapter 4

1. Bartelink, DL. Role of abdominal pressure in relieving the pressure on the lumbar inter-vertebral discs. *J Bone Joint Surg* 39B:718-725, 1957.

2. Bauer, JA, Fry, A, and Carter, C. The use of lumbar-supporting weight belts while performing squats: Erector spinae electromyographic activity. *J Strength Cond Res* 13:384-388, 1999.

3. Bird, SP, and Casey, S. Exploring the front squat. *Strength and Conditioning Journal* 34(2): 27-33, 2012.

4. Cissik, J., and NSCA Education Committee. *How to Teach Cleans, Jerks, and Snatches.* Colorado Springs, CO: National Strength and Conditioning Association, 1, 11, 43, 2002.

5. Chandler, T, Wilson, G, and Stone, M. The effect of the squat exercise on knee stability. *Med Sci Sports Exer* 21(3): 299-303, 1989.

6. Chiu, LZ, and Schilling, BK. A primer on weightlifting: From sport to sports training. *Strength and Conditioning Journal* 27(1): 42, 2005.

7. Duba, J, Kraemer, WJ., and Martin, G. A 6-step progression model for teaching the hang power clean. *Strength and Conditioning Journal* 29(5): 26, 2007.

8. Duba, J, Kraemer, WJ, and Martin, G. Progressing from the hang power clean to the power clean: A 4-step model. *Strength and Conditioning Journal* 31(3): 58-66, 2009.

9. Feher, T, Dimas, P, Conroy, M, Dreschler, A, and Gattone, M. USA Weightlifting Sports Performance Coaching Course Manual Level 1. USAW Coaching Education Series, 2017.

10. Glassbrook, DJ, Brown, SR, Helms, ER, Duncan, S, and Storey, AG. The high-bar and low-bar back-squats: A biomechanical analysis. *J Strength Cond Res* 33:S1-S18, 2019.

11. Hackett, D.A., and Chow, C. The Valsalva maneuver: Its effect on intra-abdominal pressure and safety issues during resistance exercise. *J Strength Cond Res* 27:2338-2345, 2013.

12. Harman, EA, Rosenstein, RM, Frykman, PN, and Nigro, GA. Effects of a belt on intra-abdominal pressure during weightlifting. *Med Sci Sports Exer* 21:186-190, 1989.

13. Ikeda, ER, Borg, A, Brown, D, Malouf, J, Showers, KM, and Li, SL. The Valsalva maneuver revisited: Influence of voluntary breathing on isometric muscle strength. *J Strength Cond Res* 23:127-132, 2009.

14. Kushner, AM, Brent, JL, Schoenfeld, BJ, Hugentobler, J, Lloyd, RS, Vermeil, A, Chu, DA, Harbin, J, McGill, SM, and Myer, GD. The back squat: Targeted training techniques to correct functional deficits and technical factors that limit performance. *Strength Cond J* 37(2): 13-60, 2015.

15. Lander, JE, Hundley, JR, and Simonton, RL. The effectiveness of weight belts during multiple repetitions of the squat exercise. *J Strength Cond Res* 24:603-609, 1992.

16. Lander, JE, Simonton, RL, and Giacobbe, JK. Effectiveness of weight belts during the squat exercise. *Med Sci Sports Exer* 22(1): 117-126, 1990.

17. Matuschek, C, and Schmidt Bleicher, D. Influence of squatting depth on jumping performance. *J Strength Cond Res* 26(12): 3243-3261, 2012.

18. Moore, JW, and Quintero, LM. Comparing forward and backward chaining in teaching Olympic weightlifting. *Journal of Applied Behavior Analysis* 52(1): 50-59, 2019.

19. Morris, JM, Lucas, BD, and Bresler, B. Role of the trunk in stability of the spine. *J Bone Joint Surg* 43A:327-351, 1961.

20. Morris, SJ, Oliver, JL, Pedley, JS, Haff, GG, and Lloyd, RS. Taking a long-term approach to the development of weightlifting ability in young athletes. *Strength and Conditioning Journal* 42(6): 71-90, 2020.

21. Myer, GD, Kushner, AM, Brent, JL, Schoenfeld, BJ, Hugentobler, J, Lloyd, RS, Vermeil, A, Chu, DA, Harbin, J, and McGill, SM. The back squat: A proposed assessment of functional deficits and technical factors that limit performance. *Strength Cond J* 37(2): 13-60, 2015.

22. Rippetoe, M. *Starting Strength: Basic Barbell Training,* 3rd ed. Wichita Falls, TX: The Aasgaard Company, 148-165, 170-171, 2011.

23. Sogabe, A, Iwasaki, S, Gallager, PM, Edinger, S, and Fry, A. Influence of the stance width on power production during the barbell squat. *J Strength Cond Res* 24(Suppl): 1, 2010.

24. Tillaar, RVD, and Saeterbakken, A. The sticking region in three chest-press exercises with increasing degrees of freedom. *J Strength Cond Res* 26:2962-2969, 2012.

Chapter 5

1. Anderson, K, and Behm, DG. Trunk muscle activity increases with unstable squat movements. *Can J Appl Physiol* 30(1):33-45, 2005.

2. Anderson, T, and Kearney, JT. Muscular strength and absolute and relative endurance. *Res Q Exerc Sport* 53(1):1-7, 1982.

3. Behm, DG, Drinkwater, EJ, Willardson, JM, and Cowley, PM. The use of instability to train the core musculature. *Appl Physiol Nutr Metab* 39(1):91-108, 2010.

4. Bartelink, DL. The role of abdominal pressure in relieving the pressure on the lumbar intervertebral discs. *J Bone Jt Surg* 39B(4):718-725, 1957.

5. Cho, I, Jeon, C, Lee, S, Lee, D, and Hwangbo, G. Effects of lumbar stabilization exercise on functional disability and lumbar lordosis angle in patients with chronic lower back pain. *J Phys Ther Sci* 27(6):1983-1985, 2015.

6. Cressey, EM, West, CA, Tiberio, DP, Kraemer, WJ, and Maresh, CM. The effects of ten weeks of lower-body unstable surface training on markers of athletic performance. *J Strength Cond Res* 21(2):561-567, 2007.

7. Demers, E, Pendenza, J, Radevich, V, Preuss, R. The effect of stance width and anthropometrics on joint range of motion in the lower extremities during a back squat. *Int J Exerc Sci* 11(1):764-775, 2018.

8. Dinunzio, C, Porter, N, Van Scoy J, Cordice, D, and McCulloch, RS. Alterations in kinematics and muscle activation patterns with the addition of a kipping action during a pull-up activity. *Sports Biomech* 18(6):622-635, 2019.

9. Faigenbaum, AD, Kraemer, WJ, Blimkie, CJR, Jeffreys, I, Micheli, LJ, Nikita, M, and Rowland, TW. Youth resistance training: Updated position statement paper from the National Strength and Conditioning Association. *J Strength Cond Res* 23(suppl): 60-79, 2009.

10. Fleck, SJ, and Kraemer, WJ. *Designing Resistance Training Programs.* 4th ed. Champaign, IL: Human Kinetics, 1-62, 179-296, 2014.

11. Haff, G, and Triplett, NT. *Essentials of Strength Training and Conditioning.* 4th ed. Champaign, IL: Human Kinetics, 2016.

12. Harrison, JS. Bodyweight training: A return to basics. *Strength Cond J* 32(2):52-55, 2010.

13. Hodges, PW, and Gandevia, SC. Changes in intra-abdominal pressure during postural activation of the human diaphragm. *J Appl Physiol* 89(3):967-976, 2000.

14. Huxel Bliven, KC, and Anderson, BE. Core stability training for injury prevention. *Sports Health* 5(6):514-522, 2013.

15. Kim, D, Cho, M, Park, Y, and Yang, Y. Effect of an exercise program for posture correction on musculoskeletal pain. *J Phys Ther Sci* 27(6):1791-1794, 2015.

16. Kolar, P, Sulc, J, Kyncl, M, Sanda, J, Cakrt, O, Andel, R, Kumagai, K, and Kobesova, A. Postural function of the diaphragm in persons with and without chronic low back pain. *J Orthop Sports Phys Ther* 42(4):352-362, 2012.

17. Kolar, P, Sulc, J, Kyncl, M, Sanda, J, Neuwirth, J, Bokarius, AV, Kriz, J, and Kobesova, A. Stabilizing function of the diaphragm: Dynamic MRI and synchronized spirometric assessment. *J Appl Physiol* 109(4):1064-1071, 2010.

18. Lloyd, RS, Cronin, JB, Faigenbaum, AD, Haff, GG, Howard, R, Kraemer, WJ, Micheli, LJ, Myer, GD, and Oliver, JL. National Strength and Conditioning Association position statement on long-term athletic development. *J Strength Cond Res* 30(6):1491-1509, 2016.

19. Lorenzetti, S, Ostermann, M, Zeidler, F, Zimmer, P, Jentsch, L, List, R, Taylor, W, and Schellenberg, F. How to squat? Effects of various stance widths, foot placement angles and level of experience on knee, hip and trunk motion and loading. *BMC Sports Sci Med Rehabil* 10(1):14, 2018.

20. Morris, JM, Lucas, BD, and Bresler, B. Role of the trunk in stability of the spine. *J Bone Jt Surg* 43(3):327-351, 1961.

21. Moffroid, MT, Haugh, LB, Haig, AJ, Henry, SN, and Pope, MG. Endurance training of trunk extensor muscles. *Phys Ther* 73(1):10-17, 1993.

22. Ogard, WK. Proprioception in sports medicine and athletic conditioning. *Strength Cond J* 33(3):111-118, 2011.

23. Schoenfeld, BJ, and Contreras, BM. The long-lever posterior-tilt plank. *Strength Cond J* 35(3):98-99, 2013.

24. Sogabe, A, Iwasaki, S, Gallager, RM, Edinger, S, and Fry, A. Influence of stance width on power production during the barbell squat. *J Strength Cond Res* 24(suppl):1, 2010.

25. Tillaar, RVD, and Saeterbakken, A. The sticking region in three chest-press exercises with increasing degrees of freedom. *J Strength Cond Res* 26(11):2962-2969, 2012.

26. Tvrdy, D. The reverse side plank/bridge: An alternate exercise for core training. *Strength Cond J* 34(2):86-88, 2006.

27. Ulm, R. Stability and weightlifting: Mechanics of stabilization—part 1. *NSCA Coach* 4(3):20-26, 2016.

28. Wilson, JD, Dougherty, CP, Ireland, ML, and Davis, IM. Core stability and its relationship to lower extremity function and injury. *J Am Acad Orthop Surg* 13(5):316-325, 2005.

Chapter 6

1. Di Naso, J. Core programming. In *Developing the Core*. Willardson, JM, ed. Champaign, IL: Human Kinetics, 118-119, 2014.

2. Martarelli, D, Cocchioni, M, Scuri, S, and Pompei, P. Diaphragmatic breathing reduces exercise-induced oxidative stress. *J Evid Based Complementary Altern Med* 8(1):1-10, 2011.

3. Willardson, JM. Core anatomy and biomechanics. In *Developing the Core*. Willardson, JM, ed. Champaign, IL: Human Kinetics, 5, 2014.

Chapter 7

1. Bishop, D. Warm-up II: Performance changes following active warm-up and how to structure the warm-up. *Sports Med* 33(7):483-498, 2003.

2. Brodowicz, GR, Welsh, R, and Wallis, J. Comparison of stretching with ice, stretching with heat, or stretching alone on hamstring flexibility. *J Athl Train* 31(4):324, 1996.

3. Chaouachi, A, Castagna, C, Chtara, M, Brughelli, M, Turki, O, Galy, O, Chamari, K, and Behm, DG. Effect of warm-ups involving static or dynamic stretching on agility, sprinting, and jumping performance in trained individuals. *J Strength Cond Res* 24(8):2001-2011, 2010.

4. Davis, DS, Ashby, PE, McCale, KL, McQuain, JA, and Wine, JM. The effectiveness of 3 stretching techniques on hamstring flexibility using consistent stretching parameters. *J Strength Cond Res* 19(1):27-32, 2005.

5. Dunsky, A, and Ben-Sira, D. Do different warm-up protocols affect isometric explosive muscular contraction? *Isokinet Exerc Sci* 24(1):51-58, 2016.

6. Faigenbaum, AD, McFarland, JE, Schwerdtman, JA, Ratamess, NA, Kang, J, and Hoffman, JR. Dynamic warm-up protocols, with and without a weighted vest, and fitness performance in high school female athletes. *J Athl Train* 41(4):357, 2006.

7. Fleck, SJ, and Kraemer, WJ. *Designing Resistance Training Programs*. 4th ed. Champaign, IL: Human Kinetics, 2014.

8. Fradkin, AJ, Zazryn, TR, Smoliga, JM. Effects of warming up on physical performance: A systematic review with meta-analysis. *J Strength Cond Res* 24(1):140-148, 2010.

9. Hedrick, A. Exercise physiology: Physiological responses to warm-up. *Strength Cond J* 14(5):25-27, 1992.

10. Howley, ET, and Thompson, D. *Fitness Professional's Handbook*. 7th ed. Champaign, IL: Human Kinetics, 2016.

11. Jeffreys, I. *The Warm-Up: Maximize Performance and Improve Long-Term Athletic Development*. Champaign, IL: Human Kinetics, 2019.

12. Jeffreys, I. Warm-up and flexibility training. In *Essentials of Strength Training and Conditioning*. 4th ed. Haff, GG, and Triplett, NT eds. Champaign, IL: Human Kinetics, 317-350, 2016.

13. McArdle, WD, Katch, FI, and Katch, VL. *Exercise Physiology: Energy, Nutrition, and Human Performance*. 6th ed. Philadelphia: Lippincott Williams & Wilkins, 2007.

14. McCrary, JM, Ackermann, BJ, Halaki, M. A systematic review of the effects of upper body warm-up on performance and injury. *Br J Sports Med* 49(14):935-942, 2016.

15. McGowan, CJ, Pyne, DB, Thompson, KG, and Rattray, B. Warm-up strategies for sport and exercise: Mechanisms and applications. *Sports Med* 45(11):1523-1546, 2015.

16. Ratamess, N. *ACSM's Foundations of Strength Training and Conditioning*. London: Lippincott, Williams & Wilkins, 2012.

17. Safran, MR, Garrett, WE, Seaber, AV, Glisonn, RR, Ribbeck, BM. The role of warm-up in muscular injury prevention. *Am J Sports Med* 16(2):123-129, 1988.

18. Shellock, FG, and Prentice, WE. Warming-up and stretching for improved physical performance and prevention of sports-related injuries. *Sports Med* 2(4):267-278, 1985.

Chapter 8

1. Armstrong, N, and Welsman, JR. Training young athletes. In *Coaching Children in Sport: Principles and Practice*. Lee, M, ed. London: E. & F.N. Spon, 64-77, 1993.

2. Baar, K. Training for endurance and strength: Lessons from cell signaling. *Med Sci Sports Exerc* 38:1939-1944, 2006.

3. Balyi, I, and Hamilton, A. Long-term athlete development: Trainability in childhood and adolescence. *Olympic Coach* 16(1):4-9, 2004.

4. Basso, JC, and Suzuki, WA. The effects of acute exercise on mood, cognition, neurophysiology, and neurochemical pathways: A review. *Brain Plast* 2(2):127-152, 2017.

5. Bertelsen, SL, and Thompson, B. High school weight-training curriculum: Course development considerations. *Strategies* 30(3):10-17, 2017.

6. Beunen, G, and Malina, RM. Growth and biologic maturation: Relevance to athletic performance. *The young athlete*. Malden, MA: Blackwell Publishing, 3-17, 2008.

7. Case, MJ, Knudson, DV, and Downey, DL. Barbell squat relative strength as an identifier for lower extremity injury in collegiate athletes. *J Strength Cond Res* 24(5):1249-1253, 2020.

8. Côté, J, Baker, J, and Abernethy, B. From play to practice: A developmental framework for the acquisition of expertise in team sports. In J. Starkes and K.A. Ericsson (eds.), *Expert Performance in Sports: Advances in Research on Sport Expertise*. Champaign, IL: Human Kinetics, 89-110, 2003.

9. DeLorme, TL. Restoration of muscle power by heavy resistance exercises. *J Bone Joint Surg* 27(4):645-667, 1945.

10. DeWeese, B, Sams, M, and Serrano, A. Sliding toward Sochi. Part 1: A review of programming tactics used during the 2010–2014 quadrennial. *NSCA Coach* 1(3):30-36, 2014.

11. Eston, R, and Evans, HJ. The validity of submaximal ratings of perceived exertion to predict one repetition maximum. *J Sports Sci Med* 8(4):567-573, 2009.

12. Faigenbaum, AD, Kraemer, WJ, Blimkie, CJ, Jeffreys, I, Micheli, LJ, Nitka, M, and Rowland, TW. Youth resistance training: Updated position statement paper from the National Strength and Conditioning Association. *J Strength Cond Res* 23:S60-S79, 2009.

13. Faigenbaum, AD, and McFarland, JE. Criterion repetition maximum testing. *Strength Cond J* 36(1):88-91, 2014.

14. Faigenbaum, AD, and McFarland, J.E. Resistance training for kids: Right from the start. *ACSM's Health Fit J* 20(5):16-22, 2016.

15. Faigenbaum, AD, and Naclerio, F. Paediatric Strength and Conditioning. *Strength and Conditioning for Sports Performance*. Jeffreys, I, and Moody, J, eds. New York: Routledge, 484-505, 2016.

16. Fleck, SJ, and Falkel, JE. Value of resistance training on the reduction of sports injuries. *Sports Med* 3:61-68, 1986.

17. Goldstein, JH, ed. *Sports, Games, and Play: Social and Psychological Viewpoints*. New York: Psychology Press, 2012.

18. Goodwin, JE, and Cleather, DJ. The biomechanical principles underpinning strength and conditioning. In *Strength and Conditioning for Sports Performance*. Jeffreys, I, and Moody, J, eds. New York: Routledge, 36-66, 2016.

19. Goodwin, JE, and Jeffreys, I. Plyometric training: Theory and practice. In *Strength and Conditioning for Sports Performance*. Jeffreys, I, and Moody, J, eds. New York: Routledge, 304-340, 2016..

20. Granados, A, Gebremariam, A, and Lee, JM. Relationship between timing of peak height velocity and pubertal staging in boys and girls. *J Clin Res Pediatr Endocrinol* 7(3):235, 2015.

21. Hackett, DA, Cobley, SP, Davies, TB, Michael, SW, and Halaki, M. Accuracy in estimating repetitions to failure during resistance exercise. *J Strength Cond Res* 31(8):2162-2168, August 2017.

22. Hawley, JA. Molecular responses to strength and endurance training: Are they incompatible? *Appl Physiol Nutr Metab* 34:355-361, 2009.

23. Howard, R. What coaches need to know about the NSCA position statement on long-term athletic development. *NSCA Coach* 3(3):8-10, 2014.

24. Kraemer, WJ, Adams, K, Cafarelli, E, Dudley, GA, Dooly, C, Feigenbaum, MS, Fleck, SJ, Franklin, B, Fry, AC, Hoffman, JR, Newton, RU, Potteiger, J, Stone, MH, Ratamess, NA, and

Triplett-McBride, T. American College of Sports Medicine position stand. Progression models in resistance training for healthy adults. *Med Sci Sports Exerc* 34:364-380, 2002.

25. Lauersen, JB, Andersen, TE, and Andersen, LB. Strength training as superior, dose-dependent and safe prevention of acute and overuse sports injuries: A systematic review, qualitative analysis and meta-analysis. *Brit J Sports Med* 52:1557-1563, 2018.

26. Leichter-Saxby, M, and Law, S. *The new adventure playground movement: How communities across the USA are returning risk and freedom to childhood.* London: Notebook Publishing, 2015.

27. Lloyd, RS, Cronin, JB, Faigenbaum, AD, Haff, GG, Howard, R, Kraemer, WJ, Micheli, LJ, Myer, GD, and Oliver, JL. National Strength and Conditioning Association position statement on long-term athletic development. *J Strength Cond Res* 30(6):1491-1509, 2016.

28. Lloyd, R, Faigenbaum, AD, Stone, MH, Oliver, JL, Jeffreys, I, Moody, JA, Brewer, C, Pierce, KC, McCambridge, TM, Howard, R, Herrington, L, Hainline, B, Micheli, LJ, Jaques, R, Kraemer, WJ, McBride, MG, Best, TM, Chu, DA, Alvar, BA, and Myer, GD. Position statement on youth resistance training: The 2014 international consensus. *Brit J Sports Med* 48(7):498-505, 2014.

29. Lloyd, RS, and Oliver, JL. The youth physical development model: A new approach to long-term athletic development. *Strength Cond J* 34(3):61-72, 2012.

29a. Lloyd, RS, Meyers, RW, and Oliver, JL. The natural development and trainability of plyometric ability during childhood. *Strength Cond J* 33:23-32, 2011.

29b. Lloyd, RS, Oliver, JL, Meyers, RW, Moody, JA, and Stone, MH. Long-term athletic development and its application to youth weightlifting. *Strength Cond J* 34(4):55-66, 2012.

30. Malone, S, Hughes, B, Doran, DA, Collins, K, and Gabbett, TJ. Can the workload-injury relationship be moderated by improved strength, speed and repeated-sprint qualities? *J Sci Med Sport* 22:29-34, 2019.

31. McDonagh, MJ, and Davies, CT. Adaptive response of mammalian skeletal muscle to exercise with high loads. *Eur J Appl Physiol* 52:139-155, 1984.

32. McHenry, P. (personal communication, February 20, 2020).

33. Mills, K, Baker, D, Pacey, V, Wollin, M, and Drew, MK. What is the most accurate and reliable methodological approach for predicting peak height velocity in adolescents? A systematic review. *J Sci Med Sport* 20(6):572-577, 2017.

34. Mirwald, RL, Baxter-Jones, AD, Bailey, DA, and Beunen, GP. An assessment of maturity from anthropometric measurements. *Med Sci Sports Exerc* 34(4):689-694, 2002.

35. Morris, SJ, Oliver, JL, Pedley, JS, Haff, GG, and Lloyd, RS. Taking a long-term approach to the development of weightlifting ability in young athletes. *Strength Cond J* 42(6):71-90, 2020.

36. Naughton G, Farpour, L, Carlson, J, Bradney, M, and Van Praagh, E. Physiological issues surrounding the performance of adolescent athletes. *Sports Med* 30:309-325, 2000.

37. Pellegrini, AD, and Glickman, CD. The educational role of recess. *Principal* 68(5):23-24, 1989.

38. Pichardo, AW, Oliver, JL, Harrison, CB, Maulder, PS, and Lloyd, RS. Integrating models of long-term athletic development to maximize the physical development of youth. *Int J Sports Sci Coa* 13(6):1189-1199, 2018.

39. Pichardo, AW, Oliver, JL, Harrison, CB, Maulder, PS, and Lloyd, RS. Integrating resistance training into high school curriculum. *Strength Cond J* 41(1):39-50, 2018.

40. Plisk, SS. Effective needs analysis and functional training principles. In *Strength and Conditioning for Sports Performance*. Jeffreys, I, and Moody, J, eds. New York: Routledge, 181-200, 2016.

41. Radnor, JM, Lloyd, RS, and Oliver, JL. Individual response to different forms of resistance training in school-aged boys. *J Strength Cond Res* 31(3):787-797, 2016.

42. Reuter, BH, and Dawes, JJ. Program design and technique for aerobic endurance training. In *Essentials of Strength Training and Conditioning*. 4th ed. Haff, GG, and Triplett, NT, eds. Champaign, IL: Human Kinetics, 559-581, 2016.

43. Schoenfeld, BJ, Pope, ZK, Benik, FM, Hester, GM, Sellers, J, Nooner, JL, Schnaiter, JA, Bond-Williams, KE, Carter, AS, Ross, CL, Just, BL, Henselmans, M, and Krieger, JW. Longer interset rest periods enhance muscle strength and hypertrophy in resistance-trained men. *J Strength Cond Res* 30(7):1805-1812, 2016.

44. SHAPE America. *National Standards for K-12 Physical Education.* Reston, VA, 2013.

45. SHAPE America, National Standards for Sport Coaches: Quality Coaches, Quality Sports, 3rd ed., edited by L. Gano-Overway, M. Thompson, and P. Van Mullem (Burlington, MA: Jones & Bartlett, 2021).

46. Shaw, I, and Shaw, BS. Resistance training's role in the prevention of sports injuries. In *Sports Injuries*. The Johns Hopkins Hospital, ed. Hauppauge, NY: Nova Science, 123-136, 2015.

47. Sheppard, JM, and Triplett, NT. Program design for resistance training. In *Essentials of Strength Training and Conditioning*. 4th ed. Haff, GG, and Triplett, NT, eds. Champaign, IL: Human Kinetics, 439-469, 2016.

48. Sommerfield, LM, Harrison, CB, Whatman, CS, and Maulder, PS. (2020). Relationship between strength, athletic performance, and movement skill in adolescent girls. *J Strength Cond Res* [epub ahead of print].

49. Stone, MH, and O'Bryant, HS. Practical considerations for weight training. *Weight training: A scientific approach*. Minneapolis, MN: Bellwether Press, 1987.

50. Stone, MH, Stone, M, and Sands, WA. *Principles and Practice of Resistance Training*. Champaign, IL: Human Kinetics, 2007.

51. Stracciolini, A, Friedman, HL, Casciano, R, Howell, D, Sugimoto, D, and Micheli, L. The relative age effect on youth sports injuries. *Med Sci Sports Exerc* 48(6):1068-1074, 2016.

52. Suchomel, TJ, and Comfort, P. Developing muscular strength and power. In *Advanced Strength and Conditioning*. Turner, A, and Comfort, P, eds. New York: Routledge, 13-38, 2018.

53. Suchomel, TJ, and Comfort, P. Technical demands of strength training. In *Advanced Strength and Conditioning*. Turner, A, and Comfort, P, eds. New York: Routledge, 229-248, 2018.

54. Suchomel, TJ, and Comfort, P. Weightlifting for sports performance. In *Advanced Strength and Conditioning*. Turner, A, and Comfort, P, eds. New York: Routledge, 249-273, 2018.

55. Suchomel, TJ, Comfort, P, and Stone, MH. Weightlifting pulling derivatives: Rationale for implementation and application. *Sports Med* 45:823-839, 2015.

56. Suchomel, TJ, Nimphius, S, and Stone, MH. The importance of muscular strength in athletic performance. *Sports Med* 1419-1449, 2016.

57. Suchomel, TJ, Nimphius, S, Bellon, CR, and Stone, MH. The importance of muscular strength: Training considerations. *Sports Med* 765-785, 2018.

58. Symons, DK. Psychological age. *Encyclopedia of Child Behavior and Development*. Goldstein, S, and Naglieri, JA, eds. Boston: Springer, 1180, 2011.

59. Tanner, JM, Whitehouse, RH, Marubini, E, and Resele, LF. The adolescent growth spurt of boys and girls of the Harpenden growth study. *Ann Hum Biol* 3(2):109-126, 1976.

60. Zourdos, MC, Goldsmith, JA, Helms, ER, Trepeck, C, Halle, JL, Mendez, KM, Cooke, DM, Haischer, MH, Sousa, CA, Klemp, A, and Byrnes, RK. Proximity to failure and total repetitions in a set influences accuracy of intraset repetitions in reserve-based ratings of perceived exertion. *J Strength Cond Res* 35:S158-S165, 2021.

61. Zourdos, MC, Klemp, A, Dolan, C, Quiles, JM, Schau, KA, Jo, E, Helms, E, Esgro, B, Duncan, S, Garcia Merino, S, and Blanco, R. Novel resistance training-specific rating of perceived exertion scale measuring repetitions in reserve. *J Strength Cond Res* 30(1):267-275, 2016.

Chapter 9

1. Abt, J, Ferris, C, Irrgang, J, Lephart, S, Myers, J, Nagai, T, and Sell, T. Neuromuscular and biomechanical characteristic changes in high school athletes: A plyometric versus basic resistance program. *Br J Sports Med* 39(12):932-938, 2005.

2. Chu, D, Faigenbaum, A, and Falkel, J. *Progressive Plyometrics for Kids*. Monterey, CA: Healthy Learning, 2006.

3. Frogberg, K, Holm, R, Kotoft, B, and Wedderkopp, N. Comparison of two intervention programmes in young female players in European handball: with and without ankle disc. *Scand J Med Sci Sports* 13(6):371-375, 2003.

4. Gambetta, V. *Athletic Development*. Champaign, IL: Human Kinetics, 209-227, 2007.

5. Hayes, PR, French, D, and Thomas, K. The effects of plyometric training techniques on muscular power and agility in youth soccer players. *J Strength Cond Res* 23(1):332-335, 2009.

6. Holcomb, WR, Kleiner, DM, and Chu, DA. Plyometrics: Considerations for safe and effective training. *Strength Cond J* 20(3):36-41, 1998.

7. Landow, L. Landow performance. In NSCA TSAC Annual Conference, San Diego CA, April 26-28, 2016.

8. Lloyd, R, Meyers, R, Oliver, J. The natural development and trainability of plyometric ability during childhood. *Strength Cond J* 33(2):24, 2011.

9. Triplett, NT, Brown, V, Caulfield, S, Doscher, M, McHenry, P, Statler, T, and Wainwright, R. NSCA strength and conditioning professional standards and guidelines. *Strength Cond J* 39(6):1-24, 2017.

10. Potach, DH, and Chu, D. Program design and technique for plyometric training. In *Essentials of Strength Training and Conditioning*. 4th ed. Haff, GG, and Triplett, NT, eds. Champaign, IL: Human Kinetics, 471-520, 2016.

11. Shiner, J, Bishop, T, and Cosgarea, A. Integrating low-intensity plyometrics into strength and conditioning programs. *Strength Cond J* 27(6):10-20, 2005.

12. Wathen, D. Literature review: Explosive/plyometric exercises. *Strength Cond J* 15(3):17-19, 1993.

Chapter 10

1. Alexander, RM. Mechanics of skeleton and tendons. In *Handbook of Physiology, Section 1: The Nervous System*, Brookhardt, JM, Mountcastle, VB, Brooks, VB, and Greiger, SR, eds. Bethesda, MD: American Physiological Society, 17-42, 1981.

2. American Academy of Pediatrics. Intensive training and sports specialization in young athletes. *Pediatrics* 106(1):154-157, 2000.

3. DeWeese, BH, and Nimphius, S. Program design and technique for speed and agility training. In *Essentials of Strength Training and Conditioning*. 4th ed. Haff, GG, and Triplett, NT, eds. Champaign, IL: Human Kinetics, 521-556, 2016.

4. Fields, J, and Jones, MT. Age and sex considerations. In *Developing Agility and Quickness*. 2nd ed. Dawes, J, ed. Champaign, IL: Human Kinetics, 67-76, 2019.

5. Graham, G. Assessment of speed. In *Developing Speed*. Jeffreys, I, ed. Champaign, IL: Human Kinetics, 61-77, 2013.

6. Herda, TJ, and Cramer, JT. Bioenergetics of exercise and training. In *Essentials of Strength Training and Conditioning*. 4th ed. Haff, GG, and Triplett, NT, eds. Champaign, IL: Human Kinetics, 43-64, 2016.

7. Jeffreys, I. The nature of speed. In *Developing Speed*. Jeffreys, I, ed. Champaign, IL: Human Kinetics, 5-18, 2013.

8. Lloyd, RS, and Faigenbaum, AD. Age- and sex-related differences and their implications for resistance exercise. In *Essentials of Strength Training and Conditioning*. 4th ed. Haff, GG, and Triplett, NT, eds. Champaign, IL: Human Kinetics, 135-154, 2016.

9. Miller, B. *Return to sprinting from injury*. Presented at the NSCA Maryland State Clinic, Towson, MD, February 15, 2020.

10. Preparticipation Physical Evaluation Task Force, American Academy of Family Physicians, American Academy of Pediatrics, American College of Sports Medicine, American Medical Society for Sports Medicine, American Orthopaedic Society for Sports Medicine, and American Osteopathic Academy of Sports Medicine. *Preparticipation Physical Evaluation*. 4th ed. Elk Grove Village, IL: American Academy of Pediatrics, 2010.

11. Roozen, M. Change of direction speed drills. In *Developing Agility and Quickness*. 2nd ed. Dawes, J, ed. Champaign, IL: Human Kinetics, 99-131, 2019.

12. Sanders, GJ, Turner, Z, Boos, B, Peacock, CA, Peveler, W, and Lipping, A. Aerobic capacity is related to repeated sprint ability with sprint distances less than 40 meters. *Int J Exerc Sci* 10(2):197-204, 2017.

13. Sheppard, J. Technical development of linear speed. In *Developing Speed*. Jeffreys, I, ed. Champaign, IL: Human Kinetics, 31-60, 2013.

14. Smith, AD, and Micheli, L. The prevention of sport injuries of children and adolescents. *Med Sci Sports Exerc* 25(8):1-7, 1993.

15. Triplett, NT, Brown, V, Caulfield, S, Doscher, M, McHenry, P, Statler, T, and Wainwright, R. NSCA strength and conditioning professional standards and guidelines. *Strength Cond J* 39(6):1-24, 2017.

16. Viola, M. *Speedwork basics: Change of direction.* Presented at the NSCA Maryland State Clinic, Towson, MD, February 15, 2020.

Chapter 11

1. American College of Sports Medicine. *ACSM's Guidelines for Exercise Testing and Prescription,* 11th ed. Philadelphia: Wolters Kluwer, 126, 148, 2022.

2. Banz, WJ, Maher, MA, Thompson, WG, Bassett, DR, Moore, W, Ashraf, M, Keefer, DJ, and Zemel, MB. Effects of resistance training versus aerobic training on coronary artery disease risk factors. *Exp Bio & Med* 228(4):434-440, 2003.

3. Billat, LV. Use of blood lactate measurements for prediction of exercise performance and for control of training. *Sports Med* 22(3):157-175, 1996.

4. Borg, G. Psychophysical bases of perceived exertion. *Med Sci Sports Exerc* 14(5):363-367, 1982.

5. Bushman, BA. Determining the I (intensity) for a FITT-VP aerobic exercise prescription. *ACSM's Health & Fit J* 18(3):4-7, 2014.

6. Chen, L, and Tang, L. Effects of interval training versus continuous training on coronary artery disease: An updated meta-analysis of randomized controlled trials. *Physiother Theory Prac*, 1-10, 2020.

7. Chen, MJ, Fan, X, and Moe, ST. Criterion-related validity of the Borg ratings of perceived exertion scale in individuals: A meta-analysis. *J Sports Sci* 20(11):873-899, 2002.

8. Chtara, M, Chaougachi, A, Levin, GT, Chaouachi, M, Chamari, K, Amri, M, and Laursen, PB. Effect of concurrent endurance and circuit resistance training sequence on muscular strength and power development. *J Strength Cond Res* 22(4):1037-1045, 2008.

9. Contro, V, Pieretta Mancuso, E, and Prioa, P. Delayed onset muscle soreness (DOMS) management: Present state of the art. *Trends Sport Sci* 3: 121-127, 2016.

10. Cornelissen, VA, and Fagard, RH. Effects of endurance training on blood pressure, blood pressure-regulating mechanisms, and cardiovascular risk factors. *Hypertension* 46(4):667-675, 2005.

11. Drake, JC, Wilson, RJ, and Yan, Z. Molecular mechanisms for mitochondrial adaptation to exercise training in skeletal muscle. *FASEB J* 30(1):13-22, 2016.

12. Duarte, R, Batalha, N, Folgado, H, and Sampaio, J. Effects of exercise duration and number of players in heart rate responses and technical skills during futsal small-sided games. *The Open Sports Sci J* 2(1):37-41, 2009.

13. Eleckuvan, MR. Effectiveness of fartlek training on maximum oxygen consumption and resting pulse rate. *Int J Phys Educ Fit Sports* 3(1):85-88, 2014.

14. Elliot, MC, Wagner, PP, and Chiu, L. Power athletes and distance training. *Sports Med* 37(1):47-57, 2007.

15. Eston, R. Use of ratings of perceived exertion in sports. *Int J Sports Physiol Perform* 7(2):175-182, 2012.

15a. Hagerman, P. Aerobic endurance training program design. In *NSCA's Essentials of Personal Training.* 2nd ed. Coburn, JW, and Malek, MH eds. Champaign, IL: Human Kinetics, 395, 2012.

16. Hennessy, LC, and Watson, AW. The interference effects of training for strength and endurance simultaneously. *J Strength Cond Res* 8(1):12-19, 1994.

17. Hermassi, S., Laudner, K, and Schwesig, R. The effects of circuit training on the development of physical fitness and performance-related variables in handball players. *J Hum Kinet* 71:191-203, 2020.

18. Hill-Haas, SV, Dawson, B, Impellizzeri, FM, and Coutts, AJ. Physiology of small-sided games training in football. *Sports Med* 41:199-220, 2011.

19. Hrelijac, A. Impact and overuse injuries in runners. *Med Sci Sports Exerc* 36(5):845-849, 2004.

20. Jeffreys, I. The use of small-sided games in the metabolic training of high school soccer players. *Strength Cond J* 26(5):77-78, 2004.

21. Jiaquan, X, Murphy, SL, Kochanek, KD, and Arias, E. National Center for Health Statistics: Mortality in the United States, 2018. January 2020. www.cdc.gov/nchs/products/databriefs/db355.htm#:~:text=Data%20from%20the%20National%20Vital,2017%20to%20723.6%20in%20 2018. Accessed May 17, 2021.

22. Katzmarzyk, P, Malina, R, and Beunen, G. The contribution of biological maturation to the strength and motor fitness of children. *Ann Hum Biol* 24(6):493-505, 1997.

23. Kavanaugh, A. The role of progressive overload in sports conditioning. *NSCA's Perf Train J* 6(1):15, 2007.

24. Kenney, LW, Wilmore, JH, and Costill, DL. *Physiology of sport and exercise*. 7th ed. Champaign, IL: Human Kinetics, 2019.

25. Klika, B, and Jordan, C. High-intensity circuit training using body weight: Maximum results with minimal investment. *ACSMs Health Fit J* 17(3):8-13, 2013.

26. Koutsandréou, F, Wegner, M, Niemann, C, and Budde, H. Effects of motor versus cardiovascular exercise training on children's working memory. *Med Sci Sports Exerc* 48(6):1144-1152, 2016.

27. Kropa, J, Close, J, Shipon, D, Hufnagel, E, Terry, C, Olier, J, and Johnson, B. High prevalence of obesity and high blood pressure in urban student-athletes. *J Pediatr* 178:194-199, 2016.

28. Lin, YY, and Lee, SD. Cardiovascular benefits of exercise training in postmenopausal hypertension. *Int J Mol Sci* 19(9):2523, 2018.

29. Lloyd, RS, Oliver, JL, Faigenbaum, AD, Myer, GD, and Croix, MB. Chronological age vs. biological maturation: Implications for exercise programming in youth. *J Strength Cond Res* 28(5):1454-1464, 2014.

30. MacDougall, JD. Morphological changes in human skeletal muscle following strength training and immobilization. In *Human Muscle Power*. Jones, N, McCartney, N, and McComas, A, eds. Champaign, IL: Human Kinetics, 269-285, 1986.

31. MacInnis, MJ, and Gibala, MJ. Physiological adaptations to interval training and the role of exercise intensity. *J Physiol* 595(9):2915-2930, 2017.

32. Mayorga-Vaga, D, Viciana, J, and Cocca, A. Effects of a circuit training program on muscular and cardiovascular endurance and their maintenance in schoolchildren. *J Hum Kinet* 37:153-160, 2013.

33. McHugh, C, Hind, K, Davey, D, and Wilson, F. Cardiovascular health of retired field-based athletes: A systematic review and meta-analysis. *Orthop J Sports Med* 7(8):2325967119862750, 2019.

34. National Collegiate Athletic Association. Probability of competing beyond high school. https://ncaa.org/about/resources/research/probability-competing-beyond-high-school. Accessed March 3, 2020.

35. Ntoumanis, N, Thogersen-Ntoumani, C, Quested, E, and Hancox, J. The effects of training group exercise class instructors to adopt a motivationally adaptive communication style. *Scand J Med Sci Sports* 27(9):1026-1034, 2017.

36. Potach, DH, and Chu, DA. Program design and technique for plyometric training. In *Essentials of Strength Training and Conditioning*. 4th ed. Haff, GG, and Triplett, NT eds. Champaign, IL: Human Kinetics, 471-520, 2016.

37. Powers, SK, and Howley, ET. *Exercise Physiology: Theory and Application to Fitness and Performance*. 10th ed. New York: McGraw Hill, 294-296, 2018.

38. Reuter, BH, and Dawes, JJ. Program design and technique for aerobic endurance training. In *Essentials of Strength Training and Conditioning*. 4th ed. Haff, GG, and Triplett, NT eds. Champaign, IL: Human Kinetics, 559-582, 2016.

39. Roeh, A, Kirchner, SK, Malchow, B, Maurus, I, Schmitt, A, Falkai, P, and Hasan, A. Depression in somatic disorders: Is there a beneficial effect of exercise? *Front Psychiatry* 10:141, 2019.

40. Roig, M, Nordbrandt, S, Geertsen, SS, and Nielsen, JB. The effects of cardiovascular exercise on human memory: A review with meta-analysis. *Neurosci Biobehav Rev* 37(8):1645-1666, 2013.

41. Rosenblat, MA, Perrotta, AS, and Thomas, SG. Effect of high-intensity interval training versus sprint interval training on time-trial performance: A systematic review and meta-analysis. *Sports Med* 50(6):1145-1161, 2020.

42. Sabag, A, Najafi, A, Michael, S, Esgin, T, Halaki, J, and Hackett, D. The compatibility of concurrent high intensity interval training and resistance training for muscular strength and hypertrophy: A systematic review and meta-analysis. *J Sports Sci* 36(21):2472-2483, 2018.

43. Selye, H. The general adaptation syndrome and the diseases of adaptation. *J Clin Endocrinol Metab* 6:117-230, 1946.

44. Sheppard, JM, and Triplett, TN. Program design for resistance training. In *Essentials of Strength Training and Conditioning.* 4th ed. Haff, GG, and Triplett, NT eds. Champaign, IL: Human Kinetics, 439-470, 2016.

45. Stiefel, EC, Field, L, Replogle, W, McIntyre, L, Igboechi, O, and Savoie III, FH. The prevalence of obesity and elevated blood pressure in adolescent student athletes from the state of Mississippi. *Orthop J Sports Med* 4(2): 2325967116629368, 2016.

46. Tabata, I, Nishimura, K, Kouzaki, M, Hirai, Y, Ogita, F, Miyachi, M, and Yamamoto, K. Effects of moderate-intensity endurance and high-intensity intermittent training on anaerobic capacity and VO2max. *Med Sci Sports Exerc* 28(10):1327-1330, 1996.

47. Tanaka, H. Effects of cross-training. *Sports Med* 18(5):330-339, 1994.

48. Vandoni, M, Codrons, E, Marin, L, Correale, L, Biglisassi, M, and Buzzachera, CF. Psychophysiological responses to group exercise training sessions: Does exercise intensity matter? *PloS ONE* 11(8):e0149997, 2016.

Index

About the NSCA

The National Strength and Conditioning Association (NSCA) is the world's leading organization in the field of sport conditioning. Drawing on the resources and expertise of the most recognized professionals in strength training and conditioning, sport science, performance research, education, and sports medicine, the NSCA is the world's trusted source of knowledge and training guidelines for coaches and athletes. The NSCA provides the crucial link between the lab and the field.

About the Editors

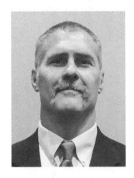

Patrick McHenry, MA, CSCS,*D, RSCC, earned a master's degree in physical education from University of Northern Colorado and a bachelors in elementary education. He has been a frequent presenter at local, state, national, and international conferences, including the national conference of the National Strength and Conditioning Association (NSCA).

McHenry was the *American Football Monthly* Regional Strength Coach of the Year in 2004, NSCA's High School Coach of the Year in 2005, and recipient of the *Strength and Conditioning Journal* Editorial Excellence Award in 2006. He also received the Strength of America Award from the President's Council on Fitness, Sports and Nutrition and was named Colorado High School Physical Education Teacher of the Year in 2012.

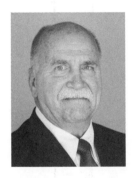

Mike Nitka, MS, CSCS,*D, RSCC*E, FNSCA*E, played football and earned a bachelor of science degree and master of science degree in health and physical education from the University of Wisconsin at La Crosse. He taught freshman physical education and junior health education at Muskego High School in Wisconsin for 38 years and coached football and wrestling, winning every level of championship Wisconsin offered (conference, regional, sectional, and state).

Nitka became an NSCA member in 1985 and, over time, earned the credentials of CSCS,*D, RSCC*E, and FNSCA*E. He presented at the 1992 NSCA national conference and discussed the concept of weight training as a unit within a high school's physical education curriculum. He served as chair of what would eventually become the NSCA's High School Special Interest Group and as a member of the NSCA Conference Committee. He was the "Coaches Corner" column editor for the NSCA's *Strength and Conditioning Journal*, with the vision to reach out to high school coaches across the country to ask them to share what they were doing in their PE classes.

Nitka was selected as the NSCA's High School Strength and Conditioning Professional of the Year in 1994 and represented the NSCA in China and Australia as a member of the NSCA Board of Directors. He contributed expertise and feedback for NSCA's informational brochure for high schools ("What's Missing? Why You Need a Qualified Strength and Conditioning Coach in Your School") and serves as an adjunct professor of exercise science at Carroll University.

About the Contributors

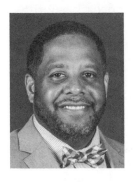

Darnell K. Clark, MPE, CSCS,*D, RSCC*D, is the director of strength and conditioning at Charlotte Country Day School. He oversees the athletic development pathways for 70 teams within 26 sports. Clark holds degrees from Northwestern University and Arizona State and is a doctoral candidate in kinesiology at the University of North Carolina at Greensboro. He is a longtime member of the National Strength and Conditioning Association, which awarded him the High School Strength and Conditioning Coach of the Year Award in 2014. He has served as the NSCA state director for North Carolina, NSCA regional coordinator for the southeast, and vice president of the NSCA Board of Directors.

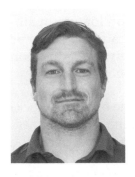

Jim Davis, EdM, MA, CSCS, RSCC*D, is a former professional football player and champion powerlifter turned nationally recognized coach, author, and speaker. Davis is a graduate of Harvard University, Northwestern University, and Knox College. He is the director of the Good Athlete Project, a nonprofit organization focused on the potential of athletics as a learning platform. He is the staff and student wellness coordinator at New Trier High School, and he is the founding director of the Illinois High School Powerlifting Association. Davis has been honored with the U.S. Marine Corps' Excellence in Leadership Award, and he was named a 2020 Semper Fidelis All-American Mentor as well as NASA Powerlifting's 2018 National Coach of the Year (and runner-up in 2019). He has presented keynote addresses internationally (including Ireland and Haiti), and his works have been published in *The Harvard Crimson*, *The Globe Post*, *Orlando Sentinel*, *World of Psychology*, *Olympic and Paralympic Coach*, Good Athlete Project blogs, and BeyondStrength.net. He is also a celebrated painter and poet.

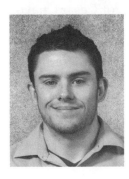

Daniel Flahie, MSEd, CSCS,*D, is the program director and an assistant professor of exercise science and health for the exercise science program, as well as the head strength and conditioning coach for all university teams with the exception of football at Mount Marty University in Yankton, South Dakota. Flahie holds both a bachelor's degree and master's degree in exercise science and is pursuing a PhD in health and human performance with a focus in gerontology.

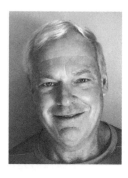

Bruce R. Harbach, MEd, CSCS,*D, is the head football coach at Schuylkill Valley High School in Reading, Pennsylvania, and a sport performance coordinator for Parisi Speed School YMCA of Sinking Spring, Pennsylvania. He taught strength and conditioning in the high school setting for over 45 years, served on the NSCA high school executive board, and is a USA Weightlifting (USAW) Level I coach. Harbach has spoken at numerous conferences, has written and published many articles, is a contributing author to books, and has designed and implemented high school strength and conditioning curriculums. He was named the NSCA's High School Strength and Conditioning Coach of the Year in 2004.

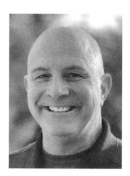

Rick Howard, DSc, CSCS,*D, FNSCA, earned his doctorate in health promotion and wellness from Rocky Mountain University of Health Professions. He is an assistant professor in applied sport science at West Chester University in Pennsylvania and a teacher at Keilir Health Academy in Ásbrú, Iceland. Howard is a fellow of the National Strength and Conditioning Association, and he contributes peer-reviewed articles, blogs, and podcasts. In addition, he presents nationally and internationally on long-term athletic development (LTAD) and the application of concepts of pediatric exercise science for coaches, personal trainers, physical education teachers, and those who wish to improve the lives of young people.

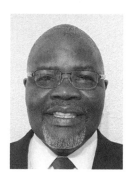

Shawn L. Jenkins, MS, ATC, CSCS, is the owner of Stockton Sports Performance and a member of the physical fitness staff for a national government organization that trains the security force. Jenkins is certified by the National Athletic Trainers' Association (NATA) as an athletic trainer (ATC) and holds the NSCA's Certified Strength and Conditioning Specialist (CSCS) certification. He holds a bachelor of arts degree in physical education from San Francisco State University and a master of science degree in kinesiology from California State University at Hayward. He was a founding member and past chair of the NSCA's diversity and inclusion committee, and he serves on the NSCA advisory committee for Northern California. He was previously the strength and conditioning coach and athletic trainer for Cesar Chavez High School in Stockton, California, and he played baseball at Louisiana State University and San Francisco State University. Jenkins is a presenter at various conferences and clinics on topics relating to sport performance and exercise prescription for youths, adolescents, and adults.

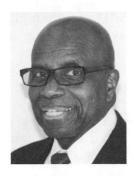

Edwin C. Jones, MA, CSCS, is a school administrator who has experience in education from elementary physical education to senior high school principal. He has served the NSCA as the first state director for the District of Columbia. He has been recognized as Region II State Director of the Year and as High School Strength and Conditioning Coach of the Year. He was the first African American to serve on the NSCA Board of Directors. Jones studied the science of strength and conditioning in Bulgaria and the USSR, from which he developed a fitness program, Total Fitness, which was instrumental in Eastern High School being honored with the Drug Free Schools National Recognition.

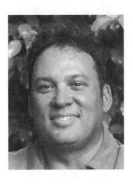

Ray Karvis, MSEd, CSCS, is the assistant director of sport performance at Dynamic Sports Training's Arizona Christian University location, where he provides training for all 18 sport programs as well as a private clientele of professional and high school athletes. Karvis has been involved in strength and conditioning since 1995 and has been a member of the NSCA since 2002. He served as the strength coach for Southern Illinois University from 2000 to 2002, for Scottsdale Community College from 2002 to 2003, and for Phoenix Christian High School from 2003 to 2009, during which time they won back-to-back state championships in 2003 and 2004. He also served as a head high school football and head track coach in Arizona. Karvis and his wife, Mandi, have been married for 25 years and reside in Phoenix.

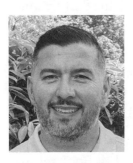

Joe Lopez, CSCS, RSCC, is the head strength and conditioning coach at Pope John XXIII High School in Sparta, New Jersey. He previously worked at Precision Sports Performance, Inception Sports Performance, and Centercourt Tennis Academy. Lopez has also served in roles with the National Strength and Conditioning Association, where he was on the high school special interest group advisory board and the New Jersey state advisory board. He is the NSCA state director for New Jersey and was honored as the State and Provincial Director of the Year in 2019. Lopez has presented at clinics and conferences at the state, regional, and national levels.

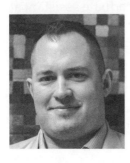

Gary S. McChalicher, EdD, CSCS, USAW, CAA, has worked as an educator and strength and conditioning coach for over 20 years. He is an athletic director and oversees K-12 health and physical education at the southeastern school district in York, Pennsylvania. McChalicher is also an adjunct professor of kinesiology at Towson University and the chairman of the NSCA's high school special interest group. He previously worked as a classroom teacher, secondary administrator, and collegiate strength and conditioning coach. McChalicher is an active competitor in Olympic weightlifting and Brazilian jiujitsu. He is married with two daughters.

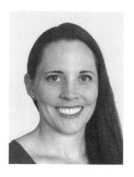

Shana McKeever, MA, LAT, ATC, CSCS,*D, is a strength and conditioning professional at Divine Savior Holy Angels High School in Milwaukee and is an adjunct professor at Carroll University in the department of human movement science. She holds a master's of art degree in kinesiology and sport studies, with a concentration in exercise physiology and performance, from East Tennessee State University. Additionally, McKeever has contributed to research investigating the use of weightlifting to enhance sport performance. Before transitioning her career to focus on performance enhancement, she served the high school population as a certified athletic trainer.

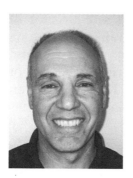

Patrick Mediate, MEd, CSCS,*D, was named the Connecticut High School Physical Education Teacher of the Year and is the strength and conditioning coordinator and assistant football coach at Greenwich High School. Mediate served on the NSCA Board of Directors and he was an NSCA Connecticut State Director, an NSCA Northeast Regional Coordinator, and a chair of the NSCA High School SIG. Mediate has received the NSCA High School Strength and Conditioning Coach of the Year award, State Director of the Year award, and President's Award, and he was a two-time NSCA Strength of America Award recipient. Mediate has hosted and presented at state, national, and international levels and was an invited guest at the 1996 Olympic games in Atlanta. He has coauthored two books on medicine ball training and an NSCA abstract paper titled "Effects of Medicine Ball Training on High School Fitness Measurements."

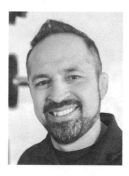

Samuel Melendrez, MS, CSCS,*D, RSCC, is in his 13th year as the full-time strength and conditioning coach at Discovery Canyon Campus High School in Colorado Springs, Colorado, where he oversees the training of student-athletes from all sports in strength and conditioning classes during the day and in before- and after-school programs. Prior to making the decision to work in the high school setting, Melendrez did internships at the Olympic Training Centers in Colorado Springs and Lake Placid, was an assistant at the U.S. Air Force Academy, and was a graduate assistant at the University of New Mexico. Melendrez was named NSCA's 2021 High School Strength and Conditioning Coach of the Year.

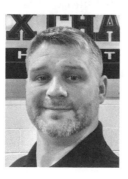

Brandon Peifer, MA, CSCS, is the head strength and conditioning coach and history teacher at Fox Chapel Area High School, where he oversees strength and conditioning for grades 7 through 12. Under his leadership, Fox Chapel was recognized by the NSCA in 2021 with the Strength of America Award. Peifer holds degrees from Clarion University of Pennsylvania and California University of Pennsylvania, and he is a USAW Level I coach. He is an NSCA member and serves on the high school special interest group executive council. Peifer is also a member of the National High School Strength Coaches Association (NHSSCA) and serves on the Pennsylvania state advisory board. He was named the Pennsylvania High School Strength and Conditioning Coach of the Year in 2020.

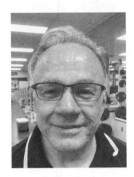

Scott Sahli, MEd, CSCS,*D, NSCA-CPT,*D, RSCC*E, USAW National Coach, is the strength and conditioning coordinator at Lakeville South High School in Lakeville, Minnesota. He is a USA Weightlifting senior coach, is a member of the NSCA conference committee, and has been the NSCA regional director for the north central region for the past six years. Previously, he coached at Northfield High School and Burnsville High School (both in Minnesota) and was the NSCA state director for Minnesota for seven years. Sahli's Olympic weightlifting teams have won 13 state championships in the last 17 years. He was selected twice as the Minnesota Strength and Conditioning Professional of the Year, and he was awarded the NSCA's High School Strength and Conditioning Coach of the Year Award in 2010. Sahli is very passionate about the importance of multisport development for young athletes.

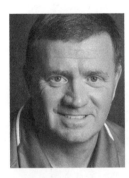

Anthony S. Smith, PhD, CSCS,*D, NSCA-CPT,*D, TSAC-F, is an associate professor of physical education at Charleston Southern University. As a professor in higher education, Smith seeks to combine knowledge from physical education and strength and conditioning to help youth sport coaches create comprehensive development programs for their athletes. His research interests include the development of expertise in sport and fitness pedagogy skills for strength and conditioning. Smith previously served as a high school basketball coach and private sport-specific trainer for young basketball players.

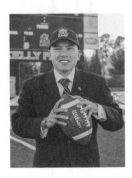

Phil Tran, JD, MSEd, CSCS,*D, is an assistant coach for varsity football and girls' varsity ice hockey at Archbishop Spalding High School in Severn, Maryland. He is the owner and head coach of PT Strength and serves as the NSCA state director for Maryland. Tran was the NHSSCA's Maryland Coach of the Year in 2019. In college, Tran played football for Baylor University, where he lettered, won Baylor football's Highest GPA Award, made the Big XII Commissioner's honor roll, earned First Team Academic All-Big XII honors, and won a postgraduate scholarship.

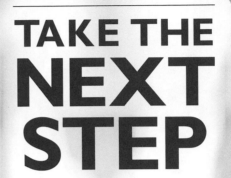

TAKE THE NEXT STEP

A continuing education course
is available for this text.
Find out more.

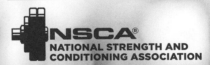

NSCA®
NATIONAL STRENGTH AND
CONDITIONING ASSOCIATION

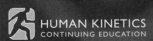

HUMAN KINETICS
CONTINUING EDUCATION

Special pricing for course components may be available. Contact us for more information.

US and International: US.HumanKinetics.com/collections/Continuing-Education
Canada: Canada.HumanKinetics.com/collections/Continuing-Education